D1651848

ORAL HYGIENE
in ORAL HEALTH

Publication Number 1001

AMERICAN LECTURE SERIES®

A Publication in

The BANNERSTONE DIVISION *of*
AMERICAN LECTURES IN DENTISTRY

Edited by

ALVIN F. GARDNER, D.D.S., M.S., Ph.D.

Bureau of Medicine
Food and Drug Administration
Washington, D.C.

No official support or endorsement by the Food and Drug
Administration or the Department of Health, Education
and Welfare is intended or should be inferred.

616.314-083

ORAL HYGIENE
in ORAL HEALTH

Edited by

HYMAN J. V. GOLDBERG, B.A., D.M.D.

Associate Professor,
School of Medicine and Dentistry,
University of Rochester,
and Dental Director,
Anthony L. Jordan Health Center
and the Rochester Health Network,
Rochester, New York

and

LOUIS W. RIPA, D.D.S., M.S.

Associate Dean and
Professor and Chairman,
Department of Children's Dentistry,
School of Dental Medicine,
State University of New York at Stony Brook,
Stony Brook, New York

With a Foreword by

ALVIN F. GARDNER, D.D.S., M.S., Ph.D.

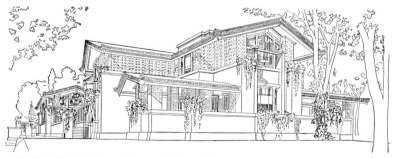

CHARLES C THOMAS · PUBLISHER
Springfield · Illinois · U.S.A.

COLGATE-PALMOLIVE LTD.
37.1 ORDSALL LANE, SALFORD 5.

3 0 APR 1979
RETURN TO TECHNICAL
INFORMATION CENTRE & LIBRARY

Published and Distributed Throughout the World by

CHARLES C THOMAS • PUBLISHER

Bannerstone House

301-327 East Lawrence Avenue, Springfield, Illinois, U.S.A.

This book is protected by copyright. No part of it
may be reproduced in any manner without written
permission from the publisher.

© 1977, *by* CHARLES C THOMAS • PUBLISHER

ISBN 0-398-03590-3

Library of Congress Catalog Card Number: 76-20674

*With THOMAS BOOKS careful attention is given to all details of
manufacturing and design. It is the Publisher's desire to present books that are
satisfactory as to their physical qualities and artistic possibilities and
appropriate for their particular use. THOMAS BOOKS will be true to those
laws of quality that assure a good name and good will.*

Library of Congress Cataloging in Publication Data

Main entry under title:

Oral hygiene in oral health.

  (American lecture series; publication no. 1001)
  Bibliography: p.
  Includes index.
  1. Mouth—Care and hygiene. 2. Dental caries.
3. Periodontal disease. I. Goldberg, Hyman J. V.
II. Ripa, Louis W. [DNLM: 1. Oral hygiene. 2. Oral
health. WU113 0635]
RK60.7.07   617.6'01   76-20674
ISBN 0-398-03590-3

Printed in the United States of America

C-1

This book is gratefully dedicated to our two families—our family of friends and our families

CONTRIBUTORS

JAMES T. BARENIE, D.D.S., M.S.

Associate Professor,
Department of Children's Dentistry,
School of Dental Medicine,
State University of New York at Stony Brook,
Stony Brook, New York

BASIL G. BIBBY, Ph.D., D.M.D.

Professor Emeritus,
School of Medicine and Dentistry,
University of Rochester,
Rochester, New York

MICHAEL BUONOCORE, D.D.S., M.S.

Research Coordinator,
Eastman Dental Center,
Associate Professor,
School of Medicine and Dentistry,
University of Rochester,
Rochester, New York

LOIS K. COHEN, Ph.D.

Special Assistant to the Director,
National Institute for Dental Research,
National Institutes of Health,
Bethesda, Maryland

ROBERT GENCO, D.D.S., Ph.D.

Associate Professor and
Director of Graduate Periodontology,
College of Dentistry,
State University of New York,
Buffalo, New York

HYMAN J. V. GOLDBERG, B.A., D.M.D.

Associate Professor,
School of Medicine and Dentistry,
University of Rochester,
and Dental Director,
Anthony L. Jordan Health Center
and the Rochester Health Network,
Rochester, New York

SAM H. HOSKINS, D.D.S., M.S.D.

Professor and Chairman,
University of Texas School of Dentistry,
San Antonio, Texas

DONALD MASTERS, D.D.S.

Associate Clinical Professor,
University of Texas School of Dentistry,
and Private Practice Limited to Periodontics
San Antonio, Texas

RUSSELL NISENGARD, D.D.S., Ph.D.

Associate Professor,
School of Dentistry,
State University of New York,
Buffalo, New York

JEANETTE E. RAYNER, B.A.

Public Health Analyst,
Division of Medicine,
Bureau of Health Manpower,
Health Resources Agency,
Department of Health, Education, and Welfare,
Bethesda, Maryland

LOUIS W. RIPA, D.D.S., M.S.

Associate Dean,
Professor and Chairman,
Department of Children's Dentistry,
School of Dental Medicine,
State University of New York at Stony Brook
Stony Brook, New York

FOREWORD

THE *American Lectures in Dentistry* series advances newer knowledge for progress of dental practice. Success in modern dental practice is dependent upon biologic as well as mechanical considerations. The interdependence of dentistry on oral biology is so great that dentists are turning to oral biologists and oral biologists to dentists in order to understand the local and systemic basis of oral disease. The oral biologic processes are currently becoming sound foundations for clinical dentistry resulting in a rather rapid extension of postgraduate instruction. Therefore, each of the books in this series unravels the oral mechanisms and provides the clinical management of many problems which have existed for decades.

The *American Lectures in Dentistry* series is charged with a striving ardor of dental wisdom, prepared by distinguished dental colleagues. Dentistry is both a science and an art which fulfills a social function. This series will, therefore, encompass clinical, oral biologic, and social topics which are most applicable to the general practitioner of dentistry. It is our hope that the efforts of the contributors will assist the dental practitioner in fulfilling his responsibility to his patients through sound judgments, proper technical knowledge, and dispatch. The *American Lectures in Dentistry* will serve as extremely practical references to aid the dental practitioner to resolve some of the problems encountered in the practice of dentistry as well as to broaden the horizons of those progressive dentists who desire the postgraduate knowledge and continuing education presented in this series. Contributors will focus attention on these aspects of dental practice causing the general practitioner the greatest concern and difficulty.

The contributors of this series will help the practicing dentist to meet the challenges of the various phases of dental practice. Their observations should be beneficial to dentists seeking to attain the best possible treatment for their patients. New oral diagnostic problems, techniques, instrumentation and therapeutic measures are emerging. It is hoped that a tradition will develop whereby the *American Lectures in Dentistry* serves the dental practitioner and dental specialist alike.

It is not humanly possible to assimilate all of the knowledge in dental school that will be needed for the practice of dentistry. In addition, new knowledge is increasing at a rapid rate. Therefore, the dental practitioner can only keep abreast of the times by showing an initiative for self-learning. It is our hope that the *American Lectures in Dentistry* will stimulate the inquiring mind and provide the dental practitioner with a foundation in basic and new knowledge, skills and attitudes of dentistry upon which he can prepare himself for dental practice in current and future years.

The modern-day dental practitioner is in need of every opportunity possible to extend his knowledge and clinical experience. It is the purpose of the *American Lectures in Dentistry* series to represent one kind of continuing education which will be readily available to him. The *American Lectures in Dentistry* series places emphasis upon the fact that dental knowledge is not a rigid, fully elaborated system of facts, but rather one that is dynamic and constantly changing as new facets of knowledge are developed into the mosaic pattern of the whole.

Doctor Hyman J. V. Goldberg and Doctor Louis W. Ripa present this highly unique monograph on *Oral Hygiene in Oral Health* for the general practitioner of dentistry. Doctors Goldberg and Ripa and their contributors have directed their discussions toward problems most frequently encountered by the general practitioner. The authors have carefully chosen their contributors in order to present the most advanced present-day philosophies in oral hygiene/oral health with broad coverage of the subject. The presentations by the various contributors allow men from diversified areas of dentistry to exchange ideas. I believe that the dental practitioners who read this monograph will conclude that the editors and their contributors have collectively enlightened dental practitioners on oral hygiene/oral health concepts and that the authors have accomplished what we set out to do in this series.

Oral Hygiene in Oral Health is a unique and welcome guide which fills a gap between clinical dentistry and basic science findings and permits rational treatment and conceptual foundations of oral hygiene/oral health in greater depth. This excellent monograph is well organized and represents a ready reference and broad guide to many of the dental practitioners' problems. It is presented in a succinct form which is understandable to the general practitioner, and will, therefore, help him to meet the duties and obligations of the profession of dentistry. The responsibility of the dentist includes diagnosis and treatment planning, seeing that the patient carries through with proper treatment, and the scheduling of a careful follow-up of the patient. The editors and contributors record some activities in the field of oral hygiene/oral health which are a part of the dental practitioner's daily practice, and some which he should recognize and appropriately refer for care.

Thanks are due to the author-editors and expert contributors of this updated review of oral hygiene/oral health for sharing with other dental practitioners the knowledge and experience so carefully collected. May it help all dentists in the daily treatment of their patients.

ALVIN F. GARDNER

PREFACE

ONE OF THE PINNACLES of professional success is an invitation to write a textbook. While we are proud of the opportunity to prepare a textbook in the field of oral hygiene, the offer left us at first with ambivalent feelings. How could we match the classical 1939 Hirschfield text? Yet an update of the material was called for as the field of oral hygiene has progressed significantly since Hirschfield's contribution. With the completion of this volume, we hope we have successfully conveyed current concepts regarding oral hygiene and its relationship to oral health.

Actually, the study of oral hygiene has experienced varying degrees of importance and relevancy; the fluctuations began prior to the Hirschfield text and continue today. Ever since early advertisements of a dentifrice manufacturer advising the public to brush their teeth three times daily and to visit their dentist twice a year, people have accepted these directives without question or scientific qualification. Many practitioners even stress the same points in giving patients preventive counseling. We questioned the scientific basis of such admonitions and sought to clarify the really complex area of oral hygiene. Consequently, when we designed our textbook, we felt that the reader should understand oral hygiene as a science and as it relates to periodontal disease and dental caries.

The relationship of oral hygiene to periodontal disease has been clearly established, but if you consider oral hygiene merely as a lavage for the oral tissues, its relationship to dental caries is somewhat ambiguous. If, however, you consider oral hygiene in its total sense to include adjunctive procedures to actual cleaning, then oral hygiene becomes significant in understanding fully the carious process—its treatment and prevention. To avoid any confusion, therefore, we have expanded the title of our book to *Oral Hygiene in Oral Health*, hoping that the entire spectrum

xiii

of oral hygiene will be placed in the proper context of oral health.

While many colleagues have contributed to the actual writing of this book, we must mention one in particular who has served as a model to both of us in the development of our careers. Basil G. Bibby has been a teacher, advisor, friend, and more. We hope that we are fulfilling his expectations.

To the other contributing authors we are extremely grateful. Each has been very patient and cooperative as we strived to complete this book.

A special word of thanks is due Ms. Norine Jones who edited the entire volume and made significant contributions to many of the chapters. While her primary training is not in dentistry, her innate brightness and skills have been extremely helpful to us. Ms. Sandra Kerr also filled a vital role by helping edit and type much of this volume. Dr. Marguerite Plume contributed in many ways to the book's development and completion. To these three very good friends we also express our deepest appreciation.

Hyman J. V. Goldberg
Louis W. Ripa

CONTENTS

ORAL HYGIENE
in ORAL HEALTH

1
OVERVIEW

Hyman J. V. Goldberg

ORAL HYGIENE has been a human concern for centuries. The preventive advantages of regular care of the teeth and gums were stressed by scientists and philosophers in some of the earliest written documents of human history. Long before the Christian era, oral hygiene was regarded so vital a health measure that some societies incorporated various oral hygiene practices into their religious rituals.[1] By studying the evolution and refinement of these early customs and beliefs, one can observe the beginnings of many of the oral hygiene methods and concepts of oral health prevalent in dental practice today. Therefore, a historical approach to the science of oral hygiene provides a unique perspective for considering the current status of oral hygiene and oral health.

In his book, *The Toothbrush: Its Use and Abuse,* Doctor Isador Hirschfield traces the development of basic oral hygiene methods from those utilized by primitive man to their modern, evolutionary counterparts. The toothpick, toothbrush, and toothpaste may seem recent in origin, but all were used by civilizations far removed in time and locale from our own.

The Toothpick

It is highly probable that primitive man used twig toothpicks to relieve the inconvenience and pressure of impacted food.[2] From such utilitarian beginnings, the toothpick achieved the added status of a decorative ornament. Gold, silver, quill, and wooden picks can be traced to Roman times;[3] and 16th and 17th century individuals wore toothpicks as charms, suspended from their necks on long chains.[4] Bronze, silver, and gold toothpicks dating from the 13th century demonstrate meticulous workman-

3

ship, and some are even studded with pearls and precious stones.[5]

Pliny, a Roman naturalist (23 to 79 AD), advocated the use of "a bone of the hare, sharp as a needle, as a toothpick; to prevent bad odors in the mouth."[6] He also maintained that it made the teeth firm to pick them with a porcupine quill.

A contemporary of Pliny, the poet Martial (40 to 101 AD), recommended toothpicks made of lentisk wood but wrote that quill toothpicks could be substituted.[7]

In *Le Citoyen Dentiste*, published in 1778, Hebert offers one of the earliest statements relating the incidence of caries to an unclean mouth.[8] He warns against leaving food between the teeth for any length of time because this neglect could soften the enamel, permitting caries to destroy the teeth. However, Aristotle (384 to 322 BC) had given a similar warning many centuries before, advising that figs and soft sweets damage the teeth since "small particles adhere between the teeth where they very easily become the cause of putrefactive processes."[9]

Dentists today often recommend the careful use of toothpicks to aid in the removal of impacted food, but the dangers of too vigorous manipulation of the toothpick were described as early as 1810 by John Fuller:

> Toothpicks of gold, silver or any hard substance, as ivory, etc., should be avoided; the constant use of them, where there is at first but a small hollow, will rapidly excavate a tooth, and induce early pain, which perhaps, if it had been let alone, would never have taken place; and by their being forced in between the teeth, they press the gums from their natural situation, and expose the roots to the cold air, which frequently produces pain in perfectly sound teeth. The same objections will apply to pins, with the addition of their being a very improper metal. Toothpicks are certainly very useful, and not to be altogether condemned; but a clean quill, or a single bundle of stiff hairs, fixed in a small ivory handle, are the best; these, as they grow soft by being kept in the mouth, where picking the teeth has become a habit, the amusement may be continued without doing mischief.[10]

The Toothbrush

The first toothbrushes were twigs or roots with the fibers

chewed or hammered into brushes at the ends.[11] Ancient literature indicates the use of such "chewsticks" was common many centuries BC. The technique persisted up to the early 19th century (when twig or root brushes were preferred) and can still be observed in parts of Asia and Africa.[12] J. R. Duval in *Dentiste de la Jeunesse* suggests that the toothbrush evolved from the ancient custom of chewing lentisk wood twigs to give a pleasant odor to the breath.[13] Duval claims that chewing lentisk and myrtle twigs was even practiced during the times of Hippocrates (5th century BC). The Romans especially valued good teeth as a sign of vigor and good health,[14] and Roman writers emphasized the use of chewsticks.[15] Ovid mentions the necessity of cleansing the teeth every morning and eliminating tartar.

Many early religious writings stress the importance of oral cleanliness and specifically emphasize the use of the toothbrush.[16] The Buddha (5th century BC) is described as "receiving water and a toothstick from the God Sakka"; serving the Buddha included bringing him water and toothbrush and washing his feet.[17] One may suppose that followers of Buddhism also practiced this form of oral hygiene.

The Jewish Talmud makes several references to "quesem," a wood chip which was divided on one end by chewing and then used as a toothbrush.[18] The Mohammedans also used toothbrushes made of wood, beaten at one end to form a fibrous brush.[19] Mohammed provided a detailed description of toothbrushing technique; the toothbrush was to be used only once and directed to the buccal surfaces, into the interdental spaces and then on the tongue. He also advised his followers, "you shall clean your mouth for this is a means of praising God."[20]

Bristle toothbrushes originated approximately 200 years ago.[21] They were added to chewsticks, sponges, and cloths as oral hygiene devices during the 18th century, but they had a difficult time gaining public acceptance. Early advertisements for American dentists provide the first illustrations of these brushes.[22] In 1789, a newspaper advertisement for Doctor Isaac Greenwood of Boston had a drawing of a toothbrush with a long brush at one end and a short one at the other end. Doctor Josiah Flagg of

Boston advertised his dental practice and dental cosmetics in 1796 with an advertisement which depicted a small rake-shaped brush and a straight bristle brush.

By the early 19th century, the bristle toothbrush was commonly used for oral hygiene and was regarded superior to chewsticks and sponges.[23] During this period, much dental literature concentrated on the size, texture, and proper manipulation of the toothbrush. John Fuller recommended using a long brush and also a rake brush for labial tooth surfaces.[24] He especially warned against violent brushing as this "abrades the gums without any better cleaning the teeth."[25] According to Fuller, proper brushing technique was to brush gently across the teeth and then up and down, allowing the brush bristles to clean interdental spaces. In addition, he advised brushing the lingual surfaces of the teeth. In 1832, Snell also recommended the use of several types of bristle brushes for adequate cleansing, a different brush for the labial, occlusal, lingual, and interdental surfaces, as well as different grades of bristles according to the area of the mouth and the condition of periodontal health.[26]

There were also early references to dental floss, one of the major preventive tools stressed today in oral hygiene instruction. In 1788, Woofendale writes: "A piece of thread introduced between them (the teeth), a brush with horse's hair, or hog's bristles, fixed in the end, in shape something like a painter's pencil; or a quill cut for this purpose; are the best I know."[27] In the early 17th century, Parmly became dissatisfied with available oral hygiene apparatus and designed his own tools.[28] Included in the kit he organized was a waxed silk thread to pass between the teeth. Commercial dental floss became available in 1882 and was made of unwaxed silk.[29]

Dentifrices

Even the idea of using special powders or mouthwashes to aid in oral prophylaxis is not new to the practice of oral hygiene, although the ingredients have changed to a large degree. The *Ebers Papyrus* is an Egyptian manuscript compiled in 1500 BC which includes all the earliest writings on medicine, probably dating to 4000 BC.[30] Many recipes for dentifrices are presented;

one recommended mixture is composed of honey, green lead, and the powder of flint stones.

During Roman times, dentifrices were very popular and were composed of such substances as burned stag's horn, pumice, ashes from the feet of a goat, and ashes of snail shells.[31] Often these ashes were mixed with bay leaves or myrrh. The Romans even used urine to strengthen their gums![32]

Avicenna (980 to 1047 AD), an Arabian physician whose doctrines were followed for 500 years, discussed oral prophylaxis and warned against dentifrices composed of coarse particles which could destroy or injure the tooth surface.[33] This same warning was repeated in the 12th century in a list of oral hygiene rules propounded by Guy de Chauliac who advised "not to clean the teeth too roughly, but to rub them with honey and burnt salt, to which, very advantageously, may be added some vinegar."[34]

The 16th and 17th centuries saw a decline in most phases of oral hygiene.[35] As with other aspects of Greek and Roman culture lost in the barbarian overthrow of Europe, much medical knowledge was lost and forgotten. Teeth were cleaned with tepid water and a cloth sponge, with the occasional use of salt. Even in the 1700's and 1800's, the ancient abrasive dentifrices were still utilized.[36] However, medical writers of the time were beginning to criticize them as being destructive to enamel. During the 1800's, some dentists began marketing their own "secret" blended toothpastes, many of which contained soap for its cleaning properties.[37] Most of the advances in dentifrice preparation have taken place in our own century.

Today oral hygiene is appreciated as the essential groundwork for any efforts to maintain oral health and adequate dentition. The current preventive movement in dentistry is based on the belief that widespread dental caries and periodontal disease can be significantly reduced, provided dentists and highly motivated patients participate in a rigorous program of oral hygiene. Despite the increase in public awareness that people do not necessarily develop dental decay and periodontal disease as a fact of life and aging, dental caries and periodontal disease are still rampant and very much a fact of life. Even with the added emphasis on oral hygiene methods and oral health provided by the media and better dental education programs, individuals still experience the ravages of dental disease. There remains a need for the dental profession to become even more involved in the understanding and elimination of these diseases.

If the dental profession is to participate actively in oral disease control and prevention, some resource manual on current concepts of oral health and oral hygiene must be available for background and consultation. Because the authors sensed a gap in dental literature concerning aspects of oral hygiene as it relates to oral health, they undertook the organization of this volume. During its conception and actual writing, this book has benefited from contributions from specialists in many areas. The authors, one a periodontist and the other a pedodontist, felt that their joint interest in community health and their somewhat different specialities provided a good foundation for pulling together and organizing the many strands of related research in the areas of oral health and oral hygiene. Due to the diverse nature of the topic, however, they invited several other specialists to share their research findings and insights in compiling various chapters.

Oral health is, of course, a multifactorial entity, and oral health status is vitally related to all areas of dental endeavor. Therefore, this volume will particularly show the relationships which exist between oral hygiene and dental diseases and the maintenance of oral health. It first presents an overview of oral hygiene. In the first chapter, "Indices for the Measurement of Oral Hygiene," various methods used for determining oral hygiene status by measurement of plaque accretions and gingival inflammation are reviewed. These indices are also evaluated with regard to both their effectiveness and applicability to specific types of research studies, i.e. clinical tests or epidemiological surveys. Using reliable indices appropriate to one's research permits comparison of findings with other studies and also aids in determination of individual patient progress when employed in an office setting.

The second chapter concerned with oral hygiene discusses various behavioral influences upon oral hygiene practices. Primarily using findings from studies of school and public health dental education programs, authors Rayner and Cohen evaluate the influential forces exerted on oral hygiene behavior by the school, parent-teacher interaction, social and socioeconomic status, family values, peer values and identification, forms of communication, and individual perception and attitude. They stress that any attempt to change an individual's oral hygiene behavior necessitates an evaluation of those forces shaping present oral hygiene behavior and a change in an individual's values concerning oral health; then an observable change in behavior is possible. The interaction of the many social, psychological, and cultural influences affecting oral hygiene especially must be taken into account since behavior change is such a complex process. For example, simply making it economically possible for an individual to obtain regular dental checkups may not result in his doing so; he might fear the dental office environment or lack appreciation for the necessity of such visits.

Patient education alone is not enough to motivate changed behavior. An understanding of the role of behavioral forces is vital as is an appreciation of how to motivate patients by identifying their individual needs and fears and by helping them fulfill their needs through improved oral hygiene.

The third chapter, "Techniques and Armamentarium Associated with Oral Hygiene," establishes that a diligent program of individual oral hygiene and proper food selection can eliminate or control dental disease. Masters and Hoskins review oral hygiene methods and evaluate them as to their effectiveness in cleaning and the potential problems they pose in patient usage. The authors then outline a personal dental care program applicable for use in the dental office with patients having existing dental problems. They base their patient education system on the premise that no therapy conducted by the dentist can maintain oral health unless effective personal oral hygiene is exercised by the patient; this must be communicated to the patient as the necessary groundwork for therapy. In addition to outlining a feasible training program for personal dental care, the authors discuss the role of the dental health educator in functioning as an auxiliary to the dentist's efforts in patient education.

The second concentration in this volume is on periodontal disease, one of the major results of inadequate oral hygiene. The first chapter in this section focuses on the influence exerted by nutrition in the etiology and management of periodontal disease and the importance of nutrition as a determinant of oral health. Also discussed is the vital role played by behavioral factors which determine present nutritional habits and affect the complex process of changing such habits.

In the second chapter focusing on periodontal disease, Nisengard and Genco review the research relating severity of periodontal disease to degree of oral hygiene efficiency, concluding that poor oral hygiene is definitely a precursor of periodontal disease as it allows plaque development near the gingival tissue. The authors also discuss current concepts of the microbial flora of the gingival crevice and its role in periodontal disease, and they review the development, structure, and location of plaque with stress on its action in periodontal disease. Emphasis is given to the pathogenicity of oral microorganisms and the modes of bacterial action in periodontal disease. Differences between etiologic bacteria and pathogenesis for gingivitis, periodontitis, and acute necrotizing ulcerative gingivitis are also discussed. In conclusion, the authors evaluate host resistance to periodontal disease and explain why plaque control by mechanical oral hygiene methods currently offers the best means for the control and prevention of periodontal disease.

The third section of the book focuses on dental caries—the etiology of the disease and how oral hygiene methods play a role in its prevention and control. The first chapter primarily deals with the alterations of tooth tissues associated with progressions of the carious lesion through the enamel, dentin, and pulp. Changes in the gross appearance of the tooth are correlated with histologic, ultrastructural, and chemical changes. Also discussed are the defense mechanisms of the tooth.

Bibby and Barenie next outline the complex relationship between foods and dental caries, specifically treating nutrient groups such as carbohydrates, proteins, fats, vitamins, phosphates, fluoride, and trace elements. Also discussed are food-saliva relationships affecting the caries process, influences of food on the oral flora and the tooth-cleaning ability of foods. The authors further recommend the basic dietary counseling information that should be incorporated into a practitioner's caries prevention program.

Stressing that it is possible to prevent or control the carious lesion by altering the internal and external environment of the tooth, Ripa discusses oral hygiene measures which are currently used in control programs. Toothbrushing, flossing, mouth rinsing, oral irrigation, and the consumption of fibrous foods are evaluated as to their therapeutic benefits.

The last chapter concerning dental caries discusses the use of fluoride and adhesives as caries-preventive measures. Fluoride studies are reviewed and the authors present factors which influence the selection and application of the available topical fluoride compounds. Professional and self-administration technics are evaluated. Also presented is a discussion of the rationale and various technics for adhesive sealants with a comparison of the relative advantages of commercially available sealants. Although these topical methods of caries control are mostly conducted in the dental office, they represent an important part of individual oral hygiene obtained through regular professional dental care.

The authors feel that this book presents the most current research and concepts concerning oral hygiene and its relationship to oral health. Since publication of the Hirschfield book in 1939, there has been no definitive volume addressed to the dental profession which adequately summarizes oral hygiene findings to date and points the way toward more successful modes of patient education and motivation. Thus, the goal of this volume is to provide both dental practitioners and students with a review of oral hygiene, not just as it specifically relates to dental caries and periodontal disease, but also as it affects oral health. Although future research will undoubtedly lead to alterations in some of the postulates of this text, the authors hope their volume will represent for many years a valuable tool in clarifying the complex area of oral health.

REFERENCES

1. I. Hirschfield, *The Toothbrush: Its Use and Abuse* (Brooklyn, Dental Items of Interest Publishing Co., Inc., 1939), p. 9.
2. Hirschfield, p. 4.
3. H. Sachs, *Kulturgeschichte der Zahnheilkunde* (Berlin, 1913).
4. Hirschfield, *The Toothbrush*, p. 6.
5. Sachs, *Kulturgeschichte der Zahnheilkunde.*
6. Hirschfield, *The Toothbrush*, p. 6.
7. Hirschfield, p. 6.
8. Hebert, *Le Citoyen Dentiste* (Lyon, 1778).
9. M. K. D. Bremner, *The Story of Dentistry* (Brooklyn, Dental Items of Interest Publishing Co., Inc., 1939), p. 31.
10. J. Fuller, *A Popular Essay on the Structure, Formation and Management of the Teeth* (London, 1810).
11. Hirschfield, *The Toothbrush*, p. 9.
12. Hirschfield, p. 13.
13. J. R. Duval, *Dentiste de la Jeunesse*, trans. from French (London, 1820).
14. Bremner, *Dentistry*, p. 25.
15. Duval, *Dentiste de la Jeunesse.*
16. Hirschfield, *The Toothbrush*, p. 9.
17. A. Coomaraswamy, *Buddha and the Gospel of Buddhism* (London, 1928), p. 37.
18. S. Grief, *Dentistry in the Bible and Talmud* (New York, 1918).
19. H. W. C. Bodecker, *Dental Cosmos*, May 1926, p. 431.
20. Bremner, *Dentistry*, p. 42.
21. Hirschfield, *The Toothbrush*, p. 18.
22. Hirschfield, p. 18.
23. Hirschfield, p. 22.
24. Fuller, *Popular Essay.*
25. Fuller, *Popular Essay.*
26. Snell, *A Practical Guide to Operations on the Teeth* (Philadelphia, 1832), pp. 197-202.
27. R. Woofendale, *Practical Observation on the Human Teeth* (Liverpool, 1788).
28. Hirschfield, *The Toothbrush*, p. 23.
29. J. H. Mosteller, "Preventive Dentistry: Fads and Facts," *J Am Coll Dent*, 40:226, 1973.
30. Hirschfield, *The Toothbrush*, p. 13.

31. Hirschfield, p. 15.
32. Bremner, *Dentistry*, p. 37.
33. Hirschfield, *The Toothbrush*, p. 16.
34. Hirschfield, p. 16.
35. Hirschfield, p. 16.
36. Hirschfield, p. 16.
37. Hirschfield, p. 17.

ORAL HYGIENE
AS A SCIENCE

2

INDICES FOR THE MEASUREMENT OF ORAL HYGIENE

Hyman J. V. Goldberg

IN ANY EFFORT to evaluate the state of oral health or the efficacy of oral hygiene methods, the clinician must utilize reliable indices for measurement. Indices provide the profession with a means of standardizing the success or failure of oral hygiene procedures in research situations and offer a basis for determining individual patient progress in the office setting. Regardless of whether they are applied in a clinical test or epidemiological survey, indices permit comparison of data. Although determining an individual patient's rate of calculus formation does not require the same degree of accuracy essential to clinical evaluation of a calculus inhibitory substance, still some mode of measurement and result comparison is vital.

In this chapter various indices for measuring plaque accretions (including calculus) and gingival inflammation will be presented with discussion of their advantages and/or disadvantages. Possible applications of the indices to epidemiological surveys, clinical studies, and evaluation of individual patient oral hygiene status will also be reviewed. Perhaps this overview will indicate reliable indices to which the profession can uniformly adhere in measuring oral hygiene, thereby facilitating comparisons of obtained results, whether they be experimental data or patient progress reports.

MEASUREMENT OF PLAQUE

Dental plaque has been the focus of many investigations concerning oral hygiene; clinicians have sought to define its nature, formation mechanism, and pathologic potential.[1] For the purposes of this review, plaque will be considered as "microbial masses, gel-like mats, organized microcolonies, microcosms, microbiotas, zooglea, or communities of microorganisms closely adherent to the tooth or restoration surfaces."[2] Plaque has the ability to remain attached to the tooth surface despite muscle action or rinsing with water.

Mandel distinguishes other soft accumulations from plaque.[3] *Materia alba* consists of the grayish-white or yellowish grouping of bacteria and cellular debris which overlies the plaque, particularly along the gingival margins. This unorganized mass results from mechanical accumulation and can be removed by vigorous rinsing or water sprays. *Debris* consists mainly of food particles and is usually easily dislodged by movement of the lip, tongue, and cheek, or by rinsing. Debris is not part of plaque, but when it becomes impacted and broken down by enzyme action, it can contribute soluble mats for the bacterial metabolic activity occurring within the plaque. *Pellicles* are either developmental (Nasmyth's membrane) or acquired. Developmental pellicles are rare in functional teeth, while the acquired pellicles are common. Acquired pellicle is a bacteria-free film composed of glycoproteins and probably lipid which is derived from the saliva and/or gingival fluid. Pellicle may cover the entire tooth surface and often becomes stained. If it is colonized by bacteria, pellicle becomes part of the plaque. *Stains* result from chromogenic bacteria, tobacco tars, and resin residues, reaction products of food component combinations, medications, etc. While dental plaque may become stained, stain is not plaque.

The extent of area covered by plaque is the most common criterion for plaque scoring.[4] In most cases, the area is assigned a number in a numerical index, derived from the mean score per tooth or tooth surface. The number of teeth examined varies from total mouth to six selected teeth, or only anterior teeth. Another procedure involves measuring the total area occupied by the plaque. A planimeter or tracings made from enlargements of Kodachrome® transparencies is used. In a modification of this technique, the transparency is projected, the areas are traced on paper, and the cutout tracings are weighed. In still another variation, grid squares are counted.

The thickness of plaque is sometimes measured and a numerical index assigned. Other studies have quantitatively assessed plaque weight by weighing deposits formed on mylar foils or removed directly from tooth surfaces.

Plaque Area Measurements: Numerical Indices

Ramfjord used area measurements as part of his periodontal disease index (PDI).[5] Six teeth are assessed: maxillary first molar, maxillary left central incisor, maxillary left first bicuspid, mandibular left first molar, mandibular right central incisor, and mandibular right first bicuspid. The interproximal, buccal, and lingual surfaces are examined. Only fully erupted teeth are scored, and missing teeth are not to be substituted. If some of the teeth to be scored are missing or unerupted, the examiner adds individual scores for each examined tooth and divides the total by the number of teeth examined. Scoring of the plaque is done after staining with Bismark brown solution. Plaque is scored according to the following criteria:

0 = no plaque present;
1 = plaque present on some, but not all, interproximal, buccal, and lingual surfaces of the tooth;
2 = plaque present on all interproximal, buccal, and lingual surfaces but covering not more than one half of these surfaces;
3 = plaque extending over all interproximal, buccal, and lingual surfaces and covering more than one half of these surfaces.

Shick and Ash[6] modified this scoring technique. Buccal and lingual, but not interproximal surfaces, of the six selected teeth are examined, and plaque scoring is restricted to the gingival half of the surfaces:

0 = absence of dental plaque;

1 = dental plaque in the interproximal spaces or at the gingival margin covering less than one third of the gingival half of the buccal or lingual surface;

2 = dental plaque covering more than one third but less than two thirds of the gingival half of the buccal or lingual surface;

3 = dental plaque covering two thirds or more of the gingival half of the buccal or gingival surface of the tooth.

The total score is divided by the number of teeth examined to obtain a mean score. Although Ramfjord's PDI is a reliable index for assessing periodontal disease, the plaque scoring technique is not so well suited for clinical studies as the modifications introduced by Shick and Ash. Shick and Ash[6] and Jamison[7] have shown that a valid representation of plaque scores for the whole mouth can be obtained using this six-tooth index. In testing the reproducibility of this scoring method, Smith and Ash[8] found that the examiners' average deviation for a single plaque score was ± 0.019 units; Rainey and Ash found a deviation of ± 0.028.

Utilizing the Shick-Ash index, Rainey and Ash[9] found that the initial plaque score on their clinical study varied from 0.75 to 1.92. None of the examined patients evidenced a mean plaque score beyond two thirds of the gingival half of the buccal or lingual tooth surface. This observation seems to justify utilization of a scoring technique that accentuates differences in the gingival half of the tooth.[10]

Stallard et al.[11] also used a partial mouth scoring technique. They examined buccal surfaces of upper right and left first molars, lingual surfaces of lower right and left first molars, and labials of upper right central and lower left central. After staining the teeth with erythrosin disclosing solution, the examiners graded plaque as follows:

0 = no stain present;

1 = stain covering not more than one third of the tooth surface;

2 = stain covering more than one third but not more than two thirds of the tooth surface;

3 = stain covering more than two thirds of the tooth surface.

A serious limitation to the numerical index of 0 to 3 such as that used by Stallard et al.[11] is that half of the scoring range (2 and 3) involves two thirds or more of the tooth surface. To be realistic, scoring techniques should reflect the fact that the plaque area of greatest concern in periodontal disease is the region close to the gingival margins.[12] The Navy Plaque Index (modified)[13] utilizes a scoring system that gives more consideration to the plaque in the gingival area. The tooth is divided into three zones—the occlusal, the middle, and the gingival zones.

> The gingival zones lies apical to an imaginary line connecting the crests of the interdental papillae and roughly parallels the marginal gingiva. This area is subdivided into a mesial, distal and middle zone, with each having a small area, not exceeding 1 mm, adjacent to the gingival tissue. The occlusal zone is coronal to the contact area or height of contour. The middle zone extends between the occlusal and gingival zones and is divided into mesial and distal areas. By assigning all areas a score of one, more emphasis is placed on plaque adjacent to the gingival tissues, inasmuch as the surface area is much smaller.[14]

Quigley and Hein[15] also recommended a numerical index that accents the gingival third of the tooth. They used a partial mouth scoring technique confined to the labial surfaces of the anterior teeth. Subjects rinsed with a basic fuchsin mouthwash, and the plaque was scored as follows:

0 = no plaque;
1 = flecks of stain at gingival margin;
2 = definite line of plaque at gingival margin;
3 = plaque covering gingival third of surface;
4 = plaque covering two thirds of surface;
5 = plaque covering over two thirds of surface.

The score was calculated as a mean amount of plaque per tooth surface per person. Although other investigators[16, 17] have employed the Quigley and Hein scoring system on labial-buccal and lingual surfaces of the whole mouth, no data on reproducibility have been presented. Problems in differentiating the one and two values could be a drawback, but Turesky et al.[17] more clearly differentiated these scores and eliminated some of the problems. They assigned values:

0 = no plaque;

1 = separate flecks of plaque at the cervical margin of the tooth;

2 = a thin continuous band of plaque (up to 1 mm) at the cervical margin;

3 = a band of plaque wider than 1 mm but covering less than one third of crown;

4 = plaque covering at least one third but less than two thirds of the crown;

5 = plaque covering two thirds or more of crown.

Other investigators have used full mouth buccal-labial and lingual surface scoring following use of basic fuchsin or erythrosine disclosing solution. Volpe et al.[18] scored with these values:

0 = no stained plaque on the tooth surface;

1 = approximately one fourth of the surface is covered with stained plaque;

2 = approximately one half of the surface is covered with stained plaque;

3 = approximately three fourths of the surface is covered with stained plaque;

4 = entire surface is covered with stained plaque.

Only deeply stained plaque was scored in an attempt to differentiate mature plaque from immature plaque or pellicle. As no data on reproducibility were presented, it is not known how accurately such a differentiation can be made.

Mandel remarks that the Ramfjord index as modified by Shick and Ash[6] possesses several characteristics which make it particularly suited for clinical studies designed to evaluate the effectiveness of agents or procedures that alter the development of plaque and its relationship to gingival disease.[19]

(1) It is efficient as it only utilizes six teeth.

(2) Although it is limited to partial dentition, it assesses both anterior and posterior teeth and lingual as well as facial surfaces. Therefore, it can be extrapolated to a total mouth evaluation.

(3) It is reproducible.

(4) Scoring is confined to the gingival half, the area of the tooth where plaque is especially involved in periodontal disease.

The Quigley and Hein index as modified by Turesky et al.[17]

has similar advantages. Particularly, it emphasizes differences in plaque accumulation in the gingival area of the tooth. Also, because the scoring values reflect relatively subtle differentiations in amounts of plaque, the index can illustrate the plaque-gingival inflammation relationship.[20] If cleansing efficiency rather than plaque-gingival relationships are being investigated, an index assessing the total tooth surface could be used. However, cleansing efficiency is still most important in the gingival third of the tooth.

Plaque Area Measurements: Total Area

Arnim[21] employed photographs of certain teeth stained with erythrosin to determine the total amount of plaque present on the labial surfaces of the four upper and lower incisor teeth. Kodachrome transparencies were enlarged four times. Outlines of the tooth surfaces and stained masses were traced on paper and their areas determined with a planimeter. Then the percentage of the surface covered by plaque was calculated.

Arnim's procedure was modified by Kinoshita et al.[22] Color slides were projected at ×65 magnification; areas of plaque and unstained tooth surface were traced on paper and cut out for gravimetric determination. Percentage of the tooth surface covered by plaque was then calculated.

Although area measurements provide more quantitative data than numerical indices, they are more time-consuming and are best employed on the incisor teeth.[23] It would be difficult to gauge accurately the amount of plaque on lingual or interproximal surfaces, even with the aid of mirrors and retractors. Ash[24] claims that "scoring from photographs often leads to erroneous conclusions." Whether the errors are greater than those with a numerical index has not yet been determined. Since there is so little data on accuracy and reproducibility, total area measurements probably have only limited applicability to clinical studies.

Plaque Thickness

Silness and Löe[25] introduced an index system focusing on plaque thickness in 1964. Löe[26] describes the procedure:

Each of the four gingival areas of the tooth is given a score from

0 to 3; this is the plaque index (PlI) for the area. The scores from the four areas of the tooth may be added and divided by four to give the PlI for the tooth. The scores for individual teeth (incisors, premolars and molars) may be grouped to designate the PlI for the groups of teeth. Finally, by adding the indices for the teeth and dividing by the number of teeth examined, the PlI for the individual is obtained.

The surface is tested by running a pointed probe across the tooth surface at the entrance of the gingival crevice after the tooth is properly dried. Investigators check to see if soft matter adheres to the point of the probe. Scoring values are as follows:

0 = gingival area of the tooth surface free of plaque;

1 = no plaque observable *in situ* by the unaided eye, but plaque is visible on the point of probe;

2 = gingival area is covered with a thin to moderately thick layer of plaque, and the deposit is visible to the naked eye;

3 = heavy accumulation of soft matter, the thickness of this plaque fills out the niche produced by the gingival margin and tooth surface; interdental areas are filled with soft debris.

Since the gingival area constitutes the measured unit, the Silness-Löe PlI may be scored for all surfaces of all or selected teeth. Thus, the PlI is applicable to large-scale epidemiological surveys as well as to the examination of smaller groups or evaluation of the individual patient.[27] Recent analyses indicate no difference in the results when only one interproximal surface is examined instead of both, provided the score is doubled and divided by four.

Two studies lend support to the validity and reliability of the PlI. Lang et al.[28] established a nearly linear correlation between the index used for facial surfaces of anterior teeth and the total area of plaque measured photographically with sodium fluorescein and a special light. When minute quantities of plaque were measured, the PlI was more consistent than the fluorescein technique. Loesche and Green[29] reported that unstained plaque scores correlated better with gingivitis and actual plaque than stained scores.

Plaque Weight

Marthaler, Schroeder, and Mühlemann[30] employed sandblasted, standardized mylar foils attached to lower lingual anterior teeth as a means of measuring total plaque weight. After exposure to various clinical conditions, the foils were dried at 110 degrees C and weighed. Deposits were removed chemically, and the foils were redried and weighed. Although this procedure is precise, it is time-consuming and probably has limited applicability to general clinical studies.[31] Removal of plaque directly from tooth surfaces and subsequent weighing is less precise but much simpler.

Two studies used plaque weight to determine the effect of dextranase. Caldwell et al.[32] scraped plaque from six tooth surfaces after a one-week period: buccal surfaces of upper right and left first molars, lingual surfaces of lower right and left first molars, labial surfaces of upper right and left central incisors. Plaque material was dried overnight at 85 degrees C and weighed. Lobene[33] scraped buccal and lingual surfaces of the maxillary right central, first premolar, and molar after a three-day period and dried the plaque at 105 degrees C for twenty-four hours. He then compared the plaque weight to the PlI scored with the Quigley and Hein method and found a poor correlation.

In plaque weight measurement, interexaminer standardization for plaque removal technique is necessary.[34] The technique does require more equipment than visualization methods and has a drawback in that it does not lend itself to daily measurements in individual subjects. Several days must elapse between sessions of harvesting and weighing the accumulated plaque.

Oral Debris

The commonly used Greene and Vermillion oral hygiene index[35] includes separate measurements for oral debris and calculus and has been mainly used in epidemiological studies. The procedure of estimating surface area covered is based on the assumption that in mouths where debris remains undisturbed for a longer period of time, more surface area will be covered by debris. In epidemiological studies, there is often no opportunity for rinsing by the subjects, so debris scores are realistic.[36] In this index, debris is regarded as the "soft foreign matter loosely attached to the teeth."[37]

Greene and Vermillion used six tooth surfaces in their studies: buccal surfaces of upper right and left first molars, labial surfaces of upper right and left central incisors. A buccal or lingual surface is considered to encompass half the tooth circumference. The following scoring system is used for the Oral Hygiene Index (OHI) to assess the measurement of oral debris:

0 = no debris or stain present;
1 = soft debris covering not more than one third of the tooth surface or the presence of extrinsic stains without debris regardless of surface area covered;
2 = soft debris covering more than one third but not more than two thirds of the exposed tooth surface;
3 = soft debris covering more than two thirds of the exposed tooth surface.

Glass[38] used a modified scoring system for debris which might have greater applicability to clinical studies. The scoring technique permits quantitation of differences within the gingival area and, therefore, may be more precise for clinical studies than the OHI.[39] The scoring is determined in this manner:

0 = no visible debris;
1 = debris visible at gingival margin—but discontinuous—less than 1 mm in height;
2 = debris continuous at gingival margin—greater than 1 mm in height;
3 = debris involving entire gingival third of tooth;
4 = debris generally scattered over tooth surface.

Podshadley and Haley[40] also introduced a modification of the OHI which is more complex than the Glass method but which may also have applicability for clinical studies.[41] Subjects use a disclosing solution and may expectorate, but no rinsing is allowed. Six teeth (the same surfaces recommended by Greene and Vermillion) are scored. The tooth surfaces are divided into five sections, each of which is assessed for stained debris and totalled for the surface score. A mean surface score is then established. The authors report that the same scores were reproduced by the same examiner on different occasions, and also by different examiners. Results were more consistent with this method than with the OHI.

Mandel comments that although plaque receives most attention in measurements of soft accumulations, the pathogenic potential of the material overlying plaque should also be considered.[42] Plaque is probably the principal culprit in dental caries and calculus formation, but not necessarily in periodontal disease. The bacteria clumps, shed epithelial cells, and disrupted leukocytes in oral debris can produce a variety of enzymes and toxic substances which can alter the integrity of the gingival tissues and initiate inflammation. Therefore, debris scoring probably has merit in clinical testing.

Clearance of Food Debris

Several investigators[43, 44, 45] have developed experimental techniques to measure the ability of a hygienic procedure, i.e. brushing, chewing apples, to clear food debris. The usual approach has been (1) to put a marker substance into a food item and have the subject chew the food, (2) to remove the loose debris by light rinsing or normal muscle action, (3) to conduct the test procedure, collect the removed debris, and analyze for the marker, and (4) to remove the residual debris by exhaustive brushing and rinsing and analyze for the marker.[46]

Cobb et al.[43] employed this procedure in several studies and used gingerbread biscuits containing copper or iron as the marker. Birch and Mumford[44] used biscuits with ferric oxide as the test material. Golden et al.[45] utilized peanut butter with radioactive serum albumin. Meaningful data has been generated by such studies, but examinations are difficult to conduct as subjects must control swallowing to prevent loss of the marker substances. Also, radioactive markers have limited appeal.

Lefkowitz and Robinson[47] suggested a more practical food debris clearance procedure. Children were given a soda cracker, followed by a hygienic procedure. They expectorated loose particles without rinsing. Examiners then applied an iodine solution which stained the cracker residue blue. Labial-buccal and lingual surfaces of all teeth were scored:

0 = no debris at gingival margin;

1 = debris extending up to 1 mm from gingival margin;

2 = debris in excess of 1 mm at gingival margin.

This test would probably have the greatest applicability for large-scale studies.[48]

MEASUREMENT OF CALCULUS

This section will review indices currently available to quantitate dental calculus and their applicability to clinical studies in particular. Early calculus clinical studies (conducted from about the mid-1940's to the late 1950's) that attempted to evaluate the effect of calculus inhibitory materials were mainly clinical impressions obtained by direct visual examination or intraoral photographs.[49] Dental instruments such as mirrors, explorers, hoes, and periodontal probes were often used to aid visual examination.

Supragingival calculus was quantitated on the basis of such categories as "absence or presence," "slight, moderate, severe," etc. The techniques used were generally rapid and subjective estimations of the absence or presence and/or amount of accumulated calculus. Little data are available concerning establishment of examiner standardization and reproducibility procedures. Although these early methods have been mostly replaced by more quantitative and reproducible means of measurement, intraoral photographs obtained under standardized conditions are a valuable visual supplement to any calculus quantitating procedure.

More recent clinical research efforts have led to the establishment of calculus-quantitating indices which are better suited to clinical testing: (1) Calculus Surface Index; (2) Probe Method of Calculus Assessment; and (3) Marginal Line Calculus Index.[51] In addition, epidemiological surveys have proved the usefulness of the PDI and the OHI. These methods all have clinical data available concerning examiner reproducibility, and all methods have been used in previous clinical studies, so data exists for comparison purposes.

Calculus Surface Index (CSI)

The CSI method developed by Ennever, Sturzenberger, and Radike[52] utilizes the four mandibular incisor teeth in the evaluation of calculus accumulation. These teeth were selected on the basis of calculus formation rate and the ease of observing calculus. In scoring, calculus is considered to be present if any amount, supragingival or subgingival, can be detected visually or by touch. If the examiner is uncertain about the presence of calculus on a given surface, the surface is scored calculus-free.

Each mandibular incisor is evaluated on the basis of four surfaces: two proximals (scored from the lingual aspect), one labial and one lingual. After the examination, the number of surfaces on which calculus has been found is assigned to each tooth. The total number of surfaces where calculus occurs is considered to be the subject's calculus score and is called the CSI.

The Calculus Surface Severity Index (CSSI) measures the quantity of calculus present on the facial, mesial, lingual, and distal surfaces of the four mandibular incisors.[52, 53] Calculus is scored on a severity scale from 0 to 3 on each of the four surfaces with a maximum possible score of 48. The scale is:

0 = no calculus present;
1 = calculus observable, but less than 0.5 mm in width and/or thickness;
2 = calculus not exceeding 1.0 mm in width and/or thickness;
3 = calculus exceeding 1.0 mm in width and/or thickness.

The CSSI method has evidenced good interexaminer reproducibility and provides a relatively rapid scoring procedure for calculus deposits.[54] It is considered particularly useful for evaluating calculus deposits that have accumulated in a short period such as one to six weeks. Although all natural teeth may be included in scoring, a study has demonstrated partial mouth scores do correlate with whole mouth scores with this method. Two other studies[56, 57] have indicated comparable calculus reductions can be obtained with either the CSI or CSSI indices when scoring a partial or a full mouth examination.

Probe Method of Calculus Assessment

The Probe Method of Calculus Assessment was developed over a seven-year period (1960-67) and provides for measurement of calculus on three constant planes.[58] Calculus is measured for the lingual surfaces of the six mandibular anterior teeth. The six teeth are assessed for calculus height, width (area), and volume (amount). Each tooth can have 9 calculus units, for a total possible score of 54 units for the six teeth.

The three measurement planes for the quantification of calculus accumulation are described as follows:

(1) The first plane is for gingival measurements and is determined by vertically positioning the probe to bisect the lingual surface of the tooth.

(2) The second plane is for distal measurements. It is obtained by positioning the probe to bisect the mesioincisal angle of the tooth and then placing the probe diagonally through the area of greatest calculus width on the distal aspect of the tooth.

(3) The third plane is for mesial measurements. It is obtained by positioning the probe to bisect the distoincisal angle of the tooth and then placing it diagonally through the area of greatest calculus width on the mesial aspect of the tooth.

Further studies were conducted to evaluate interexaminer reproducibility in the Probe Method and to compare this level of reproducibility with that for the CSI method and staining procedures using basic fuchsin solution.[59] Results showed the Probe Method offered greater interexaminer reproducibility than the other procedures. Another study of the Probe Method described and discussed probe calibration, examiner training, and proper examination procedure.[60] Additional data indicated:

(1) A statistically significant correlation existed between routinely obtained partial mouth calculus examination scores (lingual surfaces of lower anterior teeth) and full mouth scores on the same subject.

(2) The Probe Method possesses a high degree of interexaminer reproducibility.

These same correlations were verified in another study.[61]

In an independent investigation, examiners demonstrated that *in vivo* calculus scores obtained by the Probe Method correlated highly with the dry, ash, and organic weights of the same calculus directly removed from the teeth and tested.[62, 63] Again substantiating the validity of the Probe Method, a study suggested a high correlation between scores obtained with the Probe Method and simultaneously recorded gingivitis scores obtained using the modified PlI of Russell.[64]

This review indicates that the Probe Method offers a reliable method for quantitation of gingival calculus deposits, especially over relatively long periods of time.[65] Intra- and interexaminer reproducibility have been established as well as significant correlations with calculus dry weight and gingivitis. Although the method is easy to use, Volpe emphasizes that thirty to fifty examinations conducted under the guidance of an experienced investigator are essential in training a new examiner.[66] The method is also not especially rapid; five to ten minutes are required for an examination.

Marginal Line Calculus Index (MLC)

Mühlemann and Villa[67] developed this index to provide an accurate measurement of supragingival calculus accumulation in the areas closest to the gingiva. This procedure permits more precision in correlating the rate of calculus formation with inflammatory gingival disease and also permits conducting calculus inhibitory clinical studies with small groups.[68]

The MLC Index scores only that supragingival calculus formed in the cervical area along the marginal gingivae on lingual sides of the mandibular incisors. This band, paralleling the free gingiva, is divided into two parts by an axial plane bisecting the incisal edge of the incisors and directed toward the most apical position of the marginal free gingiva. The mesial and distal part of the band are scored separately; the examiner estimates the percentage of the distance covered by the calculus deposits. Percentages of 0, 12½, 25, 50, 75, and 100 are used. Whenever uncertainty arises concerning the correct percentage, the higher figure is assigned. The mesial and distal percentages for a tooth are averaged, and the means of the four teeth are then averaged for the subject's score. Before scoring, a warm stream of air is blown on the lingual surfaces until the calculus is clearly visible. The examination requires approximately five minutes.

Mühlemann and Villa provide data indicating the MLC Index has interexaminer reproducibility. However, like the Probe Method, the MLC Index requires a highly trained examiner and is a procedure best suited to small group studies.[69]

Additional Indices for Calculus Measurement

In the late 1950's and early 1960's, the Periodontal Disease Index (PDI) of Ramfjord and the Oral Hygiene Index (OHI) of Greene and Vermillion were developed to study the incidence of periodontal disease and the oral health status of various populations.[70] These indices were previously discussed in their relationship to plaque measurement. However, both indices also include calculus-quantitating components. Much data is available concerning examiner reproducibility as these indices have been utilized on a world-wide basis, especially for epidemiological surveys and to a lesser extent, for clinical studies.

Periodontal Disease Index

The Calculus Index component of the PDI utilizes six teeth: the maxillary right first molar, the maxillary left central incisor, the maxillary left first bicuspid, the mandibular left first molar, the mandibular right central incisor, and the mandibular right first bicuspid. Calculus is observed with a dental explorer and/or periodontal probe and is scored on the four surfaces of the selected teeth according to the following criteria:

  0 = absence of calculus;
  1 = supragingival calculus extending only slightly below the free gingival margin (not more than 1 mm);
  2 = moderate amount of supragingival and subgingival calculus, or subgingival calculus alone;
  3 = an abundance of supragingival and subgingival calculus.
(Subgingival calculus is emphasized because it is regarded as more influential in the pathogenesis of periodontitis than is su-

pragingival calculus.) The calculus scores for the six teeth are added and the total divided by six to provide the index for calculus.

Oral Hygiene Index

The Calculus Index component of the modified OHI (OHI-S) calls for examination of six tooth surfaces: buccal surface of the first fully erupted maxillary tooth distal to the second bicuspid on the right and left sides, lingual surface of the first fully erupted mandibular tooth distal to the second bicuspid on the right and left sides, and the labial surfaces of the upper right central incisor and lower left central incisor. Examiners use an explorer to estimate the surface area covered by supragingival calculus and to probe for subgingival calculus. Calculus scores are assigned as follows:

0 = no calculus present;
1 = supragingival calculus covering not more than one third of the exposed tooth surface being examined;
2 = supragingival calculus covering more than one third but not more than two thirds of the exposed tooth surface, or presence of individual flecks of subgingival calculus around the cervical portion of the tooth;
3 = supragingival calculus covering more than two thirds of the exposed tooth surface, or continuous heavy band of subgingival calculus around the cervical portion of the tooth.

Both the OHI-S and the PDI utilize only six teeth, and a trained examiner can accurately conduct a quantitation of calculus accumulations in a relatively short period of time.[71] Therefore, both indices are particularly suited to epidemiological studies. Volpe recommends that these indices and the Probe Method be used in long-term clinical studies (up to a year or longer) with large subject groups.[72] In such "actual length" studies, selected materials can be evaluated in clinical investigations that correspond in duration to actual calculus formation patterns.[73] In "short-term scoring procedures," a relatively large number of materials can be evaluated *in vivo* on a small group of subjects in a short period of time (one to six weeks). For such clinical studies where materials are judged for their effect on subgingival and supragingival calculus formation, Volpe recommends the CSI and MLC Index.[74]

INDICES FOR MEASUREMENT OF GINGIVAL INFLAMMATION

Gingival inflammation is the other guideline used by clinicians in determining oral hygiene status and the susceptability to periodontal disease. In this section, various indices for measuring gingival inflammation will be reviewed.

Descriptive Indices

Early in dental literature there appear descriptions of degrees of gingival inflammation.[75] Although such indices were in use up to the 1960's, they will not be discussed as they do not lend themselves well to statistical analysis or interexaminer reproducibility.

Present or Absent

Such indices do not take into account the degree of severity of gingival inflammation. However, this may not be an essential criterion since there is little available evidence to show that the severity of gingivitis is directly related to the progression of inflammation to the supporting structures of the teeth or to subsequent pocket formation.[76] Therefore, the index may be applicable to clinical studies, especially since it is simple, takes little time to conduct, is reproducible with little examiner training, and lends itself well to statistical analyses.

In one study of this nature, Arno et al.[77] examined the buccal, lingual, mesial, and distal gingivae of each tooth to determine inflammatory changes and noted whether inflammation was present or absent. Hoover and Lefkowitz[78] followed a similar approach but scored buccal and lingual papillae separately.

Numerical Indices

The PMA Index, as introduced by Schour and Massler,[79] indicates the severity of inflammation in the papillary (P), marginal (M), and attached (A) gingiva areas on a scale from 0 to

4. Originally, only the labial surface of the lower six anterior teeth was scored. Parfitt[80] modified the PMA Index by adding scoring of the buccal and lingual gingiva. The criterion he advanced are as follows:

0 = no clinical evidence of inflammation;

P,M, Or A = indicated a detectable hyperemia in the papilla, margin, or attached mucosa. This was recognized by a research worker.

1+ = denoted there was also a loss of stippling, redness, swelling, or bleeding on pressure—mild gingivitis;

2+ = denoted that severity was such that the patient might complain of symptoms such as bleeding, sensitivity, itching sensation, or tenderness; patient was usually aware of condition;

3+ = denoted presence of severe hyperemia, or obvious swelling, or that hemorrhage occurred spontaneously on slightest touch of food or toothbrush—severe gingival disease.

The presence of inflammation and its degree of severity was determined separately for each gingival area. A severity index was determined as follows:

If P or M was recorded, the score = 1. When A was recorded, there was additional score of 1. When gingival inflammation was scored (1+, 2+, etc.), this was added to the score so a recording of the PMA+++ would equal 5.

In another variation, Mühlemann and Mazor[81] scored only the papillary and marginal areas of the gingiva. The scoring was done as follows:

0 = no inflammation;

1 = bleeding from gingival sulcus on gentle probing, tissue otherwise appears normal;

2 = bleeding on probing plus a change in color due to inflammation, no swelling or edema;

3 = bleeding plus a change of color and edematous swelling;

4 = ulceration or additional symptoms.

The average Papillary-Margin Index is determined by dividing the sum of all scores by the number of areas scored.

The Ramfjord PDI (previously described for assessing plaque area and calculus deposits) also includes a numerical index for evaluating gingival inflammation. Again six teeth are scored: maxillary right first molar, maxillary left central incisor, maxillary left first bicuspid, mandibular left first molar, mandibular right central incisor, and mandibular right first bicuspid. Gingival tissue is scored as a unit around each tooth according to the following criteria:

G0 = absence of inflammation;
G1 = mild to moderate inflammatory gingival changes not extending all around the tooth;
G2 = mild to moderate gingivitis extending all around the tooth;
G3 = severe gingivitis characterized by marked redness, tendency to bleed, and ulceration.

Silness and Löe[25] evaluated six teeth for gingival inflammation: maxillary right first molar, maxillary right lateral incisor, maxillary left first premolar, mandibular left third molar, mandibular left first premolar, and mandibular right first premolar. Each gingival unit (buccal, lingual, mesial, and distal) for the six teeth is scored according to the following criteria:

0 = absence of inflammation;
1 = mild inflammation with slight change in color and little change in texture, no bleeding on probing;
2 = moderate inflammation with moderate glazing, redness, edema, and hypertrophy, bleeding on probing;
3 = severe inflammation with marked redness and hypertrophy, tendency toward spontaneous bleeding, ulceration.

Scores from the four areas are added and divided by four to equal the Gingival Index for a particular tooth. The Gingival Index for the group of teeth can be determined by adding the indices for each tooth and dividing by six.

O'Leary et al.[82] divided the entire mouth into six segments. However, their index emphasizes the severest lesion in each segment, and thus lacks necessary accuracy.[83] This approach was modified by Cohen et al.[84] who dropped the idea of six segments but still evaluated the gingiva around each tooth as a unit:

0 = no overt inflammation, gingival form consistent with periodontal health;

1 = slight inflammatory changes, blunting, loss of firmness but not encircling the tooth;

2 = slight inflammatory changes that involve both buccal and lingual aspects;

3 = presence of ulceration, spontaneous bleeding, loss of interdental continuity, or naked deviation of contour;

4 = buccal or lingual recession that exposes the root surface.

The average gingival score for a subject equals the total score divided by the units scored. Hazen remarks that in this index recession is given the highest score; this infers such a lesion results from more severe inflammatory changes.[85] However, no evidence supports this distinction.

Suomi and Barbano[86] and Suomi[87] evaluated the gingiva around all teeth. Each gingival margin and papilla is scored as follows:

0 = absence of inflammation, stippling usually noted;

1 = inflammation present with a distinct color change to red or magenta evident, may be swelling and loss of stippling, gingiva may be spongy in texture;

2 = severe inflammation with a distinct color change to red or magenta; noticeable swelling, loss of stippling and spongy consistency; either gingival bleeding on gentle probing or inflammation has spread to attached gingiva.

Each quadrant of the mouth is divided into three segments: molar, premolar, and anterior teeth. The papillae between the first molar and second premolar and the cuspid and first premolar is arbitrarily assigned to the premolar region. To obtain the mean gingival score, the examiner adds the scores of units of the three segments and divides by the number of units examined. Separate mean gingivitis scores are determined for the buccal and lingual gingival units of each segment. The investigators observed that the right and left sides of the mouth had similar patterns of involvement, but the buccal and lingual surfaces of some segments differed.

Suomi et al.[88] introduced the DHC Index which scores eight teeth: all first permanent molars, upper right central incisor, upper left first bicuspid, lower left central incisor, and lower right first bicuspid. The only substitution of teeth permitted is using the adjacent central incisor when the proper incisor is missing. Facial and lingual gingival tissues of these teeth are scored separately for inflammation with criteria based on color change and the extent of inflammation around the tooth:

  0 = no inflammation—gingiva adjacent to tooth surface is pale pink in color and firm, no swelling evident and stippling usually noted;

  1 = inflammation not encompassing all tissue adjacent to tooth surface (including papillae), gingiva in definite red or magenta color;

  2 = inflammation encompassing all tissue adjacent to tooth surface (including papillae).

Photographic Methods

Good color photographs can be very useful in evaluating gingival changes.[89] Although good intra- and interexaminer reproducibility have been claimed for this method,[90] investigators have only used labial aspects of the anterior gingiva in their examinations.[90, 91] Thus, this method of measurement is still relatively untested.

Evaluation of gingival tissue inflammation presents a complex problem to the investigator due to differences in interpretation such as those reflected in the various numerical indices. For example, Mühlemann et al. use bleeding upon gentle probing as a criterion for slight inflammation, while Silness and Löe use early color changes of the tissue and no bleeding upon probing as criteria for early tissue changes. Silness and Löe established a good correlation with their clinical index and a histologic examination of gingival tissue. Mühlemann and Son[92] did correlate average gingival fluid flow rate of the marginal gingiva with their Sulcus Bleeding Index, but they had poor correlation with individual units. Thus, the Silness and Löe approach seems most valid for use in clinical studies.[93]

DISCUSSION

Several basic considerations are involved in the decision to utilize one of the described methods for determining oral hygiene status. Especially vital is the need for intra- and interexaminer reproducibility. Reproducibility of results is a difficult objective to realize, both with many examiners and with one examiner performing an evaluation many times. Volpe further describes some basic principles to which investigators should adhere, regardless of the nature of their study.[94]

1. An investigator should be completely familiar with the methodology of a particular index. This may require direct communication with the originators of the method. In clinical or epidemiological studies, an examiner should achieve standardization of his findings by first undertaking thirty to fifty trial examinations under the supervision of a trained investigator.

2. An examiner should use all equipment and procedures specified for an index. Only in this way will comparison with other studies be possible.

3. Data should be recorded in a manner which readily lends itself to tabulation and statistical analysis.

Another area of concern is partial versus full mouth scoring. If a particular index utilizing partial mouth scoring has good correlation with full mouth scores, i.e. the Ramfjord PDI or the Greene and Vermillion OHI-S, partial mouth scoring should be sufficient, especially for large-scale surveys.[95] However, with an individual patient or in clinical therapy evaluations, scoring of all tooth surfaces is the ideal procedure.[96]

Length of time for conducting studies is also a moot point. There are no experimental data indicating proper time parameters for various kinds of investigations. However, Mandel notes that plaque reaches 90 percent of its final weight (thirty days without toothbrushing) in approximately eight days, and most subjects evidence gingival inflammation in about twenty-one days during experimental gingivitis studies.[97] Thus, investigators undertaking clinical studies to measure plaque should consider these time parameters. For example, an eight to twenty-day period would be good for mouthwash studies without brushing, but a longer time period is indicated for brushing studies where subjects are actively engaged in some form of physical plaque removal. At this point, researchers cannot say whether a thirty- to sixty-day period is adequate to determine effectiveness of oral hygiene methods or whether a one- to two-year period is really needed in order to obtain data on caries incidence and periodontal disease.

Perhaps the most fruitful contribution a clinician can make in his personal investigations is to use an established index, rather than devising a new system of measurement.[98] Operating within the confines of a proven index will provide comparison data for conducting his investigation, and his results will be suitable for comparison purposes in others' studies.

FOOTNOTES

1. I. D. Mandel, "Indices for Measurement of Soft Accumulations in Clinical Studies of Oral Hygiene and Periodontal Disease," *J Periodont Res*, 9:7, 1974.
2. Mandel, p. 7.
3. Mandel, p. 7.
4. Mandel, p. 8.
5. S. Ramfjord, "Indices for Prevalence and Incidence of Periodontal Disease," *J Periodontol*, 30:51, 1959.
6. R. A. Shick and M. M. Ash, "Evaluation of the Vertical Method of Toothbrushing," *J Periodontol*, 32:346, 1961.
7. H. D. Jamison, *Prevalence and Severity of Periodontal Disease in a Sample of a Population* (thesis, University of Michigan, School of Public Health, 1960).
8. W. A. Smith and M. M. Ash, "A Clinical Evaluation of an Electric Toothbrush," *J Periodontol*, 35:127, 1964.
9. B. Rainey and M. M. Ash, "A Clinical Study of a Short Stroke Reciprocating Action Electric Toothbrush," *J Periodontol*, 35:455, 1964.
10. Mandel, "Indices for Measurement of Soft Accumulations," p. 10.
11. R. D. Stallard, A. R. Volpe, J. E. Orban, and W. J. King, "The Effect of an Antimicrobial Mouth Rinse on Dental Plaque, Calculus and Gingivitis," *J Periodontol*, 40:683, 1969.
12. Mandel, "Indices for Measurement of Soft Accumulations," p. 10.
13. J. R. Elliot, G. M. Bowers, B. A. Clemmen, and G. H. Rovelstad, "Evaluation of an Oral Physiotherapy Center in the Reduction of Bacterial Plaque and Periodontal Disease," *J Periodontol*, 43:221, 1972.

14. Elliott et al., p. 221.
15. G. Quigley and J. Hein, "Comparative Cleansing Efficiency of Manual and Power Brushing," *JADA*, 65:26, 1962.
16. R. Lobene, "The Effect of a Pulsed Water Pressure Cleansing Device on Oral Health," *J Periodontol*, 40:667, 1969.
17. S. Turesky, N. D. Gilmore, and I. Glickman, "Reduced Plaque Formation by the Chloromethyl Analogue of Vitamin C," *J Periodontol*, 41:41, 1970.
18. A. R. Volpe et al., "Anti-microbial Control of Bacterial Plaque and Calculus and the Effects of These Agents on Oral Flora," *J Dent Res*, 48:832, 1969.
19. Mandel, "Indices for Measurement of Soft Accumulations," p. 18.
20. Mandel, p. 18.
21. S. Arnim, "The Use of Disclosing Agents for Measuring Tooth Cleanliness," *J Periodontol*, 34:227, 1963.
22. S. Kinoshita et al., "Effects of Sucrose on Early Dental Calculus and Plaque," *Helv Odontol Acta*, 10:134, 1966.
23. Mandel, "Indices for Measurement of Soft Accumulations," p. 12.
24. M. M. Ash, "A Review of the Problems and Results of Studies on Manual and Power Toothbrushes," *J Periodontol*, 35:202, 1964.
25. P. Silness and H. Löe, "Periodontal Disease in Pregnancy," *Acta Odontol Scand*, 22:121, 1964.
26. H. Löe, "The Gingival Index, The Plaque Index and The Retention Index Systems," *J Periodontol*, 38:610, 1967.
27. Mandel, "Indices for Measurement of Soft Accumulations," p. 13.
28. J. Ainamo, "Concomitant Periodontal Disease and Dental Caries in Young Adult Males," *Soum Haamaslaak Toim*, 66:301, 1970.
29. W. Loesche and E. Green, "Comparison of Various Plaque Parameters in Individuals with Poor Oral Hygiene," *J Periodontol*, 7:173, 1972.
30. T. Marthaler, H. Schroeder, and H. Mühlemann, "A Method for the Quantitative Assessment of Plaque and Calculus Formation," *Helv Odontol Acta*, 5:39, 1961.
31. Mandel, "Indices for Measurement of Soft Accumulations," p. 13.
32. R. Caldwell et al., "Effect of Dextranase Mouthwash on Dental Plaque in Young Adults and Children," *JADA*, 82:124, 1970.
33. R. Lobene, "A Clinical Study of the Effect of Dextranase on Human Dental Plaque," *JADA*, 82:132, 1970.
34. Mandel, "Indices for Measurement of Soft Accumulations," p. 20.
35. J. C. Greene and J. R. Vermillion, "The Simplified Oral Hygiene Index," *JADA*, 68:7, 1964.
36. Mandel, "Indices for Measurement of Soft Accumulations," p. 14.
37. L. W. Smith et al., "Study of Intra-examiner Variation," *J Periodontol*, 41:673, 1970.

38. R. L. Glass, "Hand and Electric Toothbrushing," *J Periodontol*, 36:323, 1965.
39. Mandel, "Indices for Measurement of Soft Accumulations," p. 15.
40. A. G. Podshadley and J. V. Haley, "A Method for Evaluating Oral Hygiene Performance," *Publ Hlth Rep*, 83:259, 1968.
41. Mandel, "Indices for Measurement of Soft Accumulations," p. 15.
42. Mandel, p. 20.
43. A. B. Cobb, D. I. Hay, and C. J. Schram, "A Method of Measuring Toothcleaning," *Brit Dent J*, III:249, 1961.
44. R. H. Birch and J. M. Mumford, "Electric Toothbrushing," *Dent Pract Dent Rec*, 13:182, 1963.
45. I. D. Golden, E. M. Collins, and P. H. Deeb, "A Comparative Study of the Clearance of Radio Iodinated Peanut Butter and Crackers from the Mouth by Two Methods of Toothbrushing," *J Periodontol*, 35: 495, 1964.
46. Mandel, "Indices for Measurement of Soft Accumulations," p. 17.
47. W. Lefkowitz and H. Robinson, "Effectiveness of Automatic and Hand Brushes in Removing Dental Plaque and Debris," *JADA*, 65:351, 1962.
48. Mandel, "Indices for Measurement of Soft Accumulations," p. 21.
49. A. R. Volpe, "Indices for the Measurement of Hard Deposits in Clinical Studies of Oral Hygiene and Periodontal Disease," *J Periodont Res*, 9:32, 1974.
50. Volpe, p. 32.
51. Volpe, p. 33.
52. J. Ennever, O. P. Sturzenberger, and A. W. Radike, "The Calculus Surface Index Method for Scoring Clinical Calculus Studies," *J Periodontol*, 32:54, 1961.
53. C. W. Conroy and O. P. Sturzenberger, "The Rate of Calculus Formation in Adults," *J Periodontol*, 39:142, 1968.
54. Volpe, "Indices for Measurement of Hard Deposits," p. 33.
55. A. G. Alexander, "Partial Mouth Recording of Gingivitis, Plaque and Calculus in Epidemiological Surveys," *J Periodont Res*, 5:141, 1970.
56. O. P. Sturzenberger, J. R. Swancar, and G. Reiter, "Reduction of Dental Calculus in Humans Through the Use of Dentifrice Containing a Crystal-Growth Inhibitor," *J Peridontol*, 42:416, 1971.
57. C. W. Conroy, O. P. Sturzenberger, B. W. Bollmer, J. R. Swancar, and E. R. Zimmerman, "The Effect of a Sodium Etidronate Dentifrice on Calculus and Gingivitis in Adults," *IADR Abstract*, No. 208, 1972.
58. Volpe, "Indices for Measurement of Hard Deposits," p. 35.
59. J. H. Manhold, A. R. Volpe, S. P. Hazen, L. Parker, and S. H. Adams "In Vivo Calculus Assessment: Part II. A Comparison of Scoring Techniques," *J Periodontol*, 36:299, 1965.

60. A. R. Volpe, L. J. Kupczak, and W. J. King, "In Vivo Calculus Assessment: Part III. Scoring Techniques, Rate of Calculus Formation, Partial Mouth Exams vs. Full Mouth Exams, and Intra-examiner Reproducibility," *Periodontics*, 5:184, 1967.

61. A. R. Volpe, L. J. Kupczak, W. J. King, H. M. Goldman, and S. M. Schulman, "In Vivo Calculus Assessment: Part IV. Parameters of Human Clinical Studies," *J Periodontol*, 40:76, 1969.

62. A. M. Sharawy, K. B. Sabharwal, S. S. Socransky, and R. R. Lobene, "A Quantitative Study of Plaque and Calculus Formation in Normal and Periodontally Involved Mouth," *J Periodontol*, 37:53, 1966.

63. A. Picozzi, S. L. Fischman, and M. Pader, "Calculus Inhibition in Humans," *IADR Abstracts*, No. 283, 1971.

64. S. L. Fischman and A. Picozzi, "Clinical Evaluation of Anti-calculus Agents—Methodology and 'Placebo' Effect," *Pharmacol Therapeut*, 1:16, 1970.

65. Volpe, "Indices for Measurement of Hard Deposits," p. 37.

66. Volpe, p. 37.

67. H. R. Mühlemann and P. Villa, "The Marginal Line Calculus Index," *Helv Odontol Acta*, 11:175, 1967.

68. Volpe, "Indices for Measurement of Hard Deposits," p. 37.

69. Volpe, p. 38.

70. Volpe, p. 42.

71. Volpe, p. 45.

72. Volpe, p. 48.

73. Volpe, p. 47.

74. Volpe, p. 47.

75. S. P. Hazen, "Indices for the Measurement of Gingival Inflammation in Clinical Studies of Oral Hygiene and Periodontal Disease," *J Periodont Res*, 9:61, 1974.

76. Hazen, p. 61.

77. A. J. Arno, A. L. Waerhaub, and A. Schei, "Incidence of Gingivitis as Related to Sex, Occupation, Tobacco Consumption, Toothbrushing and Age," *Oral Surg*, 11:587, 1958.

78. D. R. Hoover and W. Lefkowitz, "Reduction of Gingivitis by Toothbrushing," *J Periodontol*, 36:193, 1965.

79. M. Massler, I. Schour, and B. Chopra, "Occurrence of Gingivitis in Suburban Chicago School Children," *J Periodontol*, 21:146, 1950.

80. G. J. Parfitt, "Five Year Longitudinal Study of the Gingival Condition of a Group of Children in England," *J Periodontol*, 28:26, 1957.

81. H. R. Mühlemann and Z. S. Mazor, "Gingivitis in Zurich School Children," *Helv Odontol Acta*, 2:3, 1958.

82. T. J. O'Leary, W. A. Gibson, I. L. Shannon, C. F. Schuessler, and C. L. Nabers, "A Screening Examination for Detention of Gingival and Periodontal Breakdown and Local Irritants," *Periodontics*, 1:167, 1963.

83. Hazen, "Indices for Measurement of Gingival Inflammation," p. 63.
84. D. S. Cohen, L. Friedman, J. Shaprio, and G. C. Kyle, "A Longitudinal Investigation of the Periodontal Changes During Pregnancy," *J. Periodontol, 40:*563, 1969.
85. Hazen, "Indices for Measurement of Gingival Inflammation," p. 63.
86. J. D. Suomi and J. P. Barbano, "Patterns of Gingivitis," *J Periodontol,* 39:71, 1968.
87. J. D. Suomi, "Periodontal Disease and Oral Hygiene in an Institutionalized Population: Report of an Epidemiologic Study," *J Periodontol, 40:*5, 1969.
88. L. S. Smith, J. D. Suomi, J. C. Greene, and J. P. Barbano, "A Study of Intra-examiner Variation in Scoring Oral Hygiene Status, Gingival Inflammation and Epithelial Attachment Level," *J Periodontol, 41:* 671, 1970.
89. Hazen, "Indices for Measurement of Gingival Inflammation," p. 64.
90. M. Massler, H. M. Rosenberg, W. Carter, and I. Schour, "Gingivitis in Young Adult Males. Lack of Effectiveness of a Permissive Program of Toothbrushing," *J Periodontol, 28:*111, 1957.
91. D. Jackson, "The Efficacy of Two Percent Sodium Ricinoleate in Toothpaste to Reduce Gingival Inflammation," *Brit Dent J, 112:*487, 1962.
92. H. R. Mühlemann and S. Son, "Gingival Sulcus Bleeding—A Leading Symptom in Initial Gingivitis," *Helv Odontol Acta, 15:*107, 1971.
93. Hazen, "Indices for Measurement of Gingival Inflammation," p. 65.
94. Volpe, "Indices for Measurement of Hard Deposits," p. 48.
95. Mandel, "Indices for Measurement of Soft Accumulations," p. 21.
96. Hazen, "Indices for Measurement of Gingival Inflammation," p. 65.
97. Mandel, "Indices for Measurement of Soft Accumulations," p. 21.
98. Volpe, "Indices for Measurement of Hard Deposits," p. 49.

3

BEHAVIORAL FACTORS IN ORAL HYGIENE

Jeanette F. Rayner
Lois K. Cohen

INTRODUCTION

B ECAUSE THE PRACTICE of oral hygiene is, at the present time, the *sine qua non* of dental health, determination of the factors most influential in establishing mouth cleaning behavior is a major concern of dental and paradental professionals, including dental health educators. Numerous formal and informal programs of dental health education document this concern. Programs have been supported by World Health Organization, the U.S. Public Health Service, the American Dental Association and by school systems not only within the United States, but throughout the world. Nations, private groups, and individuals voice their concern. Publications dealing with school dental health education research during the past seventeen years have included over a hundred articles stressing behavioral factors in oral hygiene—and these are exclusive of studies directed only toward the general public. A seemingly endless search continues for ways of changing human behavior in the interest of dental health.

In the pages that follow, there will be an attempt to review the bulk of school and public dental health education research conducted over the past seventeen years. Both types of education are surely among the most important influencers of oral hygiene behavior. The authors will try to specify the roles exerted on behavior by the school, social or socioeconomic status, family values, peer values and identification, perception, attitudes, and various kinds of communication—e.g. fear-arousing messages or those produced for the mass media. The forces that directly or through interaction with other entities seem to motivate individuals to practice an adequate level of oral hygiene will be described.

A THEORETICAL ORIENTATION

There are several useful theories of human behavior; the major ones are the stimulus-response theories of the Behavioral School; the various reinforcement theories such as those of Hull, Guthrie, or Mowrer; the drive or tension reduction theories of Festinger, Allport, or Freud; the physiologically based theories of Hebb; and the Gestalt-oriented theories. It is with the Gestalt-oriented theories, specifically, the Lewinian field-theoretical approach, that the authors are particularly concerned. Lewin's field theory perhaps provides the most suitable frame of reference for consideration of oral hygiene behavior. This is not a new treatment; Derryberry (1960) advocated the approach as a guide to health education as did Young (1963, 1970). Because the Lewinian stance is currently accepted by many health educators, use of the theory should permit more effective interdisciplinary dialogue.

Field theory as defined by Lewin (1951) involves five essential concepts. The first concept, "the use of a constructive rather than a classificatory method," may be described as the use of a method that (1) directs one to referents in the empirical world rather than the theoretical, and (2) provides a frame of reference for the analysis of data, the identification of patterns and the interaction of events. Unlike the classificatory method, which merely identifies an entity as belonging to a particular category, Lewinian field theory involves "an interest in the dynamic aspects of events." This second concept is *most* central to the Lewinian stance; it incorporates the notion of movement, interaction and multiple effects. The third concept, "a psychological rather than a physical approach," clearly separates Lewinian theory from the more mechanistic approaches to behavior. The fourth concept, "an analysis which starts with the situation as a whole," and the fifth, "a distinction between systemic and historical problems," designate the space and time dimensions of field theory. Behavior, according to Lewin, does not depend on the effect of a single influence but rather reflects the multiple effects of various influences on the individual or group.

Field theory is based on what the individual perceives as the influences on his behavior, not necessarily on what an objective observer would define as influential. Thus, an individual's "life space" is composed of the individual and all other persons significant to him. Individuals occupy spaces, and these spaces assume positive and negative valences, depending on the effect perceived by the individual. While this description is simplistic, it does imply a dynamic theory in which action is regarded as part of the total situation and dependent on how an individual perceives that situation. Behavior, thus, cannot be understood without an analysis of the situation as a whole.

A major characteristic of Lewinian field theory is its *here* and *now* property, the time perspective of a given situation. This could be considered a limiting factor, particularly if one is trying to understand behavior from the viewpoint of past experience or future reward. Lewin states that "any type of behavior depends on the total field" at that time and not upon a "past or future field and its time perspective." A person can experience only in the present; the past and future as he "experiences" them are part of the present situation. However, both past and future may be perceived in the present in terms of expectations; to this extent they do influence behavior. Although one can perceive here and now expectations about what might happen later, there is no guarantee that his expectations will materialize. The present situation, then, has its own life space, forces, positions, barriers, and resulting behaviors, which are influenced by a person's perceptions and expectations as shaped by the past and projected into the future.

The philosophy of time perspective seems analogous to that of Heraclitus of Ephesus who said that "it is not possible to step twice into the same river." Forces, positions, and barriers in the field or life space may be likened to currents, temperatures, and molecules of water in the river. Those extant at $time_1$ (t_1) have passed downstream by $time_2$ (t_2), and a new environment of currents, temperatures, and molecules exists. This does not mean that it is impossible to study currents, temperatures, and molecules of water because there will always be a different time perspective; it simply means that one must be aware of the changing situation.

In addition to establishing the time perspective of the field, one needs to define "force," "position," and "barrier." Lewin defines a "force" as a construct which "for a given point of the life space" determines the tendency for and direction of behavior change. A force may be positive such as motivation for the practice of oral hygiene, or it can be negative in which case it is generally referred to as a "barrier" to desirable behavior. Conceivably, a situation may cause tension and a resulting shift in force from positive to negative, or the reverse. Characteristics of the life space may determine the nature of force. For example, the peer relationships of a group at one time may constitute a barrier, yet peer relationships at a later time may exert a positive influence.

"Positions" encompass the psychological phenomena involved in "group belongingness, occupational position, (or) involvement in an activity." Being a member of a particular socioeconomic status (SES) group, for example, implies the existence of a certain kind of life space or exposure to certain forces exerted by family values or life styles. Position in one socioeconomic group may expose one to a barrier, while being positioned in another may be a motivating force. In other words, position in one context may mitigate the desire for good oral hygiene, but position in another might increase the desire.

Perhaps the best descriptive statement of those social, psychological, and cultural forces which interact, impinge upon, and shape the dental health behavior of the child is found in the *School Health Education Study Report* authored by Sliepcevich (1964):

When a child enters school, he already has many attitudes and health practices which have been acquired at home. Some of these may not rest on scientific evidence and thus need modification, and some must be reinforced. Effective changes in an individual's health behavior must be related to personal goals, attitudes, values, group pressures, socioeconomic background, cultural beliefs, and perceptions of a given situation. Therefore, the methodology of health education is derived largely from the behavioral sciences, primarily sociology, social psychology and cultural anthropology. What is known about the learner and the learning process are of paramount importance.

Translating this statement into a Lewinian model gives that shown in Figure 3-1. This model, however, also describes the adult. The same social, psychological, and anthropological processes that form the child have shaped the adult. But when adult practices are considered, one must remember that different intensities of these forces may be brought to bear. Unlike the child's situation, the force of an adult's current situation, e.g. his subjective social status, may play a more significant role than any educational forces exerted at that time (Green, 1970). In other words, barriers and positive forces probably occur at different points in the model for the adult.

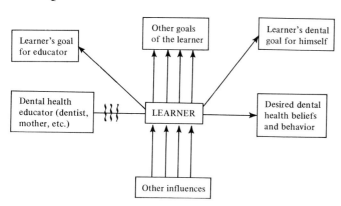

Figure 3-1

BACKGROUND OF THE DATA

Most social science-oriented investigators have selected one or two variables and have attempted to change oral hygiene behavior by concentration on these variables. In these studies, the multiple effects of individual or group situations and the interactions between many influences were not studied in any concrete fashion. This was not necessarily due to an oversight or lack of appreciation of multiple factors; it resulted from the lack of sufficiently precise information. Before study of multiple influences could occur, the influencing factors had to be identified. And to identify these factors, one had to use accepted, scientifically defined methods available at the time. Although Lewinian theory has been an accepted part of the social science armamentarium, its methods have been viewed by many researchers as being most relevant to studies of the group process, and the teaching of oral hygiene has not been generally viewed as involving group dynamics.

Hence, early attempts to change oral hygiene behavior followed two major approaches: (1) the survey method, which allowed one to discover what the influential factors were; and (2) the experimental method used by experimental or educational psychologists. The experimental method postulates an identity of influencing variables and assumes a testing rather than a discovering function. While the method is not necessarily restricted to testing hypotheses involving only a limited number of variables, dealing with few variables is both conceptually and empirically easier. Early studies on school dental health education were primarily surveys; this seems to have been the case both in the United States and abroad. American surveys (Dudding and Muhler, 1960; Lamb and Ford, 1960; Corliss, 1962) were mainly concerned with motivational factors. For example, why did children not brush their teeth? What would motivate children to do so? What health interests did children have? Were children reared in a community having a fluoridated water supply more likely to have good oral hygiene practices? Clearly, these surveys were groping for a "single handle," that is, they were exploring.

A German survey conducted about this time (Wallentin, 1960) sought the same type of information. However, unlike the American surveys, which seemed to focus their educational research on children, the German study was equally concerned with adults.

While most American researchers tended to study either children or adults, the British tended to study whole communities— adults and children—through dental health campaigns. Australian studies were directed toward assessing success in the education of parents for the sake of the children.

From 1953 to 1962, five experimental studies relevant to dental research education (Janis and Feshback, 1953; McCauley et al., 1955; Moltz and Thistelthwaite, 1955; Adams and Stanmeyer, 1960; and Dudding and Muhler, 1960) were conducted in America. Three were concerned with adults and two with children. Of the two studies using children as subjects, only one (McCauley et al., 1955) dealt with oral hygiene. The investigators attempted to determine whether actual toothbrushing in the classroom supported by a short course of instruction would result in improved oral hygiene. In the other study (Janis and Feshback, 1955), the threat of pain as the consequence of neglecting dental health was used as a fear conditioner. The focus was not actually oral hygiene but the effects of a fear-arousing stimuli as motivation. Of course, this does not necessarily prevent the findings from being useful and significant for motivating toothbrushing practices. The three studies on adults consisted of (1) an exploration of the feasibility of adult dental health education, (2) motivation of adults via rapport in the dentist-patient relationship, and (3) the effects of anxiety on learning in dental health education. The point the authors wish to emphasize is that there was a constant seeking for the "magic" factor, the one that would bring about immediate and effective results, i.e. change in behavior.

British studies during this period bore the stamp of epidemiology, but there was an equal emphasis on assaying certain behaviors, on trying to assess dental hygiene behavior by establishing a measure based on oral hygiene status. The British, more than the Americans, endorsed entire community involvement, demonstrating their recognition that factors other than the typical, pedagogically presented program of dental health education influence oral hygiene behavior. In short, from 1953 to 1963, the relationship between behavioral influences and oral hygiene practices and status was the subject of both survey and experimental research.

In 1963, researchers (Brown, 1963; Sandell, 1963; Striffler, 1963; and Tyler, 1963) stated that knowledge alone had not and would not change poor dental health behavior to good. The problem involved far more than imparting information. By 1963, the scope of behavioral influences was beginning to be defined. Interest in and realization of the need for social science research engaged the dental profession, and the magnitude of

TABLE 3-I

FREQUENCY DISTRIBUTION OF PUBLISHED STUDIES RELEVANT
TO SCHOOL DENTAL HEALTH EDUCATION

Year Published	Survey	Type of Study Essay	Experimental	Totals
1953–54			1	1
1955–56			3	3
1957				
1958			1	1
1959		1	1	2
1960	3		2	5
1961	1	3		4
1962	1	1	3	5
1953-1962 mean no.	0.5	0.5	1.1	2.1
1963	1	5	2	8
1964	1	2	1	4
1963-1964 mean no.	1.0	3.5	1.5	6.0
1965	5	1	2	8
1966	1	3	5	9
1967	1	4	11	16
1968	6	2	13	21
1969	5	1	3	9
1970*		3	7	10
1965-1970 mean no.	3.0	2.3	6.8	12.2
Totals	25	26	55	106

* Publications for this year are not complete.

the oral hygiene problem became apparent to public health administrators, health educators, social scientists, and a host of other allied health professionals. From 1964 to the present, efforts of the earlier years bore fruit. Reference to Table 3-I will show the growth and acceleration of research on school dental health education in this interim. During this time other nations became active in school dental health education, though America remained in the vanguard. In the Lewinian model (Figure 3-1), Derryberry (1960) and Young (1963, 1970) document the fact that dental health was seen as affected by the forces and tensions of its social, psychological, and environmental context.

OBJECTIVE SOCIOECONOMIC STATUS

Apart from school and public dental health education, the life space includes other important influences, which are sociocultural in character: (1) socioeconomic factors—*objective socioeconomic status* of the individual as determined by *occupation, education,* and *income;* (2) *subjective social status, identification,* and *peer relations;* (3) demographic variables—*age, sex, race,* and *ethnic origin.* These are all part of the individual's physical and social surroundings, part of his "situation as a whole." All in some measure exert force, determine positions, create or are subject to barriers. These factors are identified as "other influences" in the model of Figure 3-1. Individuals may have some limited control or no direct control over these entities in respect to changing them.

Research to date has shown that socioeconomic factors are strong influencers of dental health practices (Tyroler et al., 1965; Kegeles, 1968; Rayner, 1969, 1970; Kriesberg and Treiman, 1960; Metz and Richards, 1967; and Mobley and Smith, 1964).

Finlayson and Pearson (1967), in their study of oral hygiene practices, categorized the study population in terms of "social class school." The pertinence of socioeconomic factors to the creation or removal of barriers is rather marked in their study. Subsequent to a dental health campaign in 1961, the investigators followed 300 children over a six and one-half year time span. Their purpose was to evaluate the effectiveness of the campaign by noting either improvement or regression of the children's oral status. Each child was examined on eight occasions. Improvement in oral status was not maintained beyond the first two inspections for most of the children in the "below average" social class schools. "In the 'average' (social class) schools, significant improvement (was) maintained until 1964, while the 'above average' schools (showed) significant improvement at all times." By 1965, children attending "below average" social class schools had regressed to their precampaign oral state.

Parfit, James, and Davis (1958) surveyed the oral hygiene habits of more than 300 children from a "typical urban community in Southern England." Their findings indicated that a "picture of reasonably good oral hygiene habits emerges for a prosperous community." Davis and Land (1962), in their investigation of class-correlated practices, chose Guilford, a suburban cathedral town with a prosperous residential area of approximately 50,000 people, for the site of a dental health campaign. Guilford's "conscious sense of civic pride," the reason for its choice, emphasizes the role of class as a significant variable influencing the acquisition of oral hygiene practices.

Goose (1959) allowed for the effect of socioeconomic factors by matching a control population to the study population. The goal, of course, for the sake of determining the effects of the dental health campaign, is to remove the effect of the socioeconomic forces. Though the "situation as a whole" cannot be entirely controlled in every study, effort is usually made to nullify those aspects of the situation which could influence treatment outcome or confuse the interpretation of it. Collier and Williams (1968), McCauley et al. (1955) and Williford et al. (1967, 1967) are among those who regard such control as essential.

Roder (1969) categorized Australian children in accordance with the type of school attended—either private or "integrated government." Again the implication was that oral hygiene habits can be influenced by social class variables. Rayner (1969) studied dental hygiene and socioeconomic status and found differences between social class* groups in a white American population. Analysis† of the data revealed patterns of influence for both mothers and children of lower, middle and upper class families. Frequency of toothbrushing among lower class children was influenced by the age of the child at his first dental visit. This was not the case for children in the middle or upper categories. In respect to dental health practices in general, "lower class mothers tend to view toothbrushing as most important prior to their children's school years. Middle class mothers seem to be striving toward dental health practices and professional care as values essential to their life style. Mothers in the upper class seem to have already accepted dental health practices and professional care as part of their way of life."

Robinson et al. (1967) studied the effects of dental education and care in lower socioeconomic high school freshmen over a period of four years. They were unable to effect a change in behavior despite regular free prophylaxes, free toothbrushes and dentifrice, and four hours of instruction per year. Regular inspections during and at the end of the study showed increasing scores for Oral Hygiene Indices (OHI's) and Debris Indices (DI's) (Greene and Vermillion, 1964) in both experimental and control groups.

In keeping with these findings regarding socioeconomic status, a small family income among lower socioeconomic families is generally perceived to be a barrier to preventive dental care. Rayner (1970) found occupation and income causally related to dental visits, but no causal relationship between family income and oral hygiene practices was found when the effects of the parents' education were controlled in the analysis of research data. The relationship held for all three social classes. This is of particular interest because, in general, income is a valid indicator of socioeconomic status and usually a reliable correlate of both education and occupation. Since education has been found to

---

* Determined by father's occupation.
† Path Analysis according to Blalock (1964) and Duncan (1966).

be a predictor of toothbrushing behavior, and income correlates with education, one could expect toothbrushing behavior to be partially explained by the level of family income.

The evidence of others certainly tends in this direction. Kelley et al. (1966) reported that "oral hygiene varied markedly by levels of family income and education," but "was more closely associated with education than with income." Cohen et al. (1967) found a trend in this direction. Using data from two nationwide studies, they found that people in the higher income brackets "seem more likely to brush their teeth more frequently." Approximately 59 percent of those persons brushing two or more times per day reported incomes between three and four thousand dollars annually. The percentage of those with an annual income level of five to six thousand dollars who brushed two or more times a day was approximately 62 percent. However, approximately 72 percent brushed two or more times a day among those reporting annual incomes ranging from ten to fifteen thousand dollars. Cohen et al. point to other circumstances that may act either as barriers or forces to motivate toothbrushing behavior. For example, the number of years of formal education are highly correlated with the percentage of persons who brush twice or more daily. Thus, the importance of education is a well-documented finding.

Duany (1967), using the Decayed, Missing, Filled (DMF) score as a measure of dental health, found almost a direct relationship between the children's DMF scores and maternal education. "The mother's attitudes toward health and illness differed depending upon the mother's educational status," reported Mechanic (1964). Rayner's (1970) causal analysis of the factors influencing mothers' frequency of toothbrushing designates mothers' level of formal education as a major influencer, at least for the lower and upper socioeconomic status (SES) groups in her sample. For the middle SES group, toothbrushing frequency appears to be indirectly influenced by education, i.e. through what Rayner has called "subjective social class." These patterns reflect the differential effects of force created by the interaction of income, education, and objective social class (as defined by occupation). But perhaps of most significance for toothbrushing behavior is the interplay of external forces such as SES predictors and internal forces such as subjective social status, identification, and influence of peers. Only recently has the role of status identity as a force in oral hygiene practices received attention.

SUBJECTIVE SOCIAL STATUS

The role of status identity in preventive health behavior has been extensively and intensively studied by Green (1970), who included preventive dental visits as one form of preventive health behavior in his study. Green examined preventive health behavior in terms of the interactional forces exerted by social status, status inconsistency, and reference group norms. His research leads to a status identity model which explains the relationship between the interactional forces and preventive health behavior. Green maintains that a person tends to view himself as belonging to a specific social class—if he perceives or appreciates the idea of social stratification at all—and this perception is very much dependent on social factors such as occupation, education, income, ethnic origin, race, etc. There may be, however, discrepancies between these factors. Income and occupation may not match a person's level of education, or education and income may be disparate in regard to occupation. Prejudice against ethnic origin might be experienced, but not necessarily prevent advancement in a profession if adequate education also is present. When inconsistencies exist between ascribed status such as being born a black or Indian child and achieved status such as having acquired education and position in the community as a professional, an individual selects that aspect of his status which affords him the highest prestige, and he categorizes himself in respect to social class accordingly. He does not define his social status by "averaging" all of his attributes. Once he has defined his social status, an individual behaves in terms of the values, social pressures, and norms that he perceives as characteristic of this social class. According to Green, "In the absence of immediate threat, real or perceived, to physical well-being, preventive health actions are taken in response to social pressures and supports in the form of social norms which vary with SES." This may be a particularly useful working concept for explaining and even changing toothbrushing behavior.

In many ways the forces of social norms are reflected in oral hygiene literature, particularly that pertaining to dental health education. Peer influences, which may be strong forces or strong barriers to preventive action, may determine whether or not there is a willingness to practice what is taught. As demonstrated by Ramirez's (1969) study of dental health education for reform school boys, the influences of boyfriends may be more potent than other forces—more potent than formal education by accepted experts. Where peer group conformity is practiced to a high degree, as it tends to be in the reform school environment, willingness to change behavior depends upon peer group sanctions. The boys in Ramirez's sample failed to use a recommended disclosing wafer as an aid to toothbrushing. The barrier in this situation was mainly the peer culture, a factor in the boys' life space. Because toothbrushing, normally a private behavior, could not be private under the circumstances, Ramirez's subjects could not practice what they had been taught without opposing peer group norms, thus exposing themselves to a threatened loss of "position"—position in the Lewinian sense. Where peer sanctions are an overriding force and desired behavior is public, there should be careful evaluation of the interaction between effects of the requested behavior and peer group reactions. If peer values do not support good oral health practices, removing this barrier for an individual involves forces designed to change the practices of the peer group. The experience of Robinson et al. (1967) suggests that changing a group "en masse" is a formidable endeavor. But if the dental health educator recognizes and understands the values of the group with which he must deal, if he can put himself into the feeling state of the group, he may then be able to communicate, interpret, and anticipate the group's responses. In short, he will be better able to contend with both forces and barriers in the life space of the group. Brown (1963), Boek (1965), Kegeles (1968), and Counsell (1970), several proponents of dental health education, all advocate this approach.

Cassidy (1965) used peer group values as a force to change the oral hygiene behavior of U.S. Army recruits. Discovering the key values of newly recruited men gave him some idea of existent barriers and forces and how position could be used to motivate the men in the interest of good oral hygiene. Cassidy found that respect, well-being, and rectitude (presented here in order of their strength as motivating factors) were major values in the group and constituted major forces. Need for respect and well-being were values induced by the military environment, i.e. the current environment of Cassidy's subjects, while rectitude stemmed from earlier training. Rectitude as a value could also be induced in adult subjects through identification with the peer group. Cassidy noted, "This can be a key consideration in the oral hygiene program when the men are made to identify with the purpose of the program." In other words, once a peer group has acquired a new status identity, the force of identification can be amplified when suitable new values are defined as additional peer group norms.

Status identity and identification were found to be forces determining the toothbrushing frequency of mothers, mothers' attitudes toward toothbrushing and mothers' satisfaction in regard to their children's dental conditions (Rayner, 1970). The relatively strong infusive influence of status identity found in the total sample was not maintained in the patterns developed for each of the SES groups, but distinction of pattern is in keeping with Green's postulate. The behavior of lower SES mothers appeared least subject to status identity as far as toothbrushing behavior was concerned. This may only mean that toothbrushing behavior was not held as a value, or that status identity depended on recognition of certain status characteristics, one of which was toothbrushing. Middle SES mothers' oral hygiene practices correlated highly with status identity. Status identity for the upper SES mothers was causally related to mothers' satisfaction with their children's dental condition.

DEMOGRAPHIC FACTORS

Other forces in the life space impinging on the individual's behavior are demographic forces, i.e. those of sex, age, race, and ethnicity. In their analysis and interpretation of data from the National Health Survey, Kelley et al. (1966) found that sex and age were factors of importance to oral hygiene status. Evaluation of OHI showed that woman generally "had perceptibly cleaner teeth than men," and the "trend prevailed within each of the various age ranges." But "pronounced differences in oral hygiene" were found to exist by race. Amounts of debris and calculus on the teeth of black adults were far greater than those found on whites. A study by Robinson et al. also reflects this situation.

The evidence of SES forces on oral hygiene practices from the studies mentioned above, however, suggests that the investigators' attempts to inculcate good oral hygiene values may have been as much frustrated by racial and ethnic factors as by SES. Green (1970) considered a range of illnesses among both whites and blacks in reference to diseases for which there are *adequate preventive measures*. He noted that "a large part of the nonwhite differential is accounted for in most cases by socioeconomic differences, and therefore cannot be attributed simply to genetic differences." Kelley et al. point out that "a significantly large part of the difference observed in oral hygiene by race was accounted for by differences in income and education." Nevertheless, to dismiss genetic differences as inconsequential when compared with social forces is to deny the influence of the biological environment of the individual. It should not be forgotten that genetic differences, as biological forces, play a significant role in both the prevalence of dental disease and the occurrence of oral hygiene behavior. Susceptibility to disease may be influenced by physiological age, which in turn has been determined by the individual's genetic heritage—quite apart from his sociocultural environment. On the other hand, sociocultural factors may be important forces affecting the individual's physiological milieu. Richards and Barmes (1971) document some evidence for the interaction between disease and the sociocultural forces in their review of the literature on dental epidemiology, yet recognize that at the present time that there is considerable ambiguity at the interfaces of the social and dental sciences. Apparently, the forces associated with race, ethnicity, and genetic heritage are too much confounded with those of socioeconomic status and demographic factors to allow any inference on the basis of race or ethnicity. What seems to emerge most clearly is the interaction—in Lewinian terms—of the forces or influences of socioeconomic and other sociocultural factors on oral hygiene behavior.

DENTAL HEALTH EDUCATION

Perhaps the greatest effort to improve the dental practices of the public has been made through formalized dental health education. The forces required to overcome the barriers caused by adverse social factors are numerous, their hypothesized interactions complex, and proof of their dynamic processes not yet validated. Nevertheless, because education is a firmly entrenched institution in Western society and has repeatedly demonstrated strong associations with dental health practices, it continues to be perceived as the most effective force for altering oral hygiene practices, despite the strength of other interacting forces and barriers.

Dental health education has been part of school health education in some parts of the United States for at least thirty years as in the Tucson, Arizona school system (Bugbee, 1970). According to Dollar and Sandell (1961), there has been a "remarkable uniformity of teaching practices in all size communities, and in all geographic areas" as well. The earlier quote from Sliepcevich's report (1964) indicates that many health educators are aware of the interaction of sociocultural and psychological forces, but Young's (1963, 1970) comprehensive reviews of the literature point to a lack of such awareness among the majority of health educators. She has repeatedly drawn attention to the all-too-pervasive problem of teacher attitudes as a barrier to changing behavior. She states that "many educators assume a straight line relationship between their inputs and movements of the 'learner' towards changed beliefs and practices." An even greater barrier may be the pedagogic tendency to "treat the 'learner' as a static inert mass with no internal forces affecting the desired straight line movement toward professionally determined goals." Counsell (1970) addresses himself to the same issue, although from a somewhat oblique angle, when he maintains, "Empirical repetition of outdated methods and information leads to boredom and frustration in listeners and, if it does not interfere with learning (does not create a barrier), it interferes with acceptance of information and the promotion of changed attitudes."

The literature is rife with studies on the relationship of dental health information to attitudes and behavior (Rowntree, 1959; Lamb and Ford, 1960; Brown, 1963; Striffler, 1963; Dowell, 1965; Robinson et al., 1967; Young, 1963, 1970; Goose, 1968; Pavlid, 1968, and Roder, 1969). Young's (1969) and Cohen and Lucye's (1970) research on the effectiveness of current teaching methods in dental health education for children emphasizes the need for not only recognition of motivating forces, but the development of techniques that go "beyond information and facts and motivate for behavior" (Cohen and Lucye, 1970). Young (1969) noted that "most of the behavioral findings have indicated that students are not putting into practice knowledge they have acquired." Clearly, the barriers are not interposed between acquisition of knowledge and its translation to behavior, but between motivation and its translation to behavior. The above conclusion is *not* unanimously affirmed, even though it is one of the most consistent findings in the dental health education corpus. Gravelle et al. (1967), for example, found that high school students were able to benefit from an intensive program of dental health education. A less intensive program also improved the debris scores of the students, but not to the same degree. Detailed description of the program able to effect the change was not given, though the report suggests that behavior-changing teaching techniques were involved.

Convinced of the efficiency of dental health education as the sole factor of behavior change, Williford et al. (1967) hypothesized that education alone would influence students to improve their oral hygiene practices, hence their oral health. One hundred forty-one high school students participated in the study.

Debris scores showed a 29.9 percent reduction after completion of the course of instruction. Moreover, 65.3 percent of the students demonstrated some improvement in debris score. Improvement was also manifest in the fall of mean OHI scores and Periodontal Index (PI) scores during the pre- and post-instruction interim. Of considerable interest is the finding that no significant correlations existed between dental intelligence quotients (I.Q.) or PI scores before instruction, but a significant correlation was found following instruction.

Another apparently successful program was carried out by Fodor and Ziegler (1966) with a group of twelve and thirteen-year-old children. After exposure to disclosing tablets and a course of instruction, the subjects showed a significant decrease in plaque. It would seem that some students do translate dental health knowledge into oral hygiene behavior. Therefore, one needs to know what forces are interacting and how the usual barriers are being leveled. One interpretation could be that there were no barriers. Another might be that different forces are pressing on those who do use their knowledge, i.e. change their behavior. It could be that behavior-changing methods were used which overwhelmed the forces of knowledge, or perhaps knowledge acted as a reinforcer to behavior. In the instance cited, the use of disclosing tablets may legitimately be regarded as a behavior-changing technique. Another interpretation might be forthcoming if one approaches the problem from the semantic point of view. What is meant by "behavior change" through dental health education? Does this refer to a permanent shift, permanent in the sense of habit formation as a result of education? None of these further clarifications are explanations, but they do represent ways to tease more information from the data.

In order to identify impinging forces or barriers, it was essential to separate those studies whose findings indicated "improvement" immediately following dental health instruction from those indicating "no improvement." It was also necessary to identify those studies where subjects regressed after a period of time and those where no regression occurred. Only the experimental studies were used.

Table 3-II shows the outcome of these procedures. The studies were rank-ordered according to the ages of their subjects. Concern was for only four variables apart from age: (1) type of instruction, (2) school instruction *only,* (3) oral hygiene status *immediately* following instruction (clinically measured), and (4) oral hygiene status at follow-up (also clinically measured). The studies, of course, are not strictly comparable on any one basis, and perhaps are least comparable on the interim between

TABLE 3-II

IMPROVEMENT RELATIVE TO TYPE OF PROGRAM
AND AGE OF SUBJECTS

Study	Age	Campaign	School Only	Follow-Up
British	6-7	+		—
British	6-12	+		—
British	6-12	+≠		+o
American	6-16		+≠	+o
American	6-18		+≠	0
American	8-10		+≠	—
American	9-10		+	—
British	10-13	+	+*	—
British	11-15	+		—
Danish	11-13		+≠	—
British	12	+		—
American	12-13		+≠	0
British	12-13		+≠	+
American	13-14		+≠ʃ	0
Swedish	13-14		+	—
American	14		+≠	0
American	14		—≠ʃɪ/ʌ	0
American	14-16		—ɪ/ʌ	—
American	14-18		+	+
American	14-15		+	+
American	14-18		+	+
American	14-18		+	+
American	15-18		+	+
Swedish	18-22		+	+
American	"adults" (Naval recruits)		—≠ɪ/ʌ	0

+ = improved or maintained status.
— = no improvement or regression.
0 = no follow-up attempts.
* = both school and campaign.
o = negative follow-up for lower SES.
≠ = used erythrosin tablet or dye.
ɪ/ʌ = minority or other special population.
ʃ = use of fear-arousal techniques.

postinstruction examination and follow-up. For this reason rather crude indicators* were used. Nevertheless, the table is revealing. Only three groups failed to show improvement immediately following instruction. These three, with subjects ranging in age from fourteen to twenty-one years, proved to be unusual in some respects. One study group consisted of deprived Negro children, the second of boys in a state reform school, and the subjects of the third were young adults newly recruited to the Submarine Service. More significant than the uniqueness of the groups is the suggested force of the peer culture. The latter notion is supported by the subjects' age range, a time in which peers assume an enhanced value, and by their singular environments—life spaces in which there is likely to be particular emphasis on peer relationships. When no special circumstances intervene, teenage and adult behavior appears to be amenable to change through traditional forms of education. Yet the forces of peer culture are also operating in those who seem to be influenced by traditional education. It may be that for these individuals as well, peer behavior is the effective influence and this, rather than the traditional forms of education, tends to maximize peer culture forces in desired directions.

The picture is quite different for children under the age of fourteen. Below this age, regression or failure to sustain improvement of oral hygiene is more usual than unusual, regardless of the time interval between immediate postinstruction examination and follow-up. Specific techniques were used in the three instances where children under fourteen did maintain their improved status, suggesting that in the case of younger children, too much has perhaps been asked of traditional health education with too little understanding of the forces needed to shape desirable oral hygiene practices.

Young's statement regarding teacher attitudes and teaching techniques is a reminder that the teaching methods of health education are modeled after traditional teaching methods— primarily because school teachers provide most of the children's

---

* No follow-up = 0; improvement or sustained status after improvement = +; no improvement or regression after improvement = −.

health education. Basic to their methods is the conviction that knowledge leads to belief, belief to temporary behavior or action, and temporary action to habit. It is almost an axiom among most educators that knowledge must be antecedent to behavior change. With emphasis on knowledge, subsequent reinforcement is directed toward consolidation of knowledge, the accepted source of behavior. In social theory terms, therefore, behavior is predicated on cognitive learning.

Lewin (1951) specifies two kinds of development in the psychology of learning: (1) learning related to motivation, and (2) learning related to cognition. Habit is "interpreted as a psychological force of a character similar to motivational forces." However, research in the dental area suggests that more than motivation is needed to establish oral hygiene behavior as a habit. Learning oral hygiene must involve the acquisition of a value, a change in a value, or in Lewinian terms, "a need." For adults, this involves change in cognitive structure, but for children, cognitive learning is secondary to perception and directs motivation without an accumulation of facts or knowledge.

Table 3-II suggests that cognitive learning is appropriate for promoting good oral hygiene practices among adults but is far from satisfactory with children. Fortunately, the work of Piaget meshes with that of Lewin and strengthens the contention that children's learning of good oral hygiene habits does not necessarily entail cognitive learning, e.g. knowledge of where the bicuspids are located. According to Piaget (1969), young children learn in the form of sensory-motor manipulation. Learning is a sensory activity, a "looking," a "touching," a "seeing," a "doing" of something. Cohen and Lucye (1970) point out that children "are very interested in *how* to brush their teeth . . . that ideas retained by the child are more likely to be those obtained in a practical and useful way on the behavioral level . . . rather than on the intellectual level." In theory and in practice, one has to consider quite different points of intervention in regard to forces, barriers, and positions as they affect children's or adults' acquisition of good oral health habits.

VALUES

Rayner's (1969) causal analysis of factors influencing children's oral hygiene practices has shown that for children, behavior seems to be both the theoretical and the practical clue to effective dental health education, and that mothers' own hygiene practices are the single most important influence on their children's. This statement suggests a concept of family values. Metz and Richards's (1967) earlier study of preventive dental visits also supports the notion of family values. They found that children's dental health practices are associated with their parents'. Other studies (Kriesberg and Trieman, 1962, 1969) likewise lend credence to the role of family values in determining dental hygiene habits. Kriesberg and Trieman's (1962) "most striking finding (was) that very specific parental attitudes and practices among parents are related to this pattern (preventive dental behavior) among their children and thus in the children's later life."

Mechanic (1964), in his paper on mothers' influence on children's health attitudes and behavior, comments that "the subtlety of childhood learning is dependent more on what the parents do and how they react than the attitudes they manifest." The parents instill values. This is in keeping with Rokeach's (1969) definition of value. "A value, unlike an attitude, is an imperative to action. Values . . . have to do with modes of conduct and end states of existence . . . a value is a standard employed to influence the values, attitudes, and actions of at least some others—our children's for example." He further states that the value systems of people are shaped by social factors, i.e. norms. A more recent paper by Rokeach (1971) describes a procedure for modification of values. The authors will refer to this later when they discuss possible means to effect changes in values.

The *Modern Dictionary of Sociology* (Theodorson and Theodorson, 1969) states: "Because of the generalized nature of values, it is possible for individuals who share the same values to disagree on specific norms embodying these values." For example, few individuals would assert that keeping one's teeth is unimportant. Keeping one's teeth is considered an ideal state. However, the assertion of such a belief may or may not reflect an individual's actual behavior and may, in fact, be dependent on temporary factors inherent in the situation. Thus, it can be classified as an attitude. An individual's attitude may suggest a favorable concern about his dental health. But *value* is expressed through action when he brushes regularly, flosses regularly, and makes regularly scheduled visits to the dentist for preventive care. Action reflects a value; words, more likely than not, an attitude. Hence, one may hear vastly differing groups of individuals express the desirability of practicing good dental hygiene, yet observe quite diverse oral hygiene practices among the groups.

Green considered values in his study of preventive health behavior. Through his review of research he found that "the differences between high and low socioeconomic status were generally much smaller on questionnaire or interview items concerning attitudes and particularly, values, than on items concerning behavior." He suggested that minimal differences in values would be "all the more so in health research because of the general universality of values on health." But the "universality of values on health" refers to attitudes toward health. Only questionnaire items dealing with actual behavior reflect values. Green found greater diversity of reported behavior, thus supporting current definitions and findings on values. The reciprocity and interdependence between value and norm, the "importance" dimension of a value, i.e., whether or not the value exists for a given group and how norms have developed around it, are such that one can scarcely be studied without recourse to the other.

There are many questions regarding dental health values. For one thing, one must remember that the public tends to view dental health as different from medical health and seems to behave accordingly. For example, Roder's (1969) study of 1,000 Australian children revealed a lack of value of dental health as something desirable, a lack of the realization of serious consequences stemming from dental disease and a lack of faith in the benefits of good oral hygiene. Even more appalling was the finding that cosmetically more attractive dental prosthesis was regarded by many children as more desirable than their own teeth!

In this instance, the questionnaire findings were substantiated by the children's oral status, which *did* reflect the "importance" dimension of dental health as a value. As mentioned above, however, questionnaire responses concerning attitude and values often do not reflect what is behaviorally expressed. Rokeach refers to these kinds of responses as "opinion." To reiterate, values are more reliably indicated by behavior.

The authors have especially stressed the concept of values, but they believe it is a major factor in the formation of a child's habitual toothbrushing behavior, seeing habit as a form of behavior requiring either the acquisition of a value and norms appropriate to it, or a change in the norms of an already established value.

What forces and barriers bring about the existence of dental health as a value or change the norms of a value already existing? As an aid to describing and identifying the entities acting on values, value change, and habit, the authors present Figure 3-2, a modification of Figure 3-1. Figure 3-2 does not present a

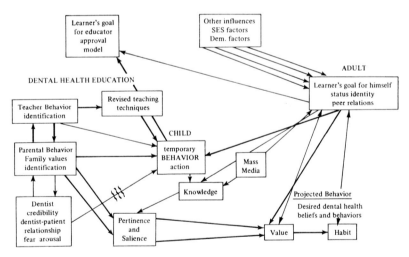

REVISED MODEL OF THE DENTAL HEALTH EDUCATION PROCESS

Figure 3-2

mathematical or causal model, though it could provide hypotheses for testing. The section under the heading, "Dental Health Education," is designed with children in mind rather than adults. The remaining part of the model has greater specificity for adults. In any case, the goal for dental public health educators as well as parents resides in the box labelled "habit." The heavy black lines represent what seem to be the major forces for accomplishing habit formation in either the child or the adult.

The particular dynamics of this revised model were suggested by the fact that children tend to regress after temporary improvement in their practices, as shown in Table 3-II and supplemented with information from other sources. Clearly, habit is the product of many forces besides the knowledge-belief-temporary action sequence. The argument of the model is that a behaviorally expressed value such as the oral hygiene practices of the mother helps establish the child's dental hygiene practices as a value.

Values are not acquired quickly, nor are they changed overnight. Chaffee's (1965) experiments on the acquisition of value change demonstrated that *salience*, or the prominence of an individual's particular behavior such that he is readily aware of it, and *pertinence*, or the relevance of the behavior for him, are essential components of value change. Exemplary dental hygiene behavior on the part of the mother may provide both salience and pertinence. Accordingly, the authors have indicated a lesser force issuing from knowledge. This condition appears to hold for both children and adults. Antonovsky and Kats (1970) in a study of preventive dental health behavior found that "a minimum amount of knowledge is adequate to allow preventive behavior; beyond this amount, any increment in knowledge has no effect." Thus, the authors feel this revised model places knowledge in a more realistic relationship to other essential variables.

PARENT-TEACHER INTERACTION

In the attempt to define major barriers, parent-teacher interaction may provide a good starting point. There is considerable evidence that mothers need to be educated as well as children, but educated for the *sake of their own well-being* as well as for their children's (Rayner, 1970). Parents need to become involved, for they make the decisions regarding their children's health, at least in the occidental countries studied. Despite this, there is a deplorable lack of parental involvement in the teaching of dental health in the schools (Sliepcevich, 1964; Guttelman, 1965). It appears that both schools and parents assign the greater part of the responsibility to the schools. Nor is this delegation of responsibility simply an attribute of the American scene. The current worldwide situation remains as it was ten years ago (Dollar and Sandell, 1961); three out of four schools have some sort of dental science program, characterized by a general uniformity of content and methodology and taught by the elementary school classroom teacher. Pincheria and Faundez (1966) reported that 99 percent of the teachers queried in their survey on dental health education in Chile felt teachers and health educators of the National Health Services ought to be responsible for the teaching of dental health practices. Sundram (1966) of Malaysia thinks the public should demand dental health education, but he also states that the dental and educational professions should be the promoters of dental health education.

A slightly different tack is taken by the British, possibly because of their National Health Service. Exclusion of the parents in dental health education is seen as a barrier to changing behavior in the children. Finlayson and Wilson (1962) present a good example of the need for commitment of both parents and children. They reported that because the adult public as well as the children were seen as recipients of dental health education, entire communities became involved. Parents were expected to contribute to their children's school dental health education. The schools, however, traditionally bore the essential burden. Rowntree (1959) emphasized the need to obtain the cooperation of parents and teachers. Using Rowntree's principles, Davis and Land (1962) designed a campaign that involved the community at every level. Schools were the main channels for reaching their population. Both the children's and parents' dental health knowledge was assessed before and after a dental health campaign in Dowell's (1965) survey study of Huddersfield. Almost every report of a dental health education campaign urges involvement of parents. Some stress that school dental health education is difficult, if not impossible, to accomplish without cooperation of parents.

Because of failure to identify the real barriers to children's preventive dental health behavior, there is failure to properly educate the parent. The Australian investigators, Jago and King (1963), gave advice regularly to mothers in regard to diet, how to supervise their children's toothbrushing practices and how to train their children. They found that educating the parents for the children's benefit, and not for the parents' sake, had little effect on the oral status of the children. The caries rates of the study and control groups demonstrated no significant difference.

Anderson's (1970) description of dental care for Swedish children offers even stronger evidence of the need for appropriate education of the parent. In Sweden, the children "are entitled to free dental care through the public dental services." Dental health education is completely divorced from parental involvement; the children view it as a school activity. The Linde and Koch (1967) study of Swedish children attributed regression of the children's toothbrushing behavior to a failure to relate toothbrushing in school to toothbrushing at home.

Review of the literature suggests that the Canadian point of view is similar to the British. Parents are regarded as a significant factor in the improvement of their children's dental health. Though not considered as information sources for their children, they are viewed as responsible agents in the youngsters' dental health education. For example, as part of a school dental health education program, Gray and Hawk (1968) sent referral cards to parents specifying the oral status of their children. Parents were then expected to respond by seeing that the children received appropriate care. The investigators concluded that motivation of parents constituted a more important element in improving the children's dental health status than did the school dental health program.

The end results of the British and Canadian approaches in

the long run correspond with the results of the American, Swedish, and other studies listed in Table 3-II. This is perhaps the clue to the kind of parental involvement required. One may hypothesize that the barriers were not and are not lack of knowledge or lack of the parental concern but lack of parental involvement in a total sense, in a value-expressed-as-a-behavior sense. This lack of parental involvement is fostered by traditional dental health education, which stresses acquisition of facts; by the usual teacher-parent relationship characterized by passing on information; and by the willingness of the school, state, or other nonfamily group to assume the parents' responsibility. However, on the operational level, one again returns to the teacher-parent interaction.

The barrier that exists between parents and teachers is the paradox encountered when parents' knowledge of dental health is viewed as an adjunct of school dental health education, while parents are simultaneously considered ineffective secondary sources. Parents are expected to reinforce what the teacher has been teaching, but they tend to be bypassed by school dental health education. This is a mistake on the part of educators since internalization of values by children is dependent upon the primary socializing agents, the mothers. The school and the teachers are the secondary agents in this case (Scott, 1970) and cannot hope to replace the parents when parent-child relationships are normal. Neglecting the parent can only weaken the potential force of school dental health education.

The viewpoint of the mental health therapists should be considered. Workers in this field are aware of how the practices of parents influence children, and they would never seriously consider attempting to change the behavior of children without attempting to change that of the parents. In fact, mental health programs have been subject to criticism because they focus on adults first and children second. Dentistry has done the opposite.

One may hypothesize that it is when teacher and parent work together for change in the parent as well as in the child that other necessary forces may come into play. These level the barrier, or resolve the paradox. But how? What actually happens in the interaction between parent and teacher when they work together?

If the interpersonal relationship develops satisfactorily, one should expect there to be identification of parent with teacher and of teacher with parent. This reciprocal identification would allow the teacher to better understand the parents' needs and help the parents acquire the norms of preventive dental health values. But what is meant by a "satisfactory interpersonal relationship?" This is crucial for a maximum influence of teachers on mothers and for maximum communication between mothers and teachers. The authors are not referring to the usual parents' school visits, when the teacher advises mothers how to deal with specific problems. The teacher in this instance is not to be perceived as an authority by the mothers but as a peer; he or she provides an example by his association with the mother. He uses his status as a "significant other" in the lives of his students' families to maximize communication and to establish a status identity for the mothers. According to Green (1970), this relationship "leads . . . in turn, to a commitment to certain norms of behavior prescribed by that status." In other words, the teacher is a major catalyst in shifting forces that change the of-no-importance dimension of a value to one that is very important. He must keep in mind that his influence on the children can be only as much as parents permit. If the relationship between teacher and parent is characterized by high identity, then the children are better able to identify with the teacher. The converse of this situation, which is currently typical of many school dental health programs, may present a problem to children whose parents do not particularly value good oral hygiene or preventive dental health practices. If a child, because of his identification with a parent who may not practice good oral hygiene, views dental health education as a criticism of his family, one could expect the internalization of his "temporary behavior" as a value and then a habit to be an impossible progression.

As shown in Table 3-II, current typical educational techniques carry enough impact to effect temporary change in children's dental hygiene behavior even though regression eventually follows. From this one must concede that present methods are not completely lacking in effectiveness. The interaction between a teacher's behavior and his teaching techniques is another point where either barriers or positive forces may occur. The literature indicates some of the characteristics of the teacher and his methods which are responsible for change.

METHODS: CHILDREN

After comparing the attitudes and knowledge scores of two groups of junior high school children following similar courses of dental health instruction, Collier and Williams (1968) found that nonsignificant (statistically) improvement occurred at one school, but significant improvement took place at the other. Improvement was objectively determined by use of oral hygiene indices and correlated with the attitudes and knowledge scores. The investigators credited the teachers for the marked improvement of one group. Teachers were described as "very enthusiastic about the project (course of instruction); they assisted in many ways to see that it progressed smoothly and continued to promote the ideas as set forth in the project after the educational phase was completed." This instance illustrates the point made by Cohen and Lucye (1970) who stress the need for teachers to motivate beyond facts and information.

The reader must not suppose that the authors discount or underestimate the need for instructional methods in behavior change because, thus far, they have accentuated sociopsychological variables. The authors feel that the interaction of socio-psychological forces prepares the field for the most effective use of specific teaching methods and materials.

Earlier in this chapter, the "perceptual mode" of learning, a theoretical position of Piaget, was postulated to be best suited to the teaching of oral hygiene practices for children. This concept helps explain the role of saliency and pertinence in the changing of a value and internalization of the value as a habit. For example, rendering plaque visible through staining techniques is in accordance with the perceptual mode of instruction. Reference to Table 3-II will show that eleven studies using children under fourteen years of age included disclosing wafers, plaque staining, or luminescence techniques as part of the program of instruction. Only five of these studies evaluated the effect of instruction by a follow-up inspection. Of these five studies, however, the subjects of three maintained their initial improvement. Three cases may not be a strong argument for assuming that plaque made visible is more impressive than other educational techniques, but such techniques do appear to increase both saliency and pertinence for children. Generally speaking, the use of disclosing tablets as an aid to education needs to be studied in conjunction with other methods and in the instruction of other groups. Is it easier, for example, to change a mother's behavior by demonstrating to her the amount of plaque on her teeth, or on her child's? Will it increase saliency and pertinence for mothers?

Another method which is seldom used in teaching oral hygiene is consistent with Piaget's theory of learning and with Lewin's field theory. The behavior-changing method advocated by Cohen and Lucye (1970) matches actual behavior in the learning situation with the desired behavior objective. Much work has been done on matching behavior, and psychologists are studying this area further. Research on matching behavior shows that imitative behavior, imitative learning, incidental learning, and modeling behavior are all involved in identification, or in Bandura's (1961) words, "an elementary prototype of identification."

Flanders (1968) reviewed the literature on imitative behavior. One of his concluding hypotheses dealt with regularity of the model's responses. He suggested that "observing a regular pattern in the model's responses will lead to increased imitation of the model by the child." Bandura and Huston (1961) and Mussen and Parker (1965) stressed the need for nurturance or emotional support for the child as a condition "facilitating such learning," another argument for the influence of the mother in the formation of habit. Only one or two of the psychological studies made any attempt to measure the length of time the imitative behavior endured. Their findings imply a possibility of endurance over time, but no proof.

McCauley et al. (1955), Linde and Koch (1967), and Bay (1968) all used some version of the matching method. The immediate results of instruction were good in the three studies, but toothbrushing behavior at home did not follow. The studies all omitted parental involvement. Obviously, the teacher must make clear to the children that toothbrushing at school is an activity which is also to be regularly and properly practiced at home. In other words, he must establish "pertinence" so that there is a transfer of behavior from one situation to another.

The success of matching behavior as a teaching device partially rests on the teacher's ability to function as a parent surrogate. Then he or she can use the powerful motivator, identification. Like the mother, his example provides pertinence and salience. Like the mother, he serves as a model. And like the mother, his approval is sought for good behavior as it is defined for the child. But it must be remembered that although the teacher is able to become a parent surrogate, this does not obviate the need for change in parental behavior. Having the educator function in this role may be effective in improving oral health practices, but his role as surrogate is limited. He is only a "secondary agent." As such, with parental cooperation, he helps create consistent situations for the children so that mutual reinforcement of the desirable behavior may occur.

The necessity for consistency in respect to pertinence and salience is illustrated by the Bay study (1968). An association was engendered in the minds of the children; toothbrushing was made pertinent by both the investigators and the children's families *while the study was in progress.* However, after the study ended, "the children resumed their previous habits of dental hygiene." Bay attributed the regression to the decreased attention to the conditions of their teeth; there was no longer any salience. Children, particularly young children, require fairly constant reminders to keep their interest level high. Thus, Bay suggested an increased frequency of dental health education and an effort to change the attitude of the children's families toward the concept of dental hygiene.

From the model, it would appear that the dentist is not regarded as a strong force or barrier in the interaction between parental behavior and children's behavior. For many adults and children, his contact with them is too limited. Those who see him frequently enough to benefit from his instruction may already hold preventive dental health practices as a value. Those who are preventively oriented are most likely to be of higher socioeconomic status and, therefore, a select group. When the dentist does interact with the dentally indigent, he may prove to be a highly creditable source for behavior change. But the literature is ambivalent on this point.

Dudding and Muhler (1960) found that "of children classified as having 'good' oral hygiene, 61 percent said they learned their oral hygiene practices from the dentist, while only 33 percent of those in the 'poor' group said that the dentist was responsible for teaching them how to brush their teeth." The real influence of the dentist, however, seems to be his impact on parents. Of the children classified as "good," 19 percent had learned from their parents of whom 80 percent had received instruction from their dentists. In a later study, Muhler (1966) was able to demonstrate improved oral hygiene indices in a sample of 150 high school students who had participated in a series of lectures given either by a dentist or a dental hygienist.

Meyers and Downs (1968), in a comparison between school dental health education programs in two public school systems, concluded that the system providing instruction by dental hygienists was the more effective. Students in this system manifested a higher level of dental health.

Williford et al. (1967) demonstrated experimentally that school dental health instruction was more effective when given by a dentist. The changed behavior was attributed to a credibility factor; the dentist was perceived as more knowledgeable and more of an authority than the school teacher. Johns and Muhler (1965) and McCauley (1955) maintained a similar stance on the basis of their study findings.

Two studies on children contradict these findings. Both involve the effectiveness of instruction given in the dentists' office. Roder (1969) investigated the brushing habits of Australian private school children. He found that despite recent dental visits, 48.1 percent could not recall toothbrushing instruction from their dentists. In Bay's (1968) investigation, dental personnel gave a group of eleven to thirteen-year-old children demonstrations of toothbrushing technique while the children were in the dentist's chair in the dental clinic. Next to the control group, the children individually instructed by the dentist showed the poorest response to instruction. This finding was interpreted in terms of the dentist-patient relationship. "Release of inhibitory emotional drives . . . when the children are seated in the dentist's chair may account for the fact that this rather traditional form of instruction apparently is not well suited for motivation of school children aged eleven to thirteen years."

How can one account for the contradictory outcomes of the two forms of instruction? In these studies, the situation, the force fields, or life spaces differ. In the dentist-patient relationship experienced in the dental office, children's emotions create a barrier which nullifies the dentist's instructional effort. In the school or lecture situation, there appears to be no barrier, but a force for promoting changed behavior. Part of the reason that no barrier seems to exist may be a result of the age of the subjects. Reference to Table 3-II shows young adults to be more amenable to traditional teaching methods, which stress acquisition of knowledge. And, as indicated above, the influence of the peer culture may also be the effective force.

Fear-arousal appeals, which have been grouped with credibility and the dentist-patient relationship in the model, may seem misplaced. However, fear arousal seems to have some characteristics which interact with credibility and the dentist-patient relationship. That is, whether or not a person finds the source of his or her information credible seems to be confused with the fear of dental treatment. For example, in his review of the literature on fear-arousal appeals, Higbee (1969) points out that "source credibility does interact with fear and this is an important variable in determining whether high-fear or low-fear is more effective." High fear appears to be effective when the credibility source is high. This may explain the improved OHI's when school dental health education is taught by a dentist.

Another point made by Higbee which may be related to the

dentist-patient relationship, particularly where children are concerned, has to do with the phenomenon of fear. He questions the notion that a fear-arousal threat is the same regardless of whether or not the thing feared has the same potential for causing fear. In his opinion, researchers have confounded two variables, "fear itself" and the "object of fear." In the dentist-patient relationship involving young patients, experiencing fear while undergoing treatment may be far more threatening than the consequences of neglect. Unpleasant as the consequences may be, a child seldom views them as probable or imminent. But the dentist, his drill and the fear associated with them are certainty, and frequency in encountering them may create a barrier in the dentist-patient relationship. Moreover, fear itself may be a block to the receptivity of the patient to instruction.

Health educators have also been concerned with threat appeals as a motivating technique. Russell and Robbins (1964) reviewed the fear-arousal literature for its implications for health education. Their conclusions were "that no particular approach —using fear or not using fear—will motivate *all* potential learners equally well." The profusion and confusion of the cumulative findings tend to support their contention. They view the "attention-getting" aspects of fear-arousal communication as most advantageous when they are properly used. A more creative approach to the use of fear-arousing stimuli may be required. Perhaps the use of fear to initiate *salience* would be sufficient. Once salience had been established, the educator could reinforce and explain by using more pleasant methods, objects, and behaviors —thereby stressing *pertinence*.

METHODS: ADULTS

The authors have not discussed the adult's experience in acquiring a value to the same depth that they have the child's experience because the adult has had experiences basically similar to the child's. For the adult, the available data point to socioeconomic and demographic factors, cultural milieu, status identity, and peer relations as most influential in shaping his oral hygiene behavior. When adults are parents, it may be easier to reach them in attempts to change oral hygiene behavior. But how does one reach adults who are not parents, who cannot be approached through their children? Should one write them off as oral hygiene "expendables?" What are the forces and barriers in their life spaces, apart from those already considered?

Mention was made earlier that Rokeach's most recent publication dealt with experimental procedures designed to *change* values. Essentially, his "experimental treatment was designed to induce feelings of self-dissatisfaction by making the subjects consciously aware that they held certain incompatible values or that they held an attitude that is incompatible with certain of their values." Note the similarity in concept between Green's status identity hypothesis and the hypothesis implied by Rokeach's procedure or technique. In both instances, the notion of incompatibility between certain values and behavior and the resulting dissatisfaction in the individual's view of himself function to change his behavior and ostensibly those values underlying the behavior. Rokeach's procedure effected value changes that were determined by use of unobtrusive measures of behavior. Results were not simply expressions of "opinion" but were expressions of action. Of considerable importance for health education is the finding that the changes in values have endured.

Rokeach's technique seems to be specific to the changing of behavior to reach consistency with the high-importance dimension of value, while Green seems to lead to either a change of values or the acquisition of new values. Green's status identity hypothesis, also supported by unobtrusive measures of behavioral effects, leads back to the source of values—which may explain why it seems relevant to new values. Green's hypothesis implies that the individual's value system is of a particular kind, shaped by various social groups but dependent upon a preferred group for its continued definition. Here, Rokeach and Green seem at opposite poles. Rokeach's procedure involves the individual with himself; the individual confronts himself in respect to his inconsistencies in value. Green's hypothesis points to a group involvement of the individual, then confrontation of the individual with himself in terms of group values. One might say that Rokeach emphasizes the "inner directedness" facets of values, while Green stresses the "other directedness" aspects.

Young (1971) and Cohen and Lucye (1970) have repeatedly pointed out that dental health information or knowledge has been insufficient in bringing about marked improvement of the public's dental health practices and status. The model in Figure 3-2 argues that knowledge is less important than holding dental health as a value. Yet review of the literature shows that adults are more prone to respond behaviorally to information than either educators or dentists have led anyone to believe. How do Rokeach's and Green's hypotheses and these observations fit together? First, the concepts suggest that information must be used in a special way—which will not be news to educators. Yet they do not contradict earlier statements regarding pertinence and salience, which involve a special use of information. The special way of using information appears to consist of exposing an individual to information in such a way as "to make him consciously aware of states of inconsistency that exist chronically within his own value-attitude system below the level of his conscious awareness," whether or not his subsequent confrontation is a self- or self-via-group orientation. Thus, a lack of self-knowledge in regard to one's own oral hygiene value system is a barrier to changed values, and consequently, behavior. Conversely, conscious awareness becomes a force for a change in oral hygiene values. Using a disclosing wafer to show an adult who values cleanliness the actual dirty state of his mouth may create the kind of inconsistency awareness required for value changes.

The dental health educator is seldom able to "capture" those adults whose values he would like to change. Persons "captive" in the armed forces comprise a limited part of the nation's population, but Cassidy's work demonstrates how necessary it is to be able to engage fully the only partially involved individual.

Meeting the problem through the mass media seems to perpetuate "superficial knowledge" of dental health which by itself has only a minor impact on value change, as demonstrated by behavior change. Although the mass media frequently aim at particular populations, there is good reason to believe that their ineffectiveness may result from a failure to provide a challenge to the individual's value system such that it penetrates below his level of conscious awareness. In other words, the message of the media is too remote from the individual's experience and too unfamiliar in terms of his life space to carry much meaning at the conscious level; thus, it misses its mark. If it fails to impress at the conscious level, there is small likelihood that it could reveal any inconsistency in the value system below the level of consciousness. The force for value change is lost, and because of this, the message may have no influence. Or, the message might elicit an adverse reaction or even create a barrier in keeping with the "inner-directed" aspect of value change.

However, the mass media are most frequently viewed as a force in the dental health education of the public. Possibly, this is because they tend to reach those persons "of somewhat greater than average education, and of somewhat better than average socioeconomic status. . . . The audience is perceived not as a mass of disconnected individuals, but rather as individuals who belong to groups and whose beliefs and attitudes are influenced by these groups" (Griffiths and Knutson, 1960). Accordingly, the message of the mass media should be a contributing factor in status identity and dental health behavior change. Yet the messages apparently fail, perhaps because even for the other-directed person they are too remote and unfamiliar to engage him effectively. In respect to failure of the message to motivate, Ratner (1963) maintained that the best target group for such communications is that containing those persons "who already visit their dentist twice a year." On the other hand, the message alone may be a sufficient reinforcer. Status identity may or may not be a force. Other forces impinge on behavior, and people do things for their own reasons (Cohen et al., 1967). Depending on the individual, good oral hygiene practices may mean "feeling good" or having "sex appeal." Their value dimension resides in the personal security provided by "feeling good" or having "sex appeal." In any case, the mass media thus far have had limited influence on changing dental hygiene practices among those most in need.

The mass media must learn to use dental health information in a special way if they are to be more than advertising vehicles. There is much potential for behavior change should the mass media experts experiment with messages geared toward salience and pertinence. Antismoking advertisements demonstrate how various messages can be designed for the different subgroups in the population such as parents of young children, "social" smokers, chain smokers, or teenagers. While advertising on a particular subject will never solve an entire problem, it can reinforce "good" behavior.

IMPLICATIONS

At the close of a chapter such as this the reader might expect a list of "things-to-do" to optimize personal oral hygiene practices. If such a list were prescribed, it could only be tentative. Although much research has been done, more is always necessary in order to prove or disprove the latest hypotheses. Each of the preceding sections has included suggestions relating (1) approaches that maximize the significance of status, peer identification or belonging to a given occupation, education, income, age, sex, race, or ethnic group; (2) formal dental health education which optimizes salience, pertinence, credibility, habit formation, long-term change, and concomitant reinforcement; (3) programs that match behavior with objectives and stress imitation of significant others such as mothers and teachers; and (4) methods such as community involvement, changing values by showing inconsistencies in currently held values, attitudes or behaviors, and more effective utilization of the mass media. The list can continue. No single approach will work on any one person or any one group of people. An entire plan is needed; planning for behavior change necessitates directing several tasks simultaneously and differentially to various target groups. This is contrary to the myth that removing the economic barrier will result in everyone going to the dentist. The economic barrier combines with other factors such as fear, inaccessibility or unavailability of services, barriers within the family context, etc., to prevent an individual from visiting the dentist. In the case of personal oral hygiene practices, forces and barriers to prescribed behaviors must be defined so that a logical strategy for counteracting undesirable behaviors may be developed. Attacking the problem without such a plan would be a fruitless effort.

EVALUATION

This entire chapter has been based on the concept of evaluation. Evaluative questions have been asked throughout: do given techniques work and why? Without such critical concern on the part of the dental health educator and practitioner, any given scheme may remain an individual's subjective opinion.

The ultimate test of effective oral hygiene is whether or not an individual or a group is free of oral disease. Clinical measurements for oral health status are described elsewhere; intermediate tests to guide the educator in assessing his plan *must* involve nothing less than clinical measurements of patients' plaque-removing performances. Amount of plaque accumulation varies with the patient, and successful removal also varies with the patient. These factors need to be considered either when the patient evaluates his own efforts or when a second person does the evaluating. Any evaluation method needs to be understood by the evaluator, for the method itself may contain biases and thereby misinform. The evaluation tool must also be amenable to standardization so that it produces valid and reliable results whenever a trained individual uses it. Evaluation of any program or practice, particularly when human behavior is to be measured, must remain anchored to empirical criteria—criteria that is real and demonstrable by scientifically valid and reliable methods. In the case of oral hygiene, where so much depends on the personal responsibility of the individual for his dental health, measuring tools that convincingly demonstrate the effectiveness of toothbrushing and flossing to the general population are also needed. Such tools exist, but there is room for improvement.

This brief mention of the need for intermediate tests and criteria for evaluation indicates one approach for evaluating the dynamics of behavioral influences on oral hygiene practices. With an adequate research plan and a valid means of assessing the effectiveness of the plan, those desiring to improve others' oral hygiene practices can expect success.

REFERENCES

Adams, R. J, and Stanmeyer, W. R.: The effects of a closely supervised oral hygiene program upon oral cleanliness. *J Periodontol, 21*:242-245, 1960.

Anderson, R., Smedby, B., and Anderson, O. D.: *Medical Care Use in Sweden and the United States—A Comparative Analysis of Systems and Behavior.* Center for Health Administration Studies, Research Series 27, The University of Chicago, 1970.

Antonovsky, A., and Kats, R.: The model dental patient: an empirical study of preventive health behavior. *Soc Sci Med, 4*:367-380, 1970.

Bandura, A., and Huston, A. C.: Identification as a process of incidental learning. *J Abnorm Psychol, 63*:311-318, 1961.

Bay, I.: Effect of instruction in toothbrushing on gingivitis and plaque in children 11-13 years old. *Tandlaegebladet, 62*:589-600, 1968.

Blalock, H. M.: *Causal Inferences in Non-experimental Research.* Chapel Hill, U of NC Pr, 1964.

Boek, W. E.: Behavioral science in dental health education. *NYS Dent J, 31*:354-362, 1965.

Brown, R. C., Jr.: Dental health education and behavioral science. The health educator's view. *NYS Dent J, 29*:414-416, 1963.

Bugbee, R. S.: An effective program in dental health education. *J Am Dent Hyg Assoc, Fourth Quarter*:40-43, 1970.

Cassidy, R. J.: *Dental Health Education Program—Determination of Operative Motivational Factors, Report Number One—Final Report.* Washington, D.C., U.S. Army Medical Research and Development Command, Office of the Surgeon General, New York, Decision Research Corporation, July 1965.

Chaffee, S. H.: *Two Sources of Value Change: Salience and Pertinence.* Paper read before the Association for Education and Journalism Convention, Syracuse, New York, August 1965.

Cohen, L. K., O'Shea, R. M., and Putnam, W. J.: Toothbrushing: public opinion and dental research. *J Oral Therap Pharm, 4*:229-246, 1967.

Cohen, L. K., and Lucye, H.: A position on school dental health education. *J Sch Health, 40*:361-365, 1970.

Collier, D. R., and Williams, J. E.: The evaluation of an educational program in preventive periodontics. *J Tenn Dent Assoc, 48*:92-103, 1968.

Corliss, J. M.: A report of the Denver research project on health interests of children. *J Sch Health, 32*:355-360, 1962.

Counsell, L. A.: The implication of the behavioral sciences for dental health education. *J Publ Health Dent, 30*:38-44, 1970.

Davis, H. C., and Land, D.: Good teeth for Guilford. A study in civic enterprise. *Brit Dent J*, 112:430-434, 1962.

Derryberry, M.: Health education: its objectives and methods. *Health Educ Mono*, Society of Public Health Educators, Inc., No. 8, 1960.

Dollar, M. L., and Sandell, P. J.: Dental programs in schools. *J Sch Health*, 31:3-15, 1961.

Dowell, T. B.: Healthy teeth for Huddersfield. *Brit Dent J*, 118:316-319, 1965.

Duany, L. F.: Children's dental health according to education level of mother. *Rev Odontol, April-October*:3-13, 1967.

Dudding, N. J., and Muhler, J. C.: What motivates children to practice good oral hygiene? *J Periodontol*, 31:141-142, 1960.

Duncan, O. D.: Path analysis: Sociological examples. *Am J Soc*, 72:1-16, 1966.

Finlayson, D. A., and Pearson, J. C. G.: Dundee dental health campaign: a study of its value six years later. *Brit Dent J*, 123:535-536, 1967.

Finlayson, D. A., and Wilson, W. A.: Dental health education—Dundee's dental health education campaign—results of survey six months later. *Brit Dent J*, 111:103-106, 1961, and 112:88-89, 1962.

Flanders, J. P.: A review of research on imitative behavior. *Psychol Bull*, 69:316-337, 1968.

Fodor, J. T., and Ziegler, J. E.: A motivational study in dental health education. *JS Calif St Dent Assoc*, 34:203-216, 1966.

Goose, D. H.: The design of a dental hygiene campaign. *Public Health*, 73: 7-13, 1959.

Goose, D. H., Goward, P. E., and Downham, D. Y.: Oral hygiene campaign in Liverpool. *Dent Pract*, 18:385-388, 1968.

Gravelle, H. R., Shackelford, M. F., and Lovett, J. T.: The oral hygiene of high school students as affected by three different educational programs, *J Public Health Dent*, 27:91-99, 1967.

Gray, A. S., and Hawk, D. R.: An evaluation of a grade one dental health program. *Can J Public Health*, 59:166-168, 1968.

Green, L. W.: Status identity and preventive health behavior. *Pacf Health Educ Rep*, No. 1, University of California, Berkeley, and University of Hawaii, Honolulu, 1970.

Greene, J. C., and Vermillion, J. R.: The simplified oral hygiene index. *JADA*, 68:7-13, 1964.

Griffiths, W., and Knutson, A. L.: The role of mass media in public health. *Am J Public Health*, 50:515-523, 1960.

Guttelman, A., Bamonte, E., and Gansberg, M.: Status of dental health education in private schools. *NYS Dent J*, 31:297-300, 1965.

Higbee, K. L.: Fifteen years of fear arousal: research on threat appeals; 1953-1968. *Psychol Bull*, 72:426-444, 1969.

Jago, J. D., and King, R. W.: The influence of dental advice in dental health in children. *Aust Dent J, 8:*323-328, 1963.

Janis, I. L., and Feshback, S.: Effects of fear-arousing communications. *J Abnorm Psychol, 48:*78-92, 1953.

Johns, C. K., and Muhler, J. C.: Can dental health education reduce permanent tooth loss? *JADA, 71:*35-38, 1965.

Kegeles, S. S.: Some changes required to increase the public's utilization of preventive dentistry. *J Public Health Dent, 28:*19-26, 1968.

Kelly, J. E., Van Kirk, L. E., and Garst, C.: Oral hygiene in adults. *Vital Health Stat, June:*1-30, 1966.

Kirk, G. S., and Raven, J. E.: *The Presocratic Philosophers.* Cambridge, Cambridge U Pr, 1962.

Kriesberg, L., and Treiman, B. R.: Socio-Economics and the Utilization of Dentist's Services. *J Am Coll Dent, 27:*147-168, 1960.

Kriesberg, L., and Treiman, B. R.: Preventive utilization of dentist's services among teenagers. *J Am Coll Dent, 29:*8-45, 1962.

Lamb, M. W., and Ford, E.: Dental health of children in the fourth grade of four elementary schools in Lubbock, Texas. *J Sch Health, 30:*15-26, 1960.

Lewin, K.: *Field Theory in Social Science,* Dorwin Cartwright (Ed.). New York, Harper and Brothers, 1951.

Linde, J., and Koch, G.: The effect of supervised oral hygiene on the gingivae of children. *J Peridont Res, 2:*215-220, 1967.

Löe, H., and Silness, J.: Periodontal disease in pregnancy. I. Prevalence and severity. *Acta Odontol Scand, 21:*533-551, 1963.

McCauley, H. B., Davis, L. B., and Frazier, T. M.: Effect on oral cleanliness produced by dental health instruction and brushing the teeth in the classroom: the 1953-1954 Baltimore toothbrushing study. *J Sch Health, 25:*250-254, 1955.

Mechanic, D.: The influence of mothers on their children's health attitudes and behavior. *Pediatrics, 30:*444-453, 1964.

Metz, A. S., and Richards, L. G.: Children's preventive visits to the dentist: the relative importance of socio-economic factors and parents' preventive visits. *J Am Coll Dent, 34:*204-212, 1967.

Mobley, E. L., and Smith, S. H.: Some social and economic factors relating to periodontal disease among young Negroes: No. 1. *JADA, 66:*486-491, 1964.

Moltz, H., and Thistelthwaite, D.: Attitude modification and anxiety reduction, *J Abnorm Psychol, 50:*231-237, 1955.

Muhler, J. C.: Practical chairside dental health education. *J Dent Child, 33:*215-218, 1966.

Mussen, P. H., and Parker, A. L.: Mother nurturance and girls' incidental imitative learning. *J Pers Soc Psychol, 2:*94-97, 1965.

Myers, S. E., and Downs, R. A.: Comparative findings in school systems with differing approaches to dental health education. *J Sch Health, 28:* 604-610, 1968.

Parfitt, G. J., James, P. M. C., and Davis, H. C.: A controlled study on the effect of dental health education on the gingival structures of school children. *Brit Dent J, 104:*21-24, 1958.

Pavlid, V.: Research into the health knowledge and behavior of school children. *Int J Health Educ, 11:*116-125, 1968.

Piaget, J., and Inhelder, B.: *The Psychology of the Child,* New York, Basic Books, 1969.

Pincheira, L., and Faundez, T.: Results of a survey on dental education. *Odontol Chilena, 15:*25-31, 1966. (See also *Oral Res Abstracts, 1:*743, 1966.)

Ramirez, A., Connor, R. B., Gibbs, R. M., Griggs, H. G., Nielson, J. O., and Reeder, O. W.: *The Effects of Different Persuasive Communications of Oral Hygiene.* Birmingham, University of Alabama, School of Dentistry, Fall 1969.

Ratner, V. M.: *Communications in Dental Health Education.* Paper read before the National Conference on Dental Health Education, Atlantic City, New Jersey, October 1963.

Rayner, J. F.: *Dental Hygiene and Socioeconomic Status.* Paper read before the 47th Annual Meeting of the International Association for Dental Research, Houston, Texas, March 1969.

Rayner, J. F.: Socioeconomic status and factors influencing the dental health practices of mothers. *Am J Public Health, 40:*1250-1258, 1970.

Richards, D. N. and Barmes, D. E.: Social factors in dental epidemiology. *Social Sciences and Dentistry: A Critical Bibliography* (Richards and Cohen, eds.) The Hague, A. Sijthoff, 1971.

Robinson, B. A., Mobley, E. L., and Pointer, M. B.: Is dental health education the answer? *JADA, 74:*124-128, 1967.

Roder, D. M.: A study of dental knowledge and behavior in 1,000 Australian school children. *Aust Dent J, 14:*327-330, 1969.

Rokeach, M.: *Beliefs, Attitudes and Values.* San Francisco, Jossey-Bass, 1969.

Rokeach, M.: Long-range experimental modification of values, attitudes and behavior. *Am Psychol, 26:*453-459, 1971.

Rowntree, F. S. D.: The Braintree Experiment. *Int J Hlth Educ, 11:*73-79, 1959, and *Brit Dent J, 107:*238-240, 1959.

Russell, R. D., and Robbins, P. R.: Health education and the use of fear: a new look. *J Sch Health, 34:*263-268, 1964.

Sandell, P. J.: Materials and methods in dental health education. *Int Dent J, 13:*154-157, 1963.

Scott, E.: Social value acquisition in preschool aged children. III. Internalization of institutionalized value expectations. *Soc Q, 2*:14-31, 1970.

Segal, D. R., Segal, M. W., and Knoke, D.: Status inconsistency and self-evaluation. *Sociometry, 33*:347-357, 1970.

Sliepcevich, E. M.: *School Health Education Study: A Summary Report.* Washington, D. C., School Health Education Study, 1964.

Striffler, D. F.: The importance of dental health education, *J Mich St Dent Assoc, 65*:318, 321-323, 1963.

Sundram, C. J.: Principles for developing dental health education programs. *Int J Health Educ, 9*:188-194, 1966.

Theodorson, G. A., and Theodorson, A. G.: *A Modern Dictionary of Sociology.* New York, T Y Crowell, 1969.

Tyler, R. W.: Implications of behavioral studies for health education. *J Sch Health, 33*:9-15, 1963.

Tyroler, H. A., Johnson, A. L., and Fulton, J. T.: Patterns of preventive health behavior in populations. *J Health Soc Behav, 6*:128-140, 1965.

Wallentin, W.: Oral hygiene and nutrition: survey of oral health conditions and breakfast contents of Westphalian school children. *Zahnaertzl Mitt, 50*:667-668, 1960. (See also *Dent Abst, 6*:240-241, 1961.)

Williford, J. W., Johns, C., Muhler, J. C., and Stookey, G. K.: Report of a study demonstrating improved oral health through education. *J Dent Child, 34*:183-189, 1967.

Williford, J. W., Muhler, J. C., and Stookey, G. K.: Study demonstrating improved oral health through education. *JADA, 75*:896-902, 1967.

Young, M. A. C.: Dental health education—whither? *JADA, 66*:821-824, 1963.

Young, M. A. C.: Studies related to some selected health problems. *Health Educ Mono, 28*:36-42, 1969.

Young, M. A. C.: Dental health education: an overview of selected concepts and principles relevant to programme planning. *Int J Health Educ, 13*: 2-26, 1970.

4

TECHNIQUES AND ARMAMENTARIUM ASSOCIATED WITH ORAL HYGIENE

Sam W. Hoskins, Jr.
Donald H. Masters

THROUGHOUT THE CENTURIES the entity, "oral hygiene," has taken on many images and meanings. To primitive man, oral hygiene was a toothpick made of bone, wood, or metal used to poke out bits of fibrous food which were both uncomfortable and socially annoying. To 20th century man, the image of oral hygiene could include all forms of gadgetry, various cleaning methods, and confusing and contradictory concepts. Oral hygiene armamentarium may range from a simple toothbrush to an oral hygiene center complete with electric implements, water sprays, special lights and mirrors, and several types of disclosing solutions—all designed by manufacturers to stimulate gadget-minded modern man in his increasing awareness of the importance of maintaining clean teeth.

In reality, any oral hygiene system worth considering must be based on needs dictated by the nature of the dental disease processes. For many centuries there has been concern about the substances which grow on the teeth and gums and their potential for harm to the dentition. When Leeuwenhoek was working with one of his first microscopes in 1683, he took samples from the gum line of his own teeth and described the appearance of the "little animals" as they moved about.

Since the days of Leeuwenhoek, many dental scientists have attempted to draw attention to the environment in which the teeth live. However, until recently the importance of controlling the dental environment has been overshadowed by a consuming passion for improved dental technology and a search for a singular antietiologic panacea for dental disease.

The latest scientist to promote interest in the oral environment is Sumter Arnim.[1-4] Stimulated by the observations of Bass and others, he has provided a wealth of information about the dental microcosm and its actions and offered suggestions for its control.[5-11] Thanks to his prolific writings and extensive cinemicrographic studies, patients and dentists alike have been able to see for themselves what goes on in the invisible world within their mouths. These studies have proved invaluable in helping people to understand that they are unwitting hosts to disease-producing microbes which, under the right conditions, thrive at the expense of the teeth and their supporting structures.

The following is a brief summary of the authors' impressions of the most salient points of the "microcosmal concept," taken from the studies of Arnim and Bass. These help shape the attitudes and methods of the modern dentist when he attempts to train patients to deal with dental disease.

1. The masses found clinging to the teeth are composed principally of motile and nonmotile microbes which often are termed, incorrectly, food debris and material alba.

2. This microcosm (bacterial plaque) is protected by a slimy, semipermeable mucoid gel—the zooglea which partially inhibits the neutralizing effect of saliva. Because of the nature of this gel the adherent masses cannot be removed effectively by water, antiseptic mouthwashes, or a coarse diet.

3. The microbial mass is relatively invisible but can be detected by staining with harmless dyes. If it is not removed every day, it will build in size and potency. Often after several days, a mineralized deposit will form within the mass and, in turn, is soon covered by active microbial colonies.

4. The microcosm forms toxic waste products which enter the gingival tissues by absorption, producing inflammatory re-

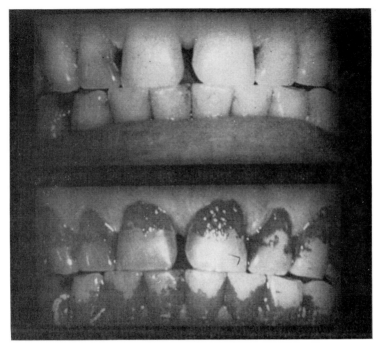

Figure 4-1. Mouth containing heavy accumulation of plaque as it appears clinically and the same mouth as it appears when a disclosing agent is used to detect and identify the "invisible" plaque (Courtesy of Doctor S. S. Arnim).

actions known clinically as periodontal disease. Adequate removal of this microbial irritant is essential to the prevention or control of periodontal disease.

5. When fed various sugars, the microbial mass can produce an acid waste which causes dissolution and ultimately cavitation in the tooth, allowing an invasion of the tooth by microorganisms.

6. The existence and potency of the microbe colonies are dependent largely upon the negligent oral hygiene habits of the host. As long as people allow the presence of the deleterious microorganisms by failure to remove them, dental disease will continue to be the most prevalent disease faced by man.

7. However, one can virtually eliminate continued dental disease by an effective system of personal dental care, including thorough daily oral hygiene and proper food selection.
8. This microcosmal concept has stood the test of time and many studies. It is now possible to say that there is a definite causal relationship between dental disease and the local dental environment.

PERSONAL DENTAL CARE ARMAMENTARIUM AND TECHNIQUES

Effective oral hygiene techniques play a vital role in the control of dental disease and should be stressed in dental office prevention programs. This section will review and evaluate the oral hygiene devices and techniques currently used for maintaining oral health.

To be acceptable, an oral hygiene technique should satisfy the following criteria.

1. It must produce effective dental cleanliness.
2. It must be safe so that by doing good it does not also do harm.
3. It must be easy to teach, easy to learn, and relatively easy to perform with consistency.

Adherence to these standards encourages objectivity in the selection of oral hygiene methods and devices.

Each major dental area or domain requires a specific device for effective dental care. The three major domains are:

1. The facial, lingual, and occlusal surfaces of the teeth—the responsibility of the toothbrush.
2. The interproximal surfaces—cleaned best by dental floss.
3. The crevicular areas (of any appreciable depths)—safely reached principally by dental irrigators.

To most patients, dental hygiene has been limited to the toothbrush, with occasional help from jabbings with toothpicks and flushing with flavored mouthwashes. Consequently, many patients have trouble accepting the fact that three different types of instruments may be necessary for adequate oral hygiene. It must be stressed that *each instrument has its own domain; one will not take the place of the other.* With practice, encouragement, and habitual use, the patient can learn to clean these domains with the specialized instruments just as he learned to use the knife, fork, and spoon to eat his meals. Even with training, however, patients tend to relapse to use of the toothbrush alone.

Detecting the Presence of the Enemy

Disclosing Dyes

Having the patient use disclosing dyes to detect microbes on the teeth has been hailed by many authorities as the most important and practical contribution to the control and prevention of dental disease. The most commonly used dye is FDC #3 red (erythrosin) which is available in tablet or liquid form and has been found to be effective and safe after many years of application.

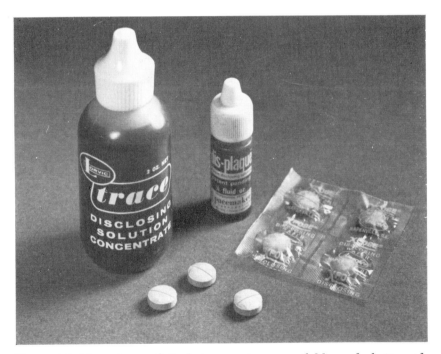

Figure 4-2. Many forms of disclosing agents are available, and obvious advantages of the different types are apparent. The tablet is probably more convenient for patient use at home and can be dissolved in water for use in a dental office.

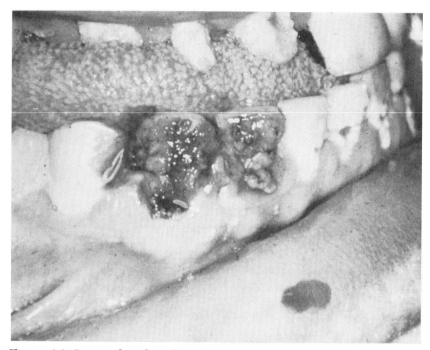

Figure 4-3. In mouths where heavy plaque accumulation is present and is visible with casual viewing, its presence is more vividly disclosed to the patient by the local application of a liquid dye.

The patient is taught to chew the fast-dissolving tablet or use a few drops of the liquid, swishing the dye through the mouth and allowing it to remain in contact with the teeth for thirty to sixty seconds. The excess water-soluble dye is removed by rinsing the mouth vigorously once or twice with water. Rinsings may be either swallowed or emptied. If the microcosm remains as bacterial plaque on the teeth, it will be stained and can be identified easily by the patient. These stains will appear most often on the surfaces between the teeth and along the gumline. Attention can then be called to the contrast between the clean and stained areas, indicating where present cleaning methods are inadequate.

Viewing Devices

The Plak-Lite® is a recent innovation, and proponents of the device claim it offers a significant improvement over both the

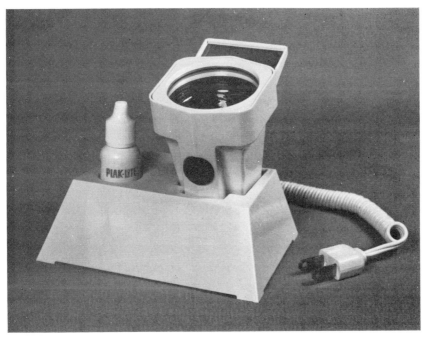

Figure 4-4. The Plak-Lite® system uses a fluorescein dye that is relatively invisible until exposed to a specially filtered light. Most conventional disclosing agents visibly stain the lips and tongue temporarily (International Pharmaceutical Co.).

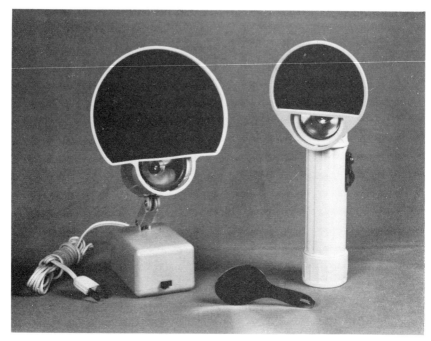

Figure 4-5. Some form of intraoral lighting method is helpful for visualization of plaque, particularly on the lingual aspects of the teeth. The 110v model (Floxite®) on the left is suitable for both dental office and home use and the flashlight model on the right is a less expensive, but more difficult to use, version for home use. The small plastic mirror provides additional intraoral viewing.

viewing system and the use of disclosing dyes. This system employs the use of fluorescein dye which is virtually invisible until it is exposed to a specially filtered light, thus overcoming the problem of prolonged staining of the lips and tongue which occurs with some disclosing agents. Since patients are always trying to turn excuses into rational reasons for behavior, perhaps this device will have motivational value.

Patients need both equipment and instructions to improve intraoral examination. Without this skill, they are far more dependent on the inspection and evaluation of the dentist. During the early part of the training period, time should be spent in teaching patients the use of a light and a reflecting system. If economics prevent the purchase of these items, a flashlight and a cosmetic mirror are of some value.

After initial skills are developed, the disclosing dye and mirror-with-light combination should be used twice a week, after the cleaning process, to determine cleaning effectiveness, and to show where increased emphasis is needed.

Facial, Lingual, and Occlusal Surfaces— Domain of the Toothbrush

Although many designs and types of toothbrushes are available, only a few can be considered acceptable performers when measured by the previous basic criteria. Because frequent, observable violations of these standards occur when stiff, potentially traumatic bristle brushes are used, there is almost a universal trend toward using the so-called soft nylon bristle brush which follows the general specification recommended by Bass in 1954.

The multitufted brush with rounded-end, small-diameter bristles (.007 to .008 inch) can be placed safely at the "critical zone" (the gingival one third of the tooth) and moved gently in a horizontal scrubbing motion which is quite effective in cleaning the teeth.

1. BASS TECHNIQUE. In the writings of Bass the "right way" to use the brush was described but never illustrated. He advocated placing the bristles at a 45 degree angle to the tooth, with the rounded-end bristles sliding into and cleaning the sulcus. The

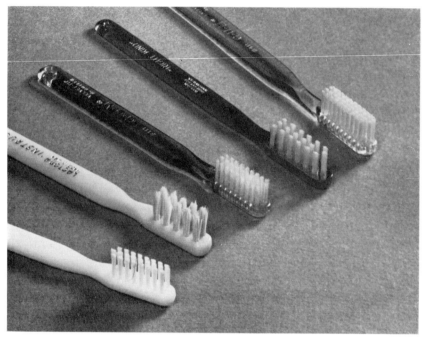

Figure 4-6. The two stiff bristle (nylon and natural) brushes on the left were frequently used in the "roll" brushing technique. Soft, multituft, round-end bristle brushes, like the three on the right, are more generally used today with techniques that direct the bristles toward the gingival sulcus to clean this "critical zone" effectively. The brush size appropriate for a specific mouth should be selected.

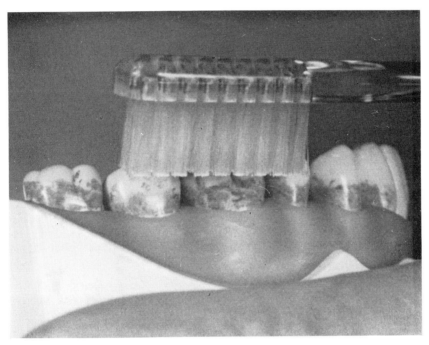

Figure 4-7. The soft, multituft bristles are directed toward the gingival sulcus at approximately a 45 degree angle to the long axis of the tooth. This permits the bristles to engage plaque in the "critical zone" (stained in this model) and avoid injury to either tooth or gingiva.

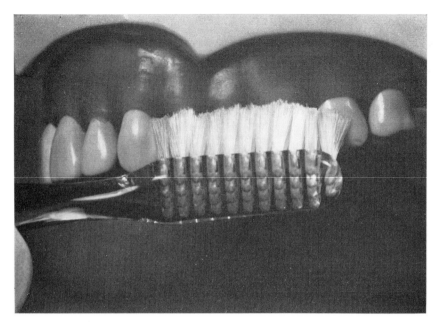

Figure 4-8. The Bass Method of brushing has several interpretations. Generally, the emphasis is to angulate the rounded-end bristles toward the gingival crevices and the "critical zone." By using a gentle, horizontal rocking motion, plaque can be removed from the region of the crevices and the side of the tooth.

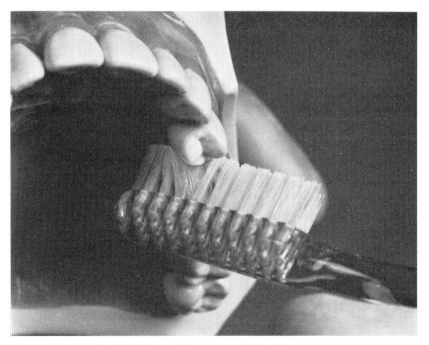

Figure 4-9. On the difficult-to-clean areas of the lingual surfaces, the horizontal rocking motion may be supplemented by a short, almost vertical sweep. This is particularly helpful in the anterior regions.

sides of the bristles are supposed to clean the supragingival tooth surface. The stroke involves limited horizontal bristle movement (less than the width of a lower incisor) and a rhythm pattern that resembles a gentle rocking motion, much like a hula skirt.

This description invites many modifications. A common method consists of placing the bristles almost parallel to the tooth and attempting to insert the inside row of bristles into the sulcus. Another variation could be described as more of a gentle, marginal scrubbing stroke with more emphasis on cleaning the "critical zone" rather than attempting to force the bristles into the sulcus. In the authors' opinion, effective sulcular brushing as described by Bass is often more wishful thinking than fact.

2. MODIFIED BASS TECHNIQUE. To improve ease of placement and to increase effectiveness of cleaning the "critical zone," many have altered the Bass technique slightly. In this modification of bristle placement, there is less emphasis on brushing into the crevice itself. Instead, there is a marginal scrubbing stroke where the bristle ends are concentrated in the gingival one third of the tooth with the outside row of bristles slightly overlapping the gingival margin. The brushing motion is essentially the same —a gentle, horizontal rocking movement.

For improved effectiveness, the lingual surfaces of the teeth are often given supplemental brushing strokes. The authors recommend following the horizontal stroke with an almost vertical short sweep, using the brush on its width rather than its length. The bristles simultaneously contact the gingival margins and tooth surface, and a short up-and-down movement is begun. The bristles enter portions of the interdental embrasures and produce a "plaid pattern" when superimposed on the previously described horizontal motion. Theoretically, this technique would not be necessary if it were not for the interference of the tongue, the incisal edges of anterior teeth, and the limited dexterity and visibility on lingual surfaces.

3. STILLMAN'S ROLL TECHNIQUE.[13] The most commonly used, and until recently the only American Dental Association-approved method of brushing, was to "brush the teeth the way they grow." The roll technique starts with the bristles pointing

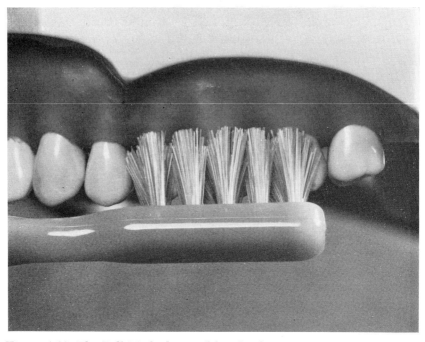

Figure 4-10. The Roll Method. Initial bristle placement is apical to the gingival margin, and the bristles are "rolled" with a sweeping motion over the gingiva and tooth toward the occlusal surface. This method is not as effective as the Bass technique in cleaning the "critical zone."

apically, more or less parallel to the tooth's long axis. The bristle ends are placed on the gingival pad. With a turning motion of the wrist, the patient sweeps the bristles over the gingival margin and tooth surface, ending off the tooth entirely. The rationale of this technique is that it is nontraumatic (which it is not), that it keeps the gums pulled coronally (an utter fallacy), and that it is easy to perform and produces effective results (questionable on both counts). Its most serious deficiency is that the bristles immediately leave the "critical zone," so that throughout most of the stroke, the area of greatest concern is brushed the least. Although this technique is still employed by many people, it is losing popularity due to its failure to satisfy the basic criteria of acceptability.

4. OTHER BRUSHING TECHNIQUES. A number of other techniques have been used during the last fifty years: Charters, the physiologic method, the original Stillman's method, and the Fones technique[14, 15] to mention a few. Most of these have been discarded because they failed to meet the more exacting requirements of modern testing. Types of toothbrushes and toothbrushing methodology, however, still remain as points of sore debate in many circles.

There is little argument over how to clean the occlusal surface. The ends of the bristles are placed on the occlusal surface, and the grooves and inclines are given a thorough scrubbing with a horizontal motion.

Powered Toothbrushes

Unless the patient has a manual infirmity, initial toothbrushing instruction is always done with the manual brush. If the patient wishes to try a powered brush after learning the fundamentals well, the proposed criteria for oral hygiene technique evaluation can be applied to determine if there is satisfactory performance. However, the use of any powered brush without instruction and follow-up testing is a highly questionable practice. Selection of the powered brush is subject to the same standards as the manual brush, and this sharply limits the choice. The powered brush must provide the same soft, rounded-tip bristles and the same gentle, back-and-forth rocking action. Many of the "automatic" brushes can be deficient in both respects and should be carefully evaluated by the clinician before being recommended.

In the authors' opinion, powered brushes should be much more closely controlled in terms of bristle standards and brush movement patterns because the intensity of application creates a potential hazard to the tissues. Also, there is a potential shock hazard with any electrically powered device which goes into the mouth. This is a fact that has been emphasized by more than one testing laboratory. Once the novelty of the automatic brush is gone, dentists face the same problem of retaining patient motivation and adherence to exacting techniques.

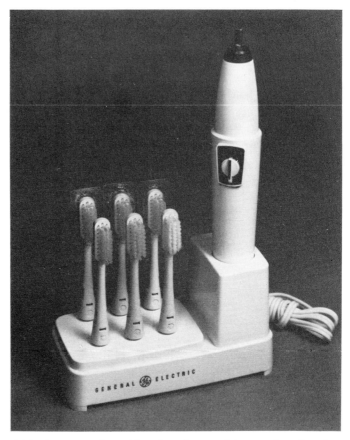

Figure 4-11. A powered toothbrush. This model provides the choice of a back-and-forth or a "roll" motion. The back-and-forth motion is more effective in cleaning the "critical zone." A choice of bristle firmness is usually provided, and a "soft bristle" brush head should be selected.

Dentifrices

Dentifrices are currently considered less important in plaque removal than in years gone by. However, they do function in two roles besides "breath sweetening": (1) They remove stains and pellicle from the tooth surfaces; and (2) they contain anticaries and desensitizing agents. Present dentifrice use by unenlightened patients can be criticized as follows:

1. Patients assume false positive results due to flavor.

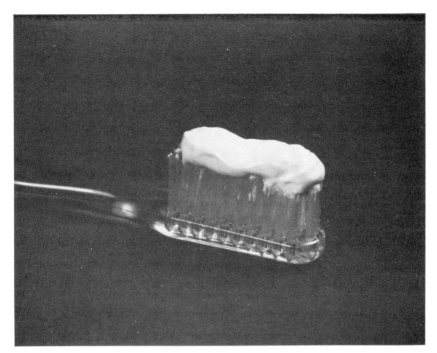

Figure 4-12. Excessive dentifrice applied to the brush interferes with the sweeping action of the bristles and creates mouth-emptying problems because of the heavy foaming.

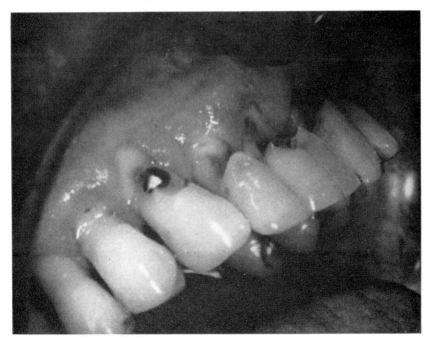

Figure 4-13. Pronounced tooth structure abrasion caused by use of a hard (stiff bristle) toothbrush, abrasive dentifrice and a vigorous scrubbing motion.

2. Excess quantities (a full stripe) render the bristles useless and increase the abrasive potential when applied to exposed root surfaces.
3. Dentifrices can increase pulpal sensitivity when used on exposed root surfaces.
4. Suds interfere with viewing the brushing technique.

In the training stage the patient should avoid the routine use of dentifrice. When it is used, only a dot should be applied and spread out with the finger. More can be added later if it is felt necessary. To remove stains and pellicle, one can use a wash cloth and an interdental cleaner in conjunction with a dentifrice. Whether dentifrices containing fluoride have a significant effect on caries will not be discussed in this chapter.

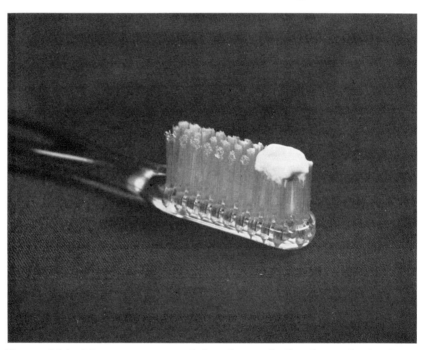

Figure 4-14. Adequate amount of dentifrice. Ideally, the teeth should be cleaned initially without the use of a dentifrice. This permits the bristles to perform the sweeping action effectively. When disclosing agents are used, it is easier to visualize the areas inadequately cleaned if no dentifrice is used. Following plaque removal, a small amount of dentifrice should be used to polish the teeth and freshen the mouth.

Interproximal Surfaces—Domain of Dental Floss

According to random surveys conducted by the authors, less than 10 percent of dental patients regularly use dental floss. In fact, most people fail to realize that cleaning the interdental surface is of any importance. Most people in our society have been taught from childhood that one *should* brush the teeth every day. After seeing the stained residue that remains between the teeth after brushing, however, it is obvious to the patient that brushing is not synonymous with cleaning. This helps to justify the emphasis on learning to clean the interdental surfaces. In spite of this increased awareness dental floss will be the last implement the patient will readily accept and master and the

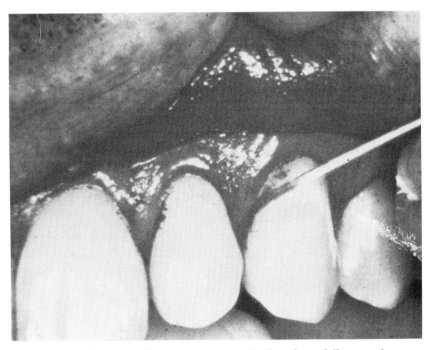

Figure 4-15. Plaque usually remains on proximal surfaces following the most careful use of the toothbrush. Dental floss, used with a scraping action, is required to clean the proximal tooth surface and into the gingival sulcus. The fingers manipulating the floss must move in the same direction to conform the floss to the curving tooth surface and to permit its introduction into the gingival sulcus.

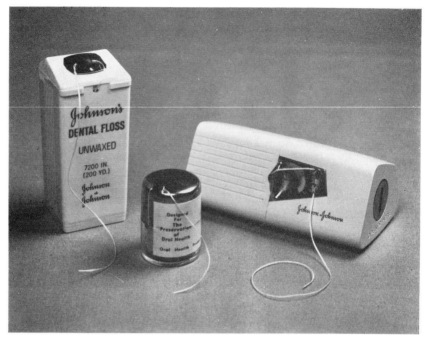

Figure 4-16. Dental floss types. A bonded form of unwaxed floss (left) provides some of the theoretical advantages of softness and filament separation of the regular unwaxed floss (center). It is of small diameter and does not shred easily, which are qualities of the waxed floss (right).

first tool to be abandoned when the patient attempts to streamline his personal dental care system.

Despite the purported superiority of multistranded unwaxed floss over waxed floss, it is usually better to use a waxed or bonded unwaxed floss during the initial training period. Since the main problems in flossing are establishment of an acceptable technique and its habitual use, the shredding of the multistranded unwaxed floss on defective restorations and calculus ledges can give the patient serious reason to discontinue doing what he already considers to be a distasteful chore.

Later, after the correction of defects, the use of multistranded unwaxed floss can be recommended. This floss does spread out over the tooth, contacting and cleaning more surface per unit of

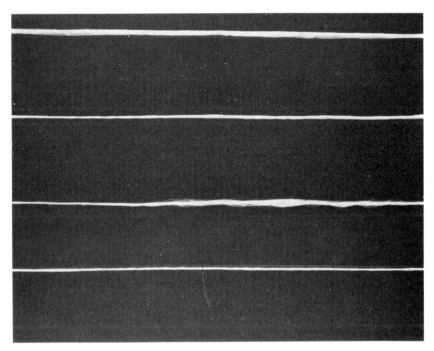

Figure 4-17. Waxed dental tape (top) is wider than dental floss, but is thick and difficult to pass through contact areas. It is seldom used in personal dental care procedures today. Regular waxed dental floss (second from top) is small enough to pass readily through contacts. When properly applied to the tooth, it effectively removes plaque without appreciable shredding of the floss. Unwaxed dental floss (third from top) contains many individual fiber elements and is purported to be more effective in plaque removal. This floss easily shreds when passed through contacts or over rough restorations or calculus projections. For this reason many patients become discouraged and discontinue its use. Bonded unwaxed dental floss (bottom) may combine the advantages of both waxed and unwaxed floss. It is softer than conventional waxed floss and conforms to the tooth surface readily. It is effective in plaque removal but does not shred easily. It is small in diameter and passes easily through most contacts.

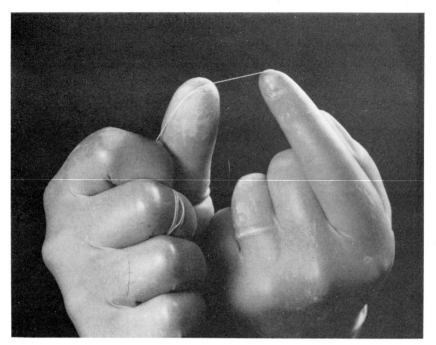

Figure 4-18. Good floss grip is essential for consistent results. The floss must be secured, enabling the thumbs and forefingers to be free to maneuver the floss in various combinations.

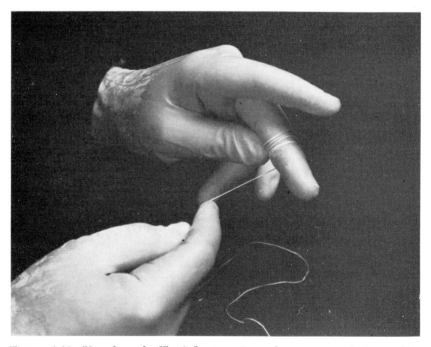

Figure 4-19. "Spool method" of flossing. Several wraps round the middle finger of both hands give anchorage for holding a minimum of eighteen inches of floss.

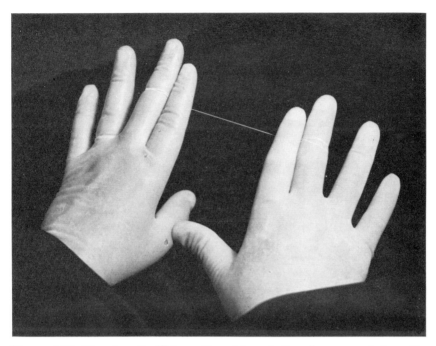

Figure 4-20. "Spool method" is continued by winding floss around the middle finger until approximately one thumb span is achieved. For reaching the most posterior areas, two thumb spans may be necessary.

movement. It is also thinner than waxed floss and can be slipped easily between the contacts. However, the authors have seen little difference in effectiveness of the two types of floss in actual tests of plaque removal.

Proper grip of the floss is essential if the patient is to develop expertise and consistency. The grip must provide both security and maneuverability. The spool method is most commonly used and is relatively easy to teach. It does tend to impair circulation to the wrapped fingers, causing discomfort and concern to some patients.

A prefabricated answer to the floss and yarn combination has been introduced to the market recently. Super Floss®* is made

* Educational Health Products Inc., 221 Mill Road, P.O. Box 24, New Canaan, Conn. 06840.

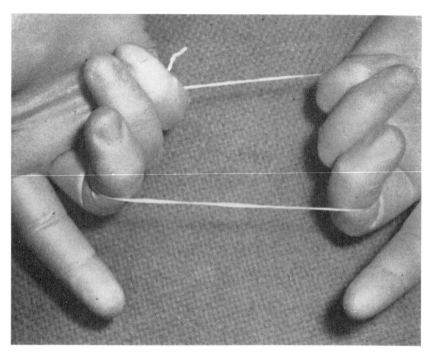

Figure 4-21. "Circle or loop method" gives excellent control without some of the disadvantages of other grips. With a little practice, the circle can be tied to the most suitable diameter for patient's needs.

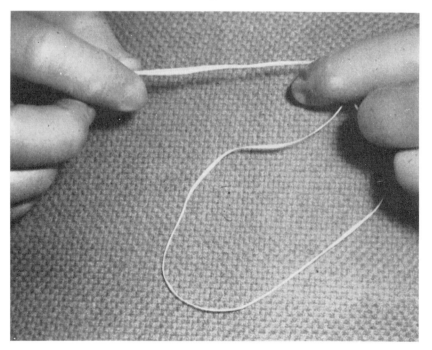

Figure 4-22. One way of beginning the circle is to use fourteen to eighteen inches of floss and tie off the desired circle diameter.

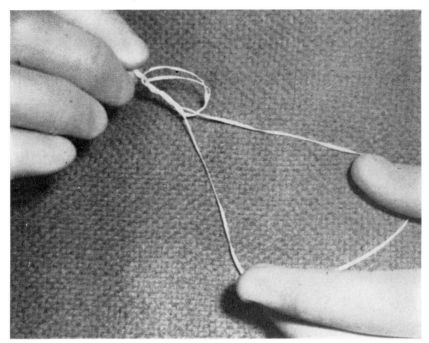

Figure 4-23. A double overhand knot secures the floss loop at the desired diameter. Although this step takes a few moments, it saves time in the long run.

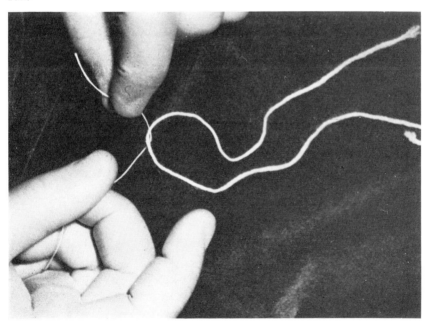

Figure 4-24. Combination of floss and yarn for interproximal cleaning. Yarn should be tight twist, two- or three-ply synthetic (baby sweater type). A single knot can be tied to secure floss around the yarn, or the floss can be passed doubled. Wetting the yarn and stripping away loose fibers improves patient acceptability.

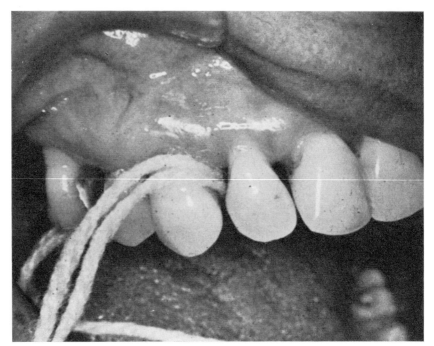

Figure 4-25. The coarse surface of the yarn easily removes surface plaque from large embrasures and long roots. Minimum movement back and forth is required. If a knot is tied, the floss can also be used for crevicular cleaning.

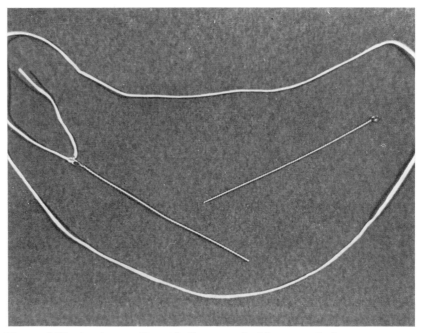

Figure 4-26. A wire needle with floss attached by a single knot is an easy way to clean difficult-to-reach interproximals cervical to splinted contacts and pontics.

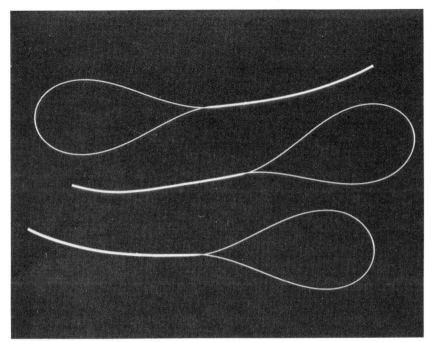

Figure 4-27. A recent innovation in threading devices is the heavy mono-filament loop which threads easily and pulls doubled floss through splinted contacts (supplied by John Butler Brush Company).

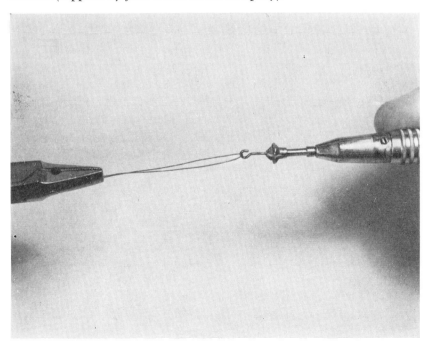

Figure 4-28. The wire needle for floss threading can be produced in the office with a jig made by soldering a hook onto a mandrel. When placed in the straight handpiece, the .010 orthodontic wire held by the pliers becomes a needle a few seconds after the rheostat is activated.

of heavy gauge nylon and has a section of teased strands resembling Velcro®. It is used for the same purpose and by the same methods as the floss and yarn combination previously described.

A recent innovation is the circle floss devised by one of the authors.[12] The circle allows easy gripping with the last three fingers of each hand and maintains maneuverability with the thumb and forefingers. Preparing the circle takes an extra moment, but it later saves both time and frustration. After passing through the contact with a slight sawing motion, the floss should enter the proximal crevice and be tucked to conform to the rounded tooth surface. Particular attention should be paid to cleaning the often-missed line angles. The principal movement is up and down along the tooth surface, using the floss as a miniature scraper. After cleaning one surface in the proximal space, the floss is moved over the gingival papilla, and the procedure is repeated on the adjacent tooth surface.

Floss can be combined with yarn in order to clean large interproximal surfaces with undulating curves.[16] The yarn should be two or three-ply nylon, dacron, or orlon, and it should be small gauge with a tight twist. It should be moistened and stripped between the fingers before use to prevent loose threads from gathering in the mouth. The leader piece of floss is slipped through the contact and the yarn drawn through the embrasure.

Frequently, periodontal patients have splinted contacts or bridgework which require extra aids such as wire, plastic or monofilament needles to assist the patient in threading the floss for cleaning. It is surprising how seldom patients are equipped for and instructed in cleaning under new fixed bridgework. A wire needle is usually superior to the flat plastic one and can be made in the office with a simple jig.

Floss-Holding Devices

There are several devices on the market for holding dental floss, possibly making the job a little easier for the patient, but not necessarily improving the effectiveness of dental floss as an interproximal cleaner. The authors have tested several of these

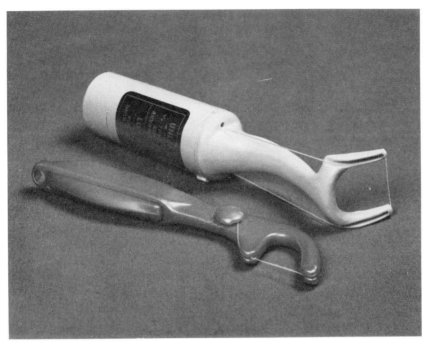

Figure 4-29. Floss-holding devices come in several sizes, shapes, and actions. The E-Z Denta-Flosser® below made by Preventive Dentistry Products Inc. and the Dentacare Floss Span® above made by Gretacor Devices appear worthy of attention.

and have found no device that is clearly outstandingly acceptable from all standpoints. The chief objection is the limitation of the preset arc in tucking around the tooth to clean line angles. However, if all attempts to obtain effective and habitual use of floss are to no avail, one should consider recommending a floss-holding device to the patient.

Auxiliary Aids for Interproximal Cleaning

1. When properly used, the toothpick can be an excellent adjunctive cleaning instrument for interproximal surfaces. However, it can be hazardous unless thorough instruction is given. If placed in a contra-angle handle such as the Perio-Aid®, the toothpick becomes an instrument which can

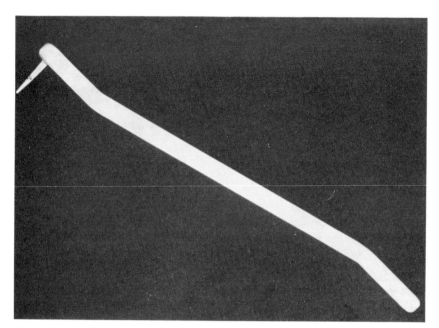

Figure 4-30. The Perio-Aid® (original model) allows versatile use of the toothpick after it is jammed into the cone-shaped holding receptacle and broken off. This instrument can clean hard-to-reach areas which cannot be managed readily with floss.

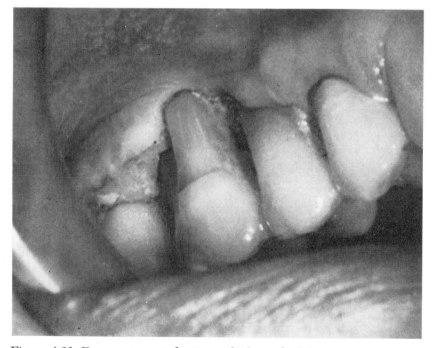

Figure 4-31. Damage to periodontium which resulted from improper use of Perio-Aid®. When auxiliary instruments such as these are prescribed, great care must be given to provide proper instruction and stress caution in their use.

be manipulated easily to clean proximal surfaces or hard-to-reach places such as line angles, furcations, and distal surfaces of terminal molars. It cannot be a consistent substitute for floss, however, because it cannot go safely into the proximal crevice. There are many instances where well-intentioned but overvigorous use of a potentially traumatic instrument such as this has produced harmful results.

2. Stimudents®, pipecleaners, Proxabrushes®, and interdental stimulators all have specific applications. The Stimudent has limited importance because its use is confined largely to the anterior segment of the mouth, and the approach is largely from the facial aspect. The pipecleaner is used occasionally for cleaning large root surfaces, under bridges, and through wide, open furcations. Interdental stimulators are comparatively poor cleaning instruments. Since the gingivae require little stimulation by artificial means, the authors seriously question the continued arbitrary use of these stimulators. A possible exception is in the attempted reduction of redundant tissue caused by edematous enlargement.

Gingival Crevice—Domain of the Dental Irrigator

When the gingival crevice or sulcus is shallow and relatively healthy it presents no serious problem when effective tooth brush and floss techniques are used. However, many people have periodontal disease which originates in the gingival crevice and destroys the crevicular epithelium and the fiber units. As the crevice deepens, it becomes filled with toxic residues as well as countless microbial bodies which float freely in the crevicular exudate. All this toxic matter tends to perpetuate the pathologic process. The gingival crevice is seldom cleansed thoroughly by any of the previously mentioned hygienic techniques. The dental irrigator is the instrument of choice since it offers the most effective and safest method of irrigating the contents of the gingival crevice. It acts as a lavage to the gingival wound, cleansing it of cellular debris, microbial masses and their toxins and other entrapped residues.

No personal dental care instrument has been viewed with such controversy as the dental irrigator. After reviewing the literature and talking with many clinicians over the years, the authors feel that much of the controversy apparently stems from a misunderstanding of what the irrigator is supposed to do.[17, 18]

The following is a listing of some of the common complaints against the dental irrigator with editorial comment by the authors, based on their experience with approximately 5000 cases where water irrigation was used.

1. *Water will not clean plaque from the teeth.* Advocates of dental irrigation have never claimed adherent plaque removal is one of its primary roles. It does reduce the thick outer layer of plaque, however.

2. *Water irrigation will cause additional injury to the dam-*

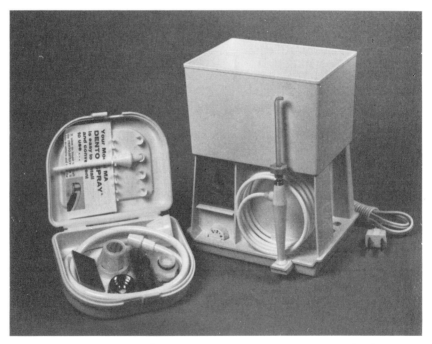

Figure 4-32. Two types of dental irrigators in common use: The faucet-attached model (Dento Spray®, Texell Mfg. Company) on the left emits a steady stream and delivers three to four times as much water in a given time period as does the pump-driven irrigator (Teledyne Water Pik®) which features a pulsating water stream.

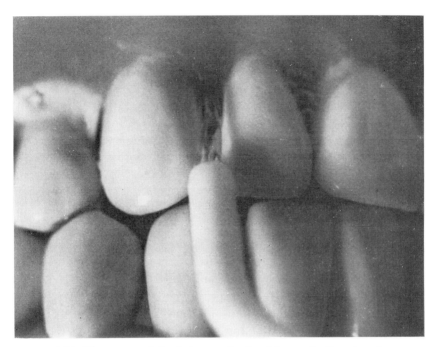

Figure 4-33. Placement of the irrigator tip should permit directing the warm water stream *into* the crevices. The feel of the tip against the side of the tooth can act as a guide since the patient cannot actually watch this action. Directions of some manufacturers mislead consumers by indicating that an irrigator is primarily an interproximal cleaning device.

aged epithelial lining of the pocket. Irrigation with high-pressure water-bullets is more likely to disturb exposed blood vessels and cause bleeding and increase tenderness than a gentle, constant stream of water. There is no evidence that any additional injury is likely.

3. *Transient bacteremias are common occurrences with water irrigators.* Transient bacteremias occur with any other tooth-cleaning device as well. Even food or gum chewing will cause microbes and their toxins to start migrating, which makes it logical to maintain a reduced population of the threatening organisms in the gingival crevice and to take proper precautions in patients with valvular heart problems.

4. *Some patients stop using floss in favor of the dental irrigator. Since water will not remove adherent plaque effectively, an increase in gingival inflammation is common.* Although this is noted occasionally, it is not the fault of the irrigator, but rather the failure of the teacher to make clear the role of irrigation and its relationship to plaque. Separating the dental areas into their various domains and identifying the instruments which clean each domain helps eliminate this problem. The existence of this tendency does not in any way condemn the proper use of water irrigation.

5. *One must use a pulsating stream to stimulate the gums and remove properly the contents of the crevices.* On the contrary, the authors have found a continuous stream of warm water under moderate pressure offers a better lavage of the wound than does the water-bullet effect which relies on high pressure rather than water volume. It is absurd to cite the need for gingival stimulation; there is already more blood in the area than is needed. Stimulation is certainly not the role of the dental irrigator.

6. *Water irrigation cannot clean deep pockets thoroughly. Improvement in external symptoms and signs does not reflect the true status of the health of the pocket.* Unless an inordinate amount of time and skill is utilized, deep pockets are difficult to clean with an irrigator. However, the authors have seen exceptions to this. There is some truth to the suspicion that many people may be fooled by the change in signs and symptoms at the upper level of the crevice while the substance in the deeper pocket continues its destructive process. Where possible, pockets should be reduced by appropriate therapy to aid in patient management.[19, 20]

The authors' experiences with patients using irrigators have produced varied results but certain impressions have been formed. It appears that the shallower the crevice, the more responsive it is to simplified hygiene techniques. However, all pockets cannot be zero depth. The therapist should be enlightened sufficiently to prescribe according to a true evaluation of the given situation and not to be influenced prejudicially by unfounded opinion. For those who are reluctant to prescribe water lavage for a periodontal patient, the authors would invite observation of a sedimentation test (originally advocated by Arnim) which may be described as follows:

1. Have the patient with periodontal pockets brush, floss, and rinse thoroughly as he is taught to do routinely each day. Save a portion of the rinsings for testing.
2. Use an irrigator (or a 15cc syringe with a blunt needle) to irrigate several pocket areas, catching the rinsings either in a beaker or a plastic liner in the lavatory.
3. Place the collections in a centrifuge tube, spin down, and examine the contents. The gross appearance of the layers of the pocket contents will show what was left behind after thorough brushing, flossing, and rinsing. Microscopic examination of the solid layer will usually prove quite informative to both the therapist and the patient.

PERSONAL DENTAL HEALTH TRAINING PROGRAM

If patients are to control dental disease effectively, many of them need professional instruction and continued guidance in mastering oral hygiene methods and establishing a personal dental care regimen. In this section the authors outline such a training program which can be conducted in the dental office for patients with existing dental problems or an interest in preventing disease.

A Practical Testing Program—Seeing Is Believing

Both dentists and patients can justify the emphasis placed on personal dental care when they see the clinical effect that retained microbes have on the dental tissues. Further, it is reassuring and reinforcing for patients to see the clinical changes which occur when polluted areas are thoroughly and repeatedly cleaned by the individual.

A suggested approach to this revealing testing program is as follows:

1. Select a few interested patients with overt signs of periodontal disease, documenting the initial clinical picture by

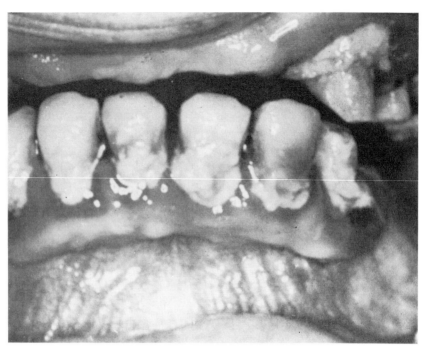

Figure 4-34. A seventy-seven-year-old patient whose personal dental care neglect of several years has resulted in gross accumulation of plaque and extensive periodontal involvement.

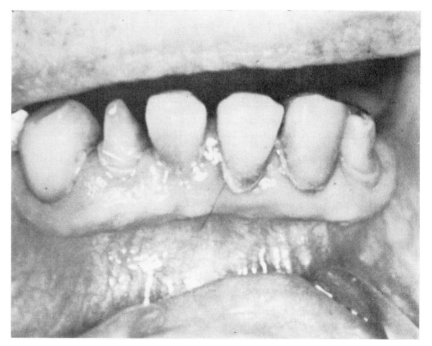

Figure 4-35. Same patient as Figure 4-34, after two weeks of effective personal dental care. No therapy was performed. All plaque removal and inflammation reduction was the result of the newly motivated patient's efforts.

some means (description, photographs, and/or phase contrast samplings).

2. Help these patients learn about the dynamic action of the microbes which help to cause dental disease and explain the role of the patient in controlling dental disease.

3. During several visits, instruct patients in the necessary techniques of daily personal dental care. Check and reinstruct them in three to seven-day intervals until definite changes in their signs and symptoms are noted. (Again, document the results.)

4. Plan and conduct regular dental treatment, depending upon the requirements of the patient.

5. Continue adjusting the hygiene regimen as may be required due to altered dental anatomy, new dental appliances, or trends toward relapsing to old hygiene habits. Compare the health status of these mouths against that of patients whose personal dental care is nonstructured.

Patients and dentists who have tried this initial emphasis on personal dental care have found the experience very rewarding. Once a dentist sees for himself that there is a positive relationship between the adherent microcosm and the continuance of dental disease, he comes to believe that the procedures controlling the cause of dental disease are at least as important as those correcting the results. He then will find a way to structure his practice around these principles, rather than making them merely adjuncts to conventional treatment.

Explaining the Program to the Patient

An effective personal dental health system must begin with communication of concepts about dental disease and its control during the initial examination and consultation. If the patient has an avowed interest in keeping his teeth indefinitely, it must be made clear that this objective can be achieved *only if dental disease can be stopped in his mouth.* This will require a high level of personal involvement. The patient must understand that his indispensible role in the treatment is to perform effective daily care of his mouth. Although merely changing the practice of

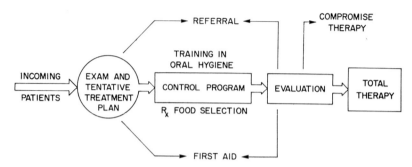

Figure 4-36. A diagram of an effective pattern of practice. Philosophically, the patient is best served by traveling along the broad horizontal line from examination to total therapy.

oral hygiene sounds insignificant, behavior modification is a complex process.

The patient should be told how the various treatment phases will be conducted as shown in the diagram of practice. There are several advantages to such a practice outline.

1. The patient is made aware of the importance the dentist places on personal dental care as it relates to the total therapy.
2. Introducing reparative therapy too hastily may destroy the patient's opportunity to experience initial signs of improvement resulting from his own efforts.
3. The total therapeutic outline is identified as being largely dependent upon effective *personal dental care*. The patient needs this understanding to identify clearly the difference between his role and that of the dentist.

This type of emphasis has given rise to the axiom that *corrective dental treatment by the dentist cannot substitute effectively for personal dental care by the patient.*

If the patient's past dental experiences have largely consisted of reparative services, this new approach may bring a variety of reactions. These will range from an occasional rejection to doubtful hesitancy by many "spoiled" patients, to enthusiastic acceptance by mature individuals who express wonder that this approach to dental care has not been presented to them before.

The dentist knows that most patients have good intentions but often have poor dental habits, and these habits are not easily changed. The varying initial reaction of patients to the program, therefore, often is not completely indicative of future personal performance. It does help to separate those crisis-oriented patients, who only want to continue bringing their "sick mouth" to the dentist for repair, from those patients who are truly interested in preserving their dentition for a lifetime and are

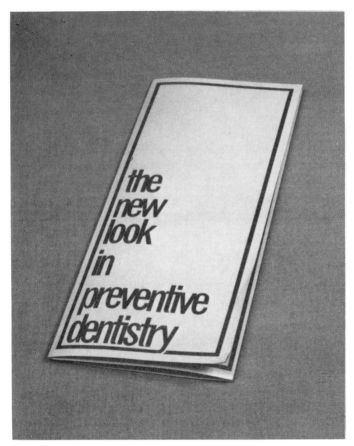

Figure 4-37. Many practitioners prefer to provide written information that outlines their concept of dental care to orient the patient and welcome him to the office. Such a pamphlet can be used to define the responsibility of both the dentist and the patient.

willing to become personally involved. The dentist is better able to make final treatment recommendations for a mouth extensively involved in disease after he has viewed the patient's performance in the personal dental care program. Such observations can eliminate much speculation as to future success.

If a choice has to be made, the allotted time of the initial visit can be utilized best by explaining to the patient basic dental problems and the concepts that will serve as guides in their solutions. There can be time later for more comprehensive examination and discussion of the details of professional care with the patient. The dental disease control program is described as usually having three essential parts:

1. THE INTRODUCTION. Initial information and technique training are provided. The objective is to reach a level of accomplishment acceptable to both the standards of the dentist and the requirements of the patient's problems before proceeding with corrective dental treatment. This training period may vary from three to eight weeks, depending upon the complexity of the situation.

2. MODIFICATION. Alteration and reinforcement of the oral hygiene techniques and practices is usually necessary during reparative treatment and before dismissal. These changes become necessary due to altered anatomic conditions and relapses in a patient's hygiene skills and habits.

3. CONTINUOUS MAINTENANCE. The patient is entitled to know that a continuous specified dental hygiene system will be necessary throughout life if dental health is to be maintained. Personal dental care should be augmented by interval examination and care by the dentist or his auxiliary.

A summary of these points needs to be covered at the initial consultation.

1. The concept of personal dental care training.
2. The order of procedure of this program and the personal involvement which it requires, relating this to the patient's stated objectives for his dental future.
3. The cost of this initial phase based on a predicted number of visits and concomitant response.

4. If certain concepts are to be relayed through use of audio-visuals, written materials, etc., the patient should be fore-warned. If a dental auxiliary will act as a dental health educator, the role of the auxiliary should be explained and, if possible, the auxiliary should be introduced to the patient.

5. Reinforcers can be used, such as samples of the patient's plaque viewed under the phase contrast microscope, or written material such as a reprint from the literature, or a pamphlet prepared by the dentist himself.

UTILIZING A DENTAL HEALTH EDUCATOR

In the authors' opinion, once the dental therapist is convinced that personal dental care training must be an integral part of therapy, he faces a fundamental fact: he cannot continue indefinitely to conduct this program personally for reasons of both time and economics. He must expand his system of delivery to include an auxiliary, who functions as an extension of the dentist. The experience of many dentists seems to establish the validity of this principle. The authors have found that the dental auxiliary who becomes a dental health educator (DHE) can be effective, efficient, and an economic asset to both patient and dentist.[21] However, some dentists find it difficult to initiate this step.

Certain criteria help to make this system workable:

1. A qualified person must be chosen and trained to do the job.

2. The *dentist* must introduce the patient to the rationale and the conduct of the dental disease control program.

3. The *dentist must transfer his authority* in dental health education to the DHE in a fashion acceptable to the patient. (Personal introduction is always best.) The patient should be told that although the dentist may not conduct the training at each visit, he is kept informed of the progress and can alter the prescription as needed.

4. The patient should be assured that the health education program is not *prefabricated*, but rather that it is specifically *prescribed* for his needs and may not be precisely what oth-

er patients are taught. The DHE, then, is helping to fill the prescription ordered by the dentist.

The Equipment and Facilities for Dental Health Education

Presuming the dentist can find and train a person to be a dental health educator, the next step is the procurement of the necessary equipment and facilities for the personal dental care training program.

It is ideal to have a room designed for dental health education. The room does not have to be a full size operatory, but it should contain all necessary equipment and supplies. The learning environment can be enhanced by surrounding the patient with posters and reinforcing messages which relate to the procedure and concepts being taught. It may be helpful to simulate

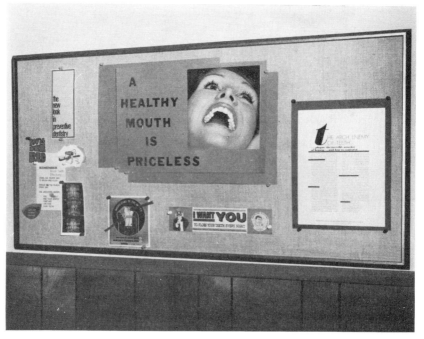

Figure 4-38. Example of creating a learning environment in the room used for training. The bulletin board can be changed periodically to add interest items as well as bits of information to reinforce the training program.

a bathroom scene—a cabinet, lavatory and lighted mirror. This way patients can be instructed in a setting similar to what they will use at home. (Actually, personal dental care techniques, except the use of toothpaste and irrigation, can be performed other than in a bathroom situation.)

If an audiovisual projector is used, it should be simple to operate and should preferably have an automatic cut-off. The phase contrast microscope can be a valuable adjunct in patient education and training. The dentist will also find it useful in diagnosis to interpret the samples and relate them to the disease state.

If a treatment room has to be used for several purposes, a mobile cart or cabinet can be used to carry all the necessary items for the personal dental care training. Then any operatory can be used for the program. This has some disadvantages, but space problems are commonly encountered and do not justify denying patients these services. *If a dentist wants his patients trained in personal dental care, he will find a way to overcome every obstacle.*

Pattern for a Typical Dental Health Education Program

As previously stated, the dental disease control program is divided into three main phases: introduction, modification, and continuous maintenance.

The DHE plays the most prominent role in the introductive phase; however, at times he or she can be helpful in altering or reinforcing patients' skills and habits. Patients on a continuous recall program sometimes can be served better by short interval visits with the DHE to receive help in hygiene skills than by "regular" four to six-month visits for scaling and polishing. The dentist must determine the need of the individual patient and order the prescription accordingly.

Outline of the Introductory Phase

As previously stated, the dentist must prepare the patient to accept an organized system of personal dental care which is taught in the office by the DHE, according to prescription by the dentist. A typical introductory prescription for training a patient with *moderate to advanced periodontal disease is as follows:*

Training Visit One

The patient views an elementary film illustrating the living plaque and its effect on dental tissues. Before the viewing, the patient is told what points to watch for and why he will benefit from watching the film. These points are then discussed with him at the end of the film.

The patient is shown how disclosing dye can be used to reveal the adherent plaque on the teeth. There is a demonstration of the use of an intraoral and extraoral mirror and light system to reveal the plaque in its various hiding places. This is a very important step; as much time as necessary should be allotted so the patient can reach a high level of accomplishment. The more proficient the patient is at detection of plaque, the less dependent he becomes on interval care by the dentist.

Use of a polished-end bristle brush is taught by the DHE, first brushing a large-scale model. He explains brush position, grip, the rhythm of the stroke, and points of brushing emphasis. The patient brushes the model, and the technique is critiqued before he begins in the mouth. He then brushes in the mouth, and a critique is given. The lighted mirror is used to reveal any remaining plaque. This helps to demonstrate that the brush has some definite limitations.

The patient is dismissed after the DHE summarizes what has been accomplished at this visit, the concepts learned, and the techniques that were taught. Giving the patient illustrations of the techniques to take home can help reinforce this skill.

Training Visit Two *(approximately three to seven days later)*

Disclosing dye is used. The mouth is viewed in the lighted mirror and checked by both the DHE and the patient. Brushing technique is demonstrated by patient and altered as necessary by the DHE.

The areas of residual plaque are pointed out as being outside

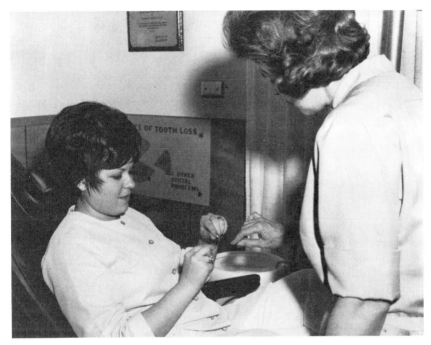

Figure 4-39. The dental health educator demonstrates floss grip and action before allowing the patient to mimic the example. The patient then has formed mental images before having sensate experience.

the domain of the brush. Dental floss use is explained and techniques for manipulating the floss are demonstrated first on the model and then in the mouth; the techniques are adjusted according to individual needs. If other interproximal cleaners are indicated, these can be introduced. Again, when the patient leaves, illustrations of the floss technique can be helpful as a reinforcer.

Training Visit Three *(approximately seven days later)*

Disclosing dye, lighted mirror, brushing, and flossing techniques are viewed and adjusted if necessary. Time is spent in reinforcing these skills if any technique deficiency is noted.

The dental irrigator is demonstrated (dry) on the model with just the tip being placed in proper position, and the patient is in-

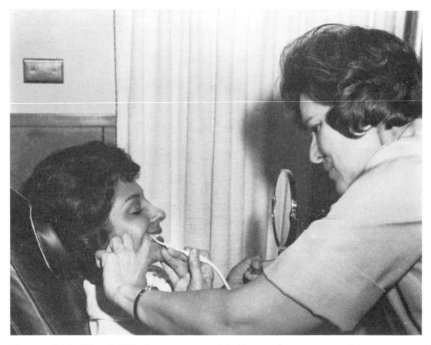

Figure 4-40. The DHE demonstrates "dry" tip placement and has the patient repeat this procedure before actually doing a "wet" demonstration.

structed in a safe, well-directed irrigation technique. The tip is placed in the patient's mouth; he is asked to proceed as though water were being used. The appliance is then hooked up to the water supply, and the patient is instructed at the lavatory. Although this is a somewhat messy process, it is a very important step in the training system.

If other auxiliary aids are indicated, they can be introduced at this appointment. Also, this is a good time to begin discussing food selection habits and fulfilling the dietary prescription.

Training Visit Four *(approximately seven days later)*

All preceding techniques are checked, and the patient is reinstructed as necessary. For example, patients often continue to rely too much on the brush and do not place enough emphasis on floss or the dental irrigator. This dependency on old habits is common and hard to alter. Any vivid examples or illustrations which will turn the patient's mind toward an expanded view of dental hygiene are in order.

Training Visit Five *(two to three weeks later)*

The DHE evaluates each technique and habit and reports the progress to the dentist. The course of action from this point de-

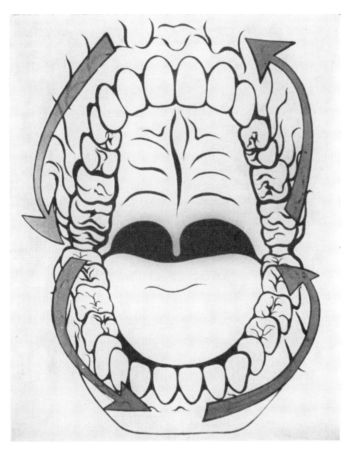

Figure 4-41. The pattern of cleaning is important. The above illustration from the *Toothkeeper* (a program of dental health education for elementary grades by Health Education Division, Den-tal-ez Mfg. Company) gives a simple set of directions. Brush around the mouth in a circle, first on the facial, then on the lingual (twice in a plaid pattern is optional) and finally on the occlusal. Then use floss and the irrigator in the same sequence. This prevents inadequate cleaning caused by skipping around in a random pattern.

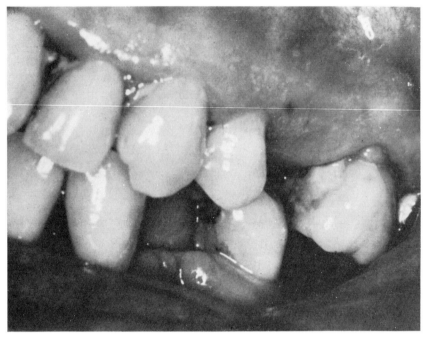

Figure 4-42a. Dental care behavior is hard to change as evidenced by the case above which demonstrates a pattern of plaque and calculus collection before treatment. (Note the exceptionally clean facial surface where patient spends all her time brushing.)

pends on the original treatment outline. (If gross, obstructive calculus deposits exist, some preliminary scaling may be undertaken after visit two or visit three to assist the hygiene techniques.) During the introductory phase, the DHE should be cautioned against unduly admonishing the patient. If a poor result continues, a direct confrontation with the patient is more effective than scolding or criticizing. The patient should be asked frankly why he thinks certain areas still remain uncleaned. If the skill is obviously satisfactory, then the fault is with inadequate or inconsistent habits. If fundamental conditions are not being met by this time, the DHE may find it helpful to ask the doctor to check the patient and offer advice on improving effectiveness.

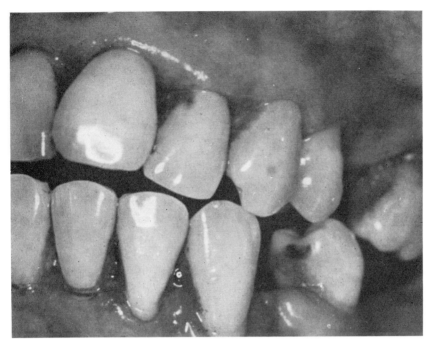

Figure 4-42b. After three months of instruction and subsequent instrumentation, the patient's visits were interrupted by a four-week absence which resulted in a relapse to her previous routine of brushing "clean spots" and not flossing regularly.

When attempting to train patients with long-standing bad hygiene practices, one should not be discouraged by initial failure to achieve a high level of personal performance. As Arnim has said, "Actually it is easy to maintain dental health throughout a lifetime; the difficult problem is to convince people that it is a worthwhile undertaking."

Modification

After the patient has met the requirements of personal care training in the introductory phase, corrective treatment can be pursued. However, corrective treatment often results in changing dental architectural form, necessitating personal care requirements different from those taught in the introduction. For

example, altered gingival margins, large open embrasures or furcations, and stationary bridges usually require modification of
brushing and flossing. As soon as possible after making the alterations, the dentist should "customize" appropriate hygiene
techniques to prevent the ill effects of "lag time."

Maintenance—The Real Test

When the patient has been trained in personal dental care and
has received the necessary corrective therapy, he should be ready
for release from active treatment. The problem now is maintaining dental health and the results of professional care. No
dental care system can control all etiologic contingencies. But the
patient who follows the described system should expect *to increase
the probability of keeping his teeth for a lifetime.*[22] However,
every therapist is well acquainted with the meaning of this axiom: "In spite of impending rewards, patients tend to relapse to
the comfort of old habits rather than accept the discipline of
the new." Regular checking of patient oral hygiene status and
reinforcement of the acquired oral hygiene techniques is a necessary element in the patient's total therapy. One should never
feel complacent about dental health. The threat of dental disease will remain as long as the teeth remain. The team approach
with both patient and dentist interacting and playing their respective roles is the modern answer to the management of dental disease. Neither can be successful alone because "dental
health, like success, is not a destination, but a continuous jour-
ney."

REFERENCES

1. S. S. Arnim, "Thoughts Concerning Cause, Pathogenesis, Treatment
   and Prevention of Periodontal Disease," *J Periodontol,* 29:217,
   1958.
2. S. S. Arnim, "Microcosms of the Human Mouth," *J Tenn Dent Assoc,*
   39:3, 1959.
3. S. S. Arnim, "The Use of Disclosing Agents for Measuring Tooth Cleanliness," *J Periodontol,* 34:227, 1963.
4. S. S. Arnim, C. C. Diericks, and E. S. Pearson, Jr., "What You Need to
   Know and Do to Prevent Dental Caries and Periodontal Disease,"
   J N Car Dent Soc, 46:296, 1963.

5. C. C. Bass, "The Optimum Characteristics of Toothbrushes for Personal Oral Hygiene," *Dent Items of Int*, 70:696, 1948.
6. C. C. Bass, "The Optimum Characteristics of Dental Floss for Personal Oral Hygiene," p. 921.
7. C. C. Bass, "The Necessary Personal Hygiene for Prevention of Caries and Periodontoclasia," *J La Med Soc, 101*:52, 1948.
8. C. C. Bass, "An Effective Method of Personal Oral Hygiene," *J La Med Soc, 106*:100, 1954.
9. L. S. Parmly, *A Practical Guide to Management of the Teeth Comprising a Discovery of the Origin for Decay of the Teeth with its Prevention and Cure* (Philadelphia, Collins and Croft, 1819).
10. S. W. Merritt, *Periodontal Diseases, Diagnosis and Treatment* (New York, Macmillan, 1933).
11. T. B. Hartzell, "Important Factors in the Etiology and Control of Periodontoclasia," *JADA, 14*:899, 1927.
12. D. H. Masters, "Oral Hygiene Procedures for the Periodontal Patient," *Dent Clin N Am, 13*:3, 1969.
13. P. R. Stillman, "Physical Culture for the Gums," *Dent Cosmos, 56*:1042, 1924.
14. W. J. Charters, "The Ideal Method of Brushing the Teeth and Standardizing the Toothbrush," *JADA, 7*:155, 1919.
15. A. C. Fones, "Instructions for Home Care of the Teeth," *Dent Items of Int, 37*:365, 1915.
16. J. Smith, T. W. O'Connor, and W. Radentz, "Oral Hygiene of the Interdental Area," *Periodontics, 1*:204, 1963.
17. W. J. Killoy, *The Quality, Nature and Time Required for Recurrence of the Microbial Mass Irrigated from the Periodontal Pocket*, master's thesis (University of Texas, June 1968).
18. C. F. Sumner, III and P. J. Crumley, "Effectiveness of a Water Pressure Cleaning Device," *Periodontics, 3*:193, 1965.
19. H. M. Goldman and D. W. Cohen, *Periodontal Therapy*, 4th ed. (St. Louis, Mosby, 1968).
20. J. F. Prichard, *Advanced Periodontal Disease* (Philadelphia, Saunders, 1972).
21. D. H. Masters, "The Utilization of the Dental Health Educator in Private Practice," *J Tenn Dent Assoc, 52*:4, 1972.
22. Richard I. Evans, Lectures, Preventive Dentistry Course, Dental Science Div., School of Aerospace Medicine, Brooks AFB, Texas, 1970-1976.

RELATIONSHIP OF ORAL HYGIENE TO PERIODONTAL STATUS

5

INTERACTION OF NUTRITIONAL FACTORS IN ORAL HYGIENE AND ORAL HEALTH

Hyman J. V. Goldberg

THE INTAKE of the right kinds of food is vital to individual health and performance. An individual's diet serves several purposes: (1) It provides material for the building and maintenance of body tissues; (2) it furnishes fuel for energy; and (3) it supplies substances that serve to regulate body processes.[1] While one particular food may fulfill all these functions or only one function, all three functions must be supported by the diet in order to maintain health.

Nutrients are those chemical substances found in foods which fulfill our bodily needs. Six are necessary for adequate functioning: carbohydrates, proteins, fats, vitamins, minerals, and water.[2] Carbohydrates, fats, and protein are energy nutrients and can be used interchangeably to supply energy for work and heat, depending on which is most plentiful in the diet.[3] Protein, minerals, and water are used in the composition and maintenance of body tissues. Vitamins are present in foods in only minute quantities, but they are important in regulating body processes. Both minerals and vitamins serve as regulators by promoting oxidative processes, nerve and muscle functioning, and tissue vitality.

145

Water also serves in a regulatory capacity as it holds substances in solution in the digestive juices, blood, and tissues, and it helps regulate body temperature, excretion, and circulation.

Nutritional status can be considered as a cellular condition since it is at the cellular level that nutrients are required.[4] Obtaining, selecting, digesting, and absorbing food are all preliminary stages leading to cellular activity. The cells comprising various tissues differ in structure and composition, depending on the kind of tissue. There is also a difference in the kinds and rates of chemical reactions which take place in the various types of cells. These different cells, with specialized structure and function, have varying nutrient requirements. For example, bone cells require large amounts of calcium and phosphorus, while red blood cells need iron. Each variety of cell must maintain its own specific relationship to its environment and source of nutrients, the extracellular fluid.

Throughout life, every individual continues to need the six basic nutrients for optimal health and body functioning, although the specific amounts needed may vary with age. Nutritional illness knows no boundaries. While people are uncomfortably familiar with the bloated bellies and gaunt faces of the Biafran children, their own children may be regularly consuming empty calories. Their grandparents, living alone and finding it difficult both to cook and chew good foods, may be subsisting on a diet of cream pies and coffee. The underprivileged poor, meanwhile, often consume low-cost foods which are filling but lack nutritional value. Malnutrition is, perhaps, most unfortunate when it occurs during the prenatal or postnatal period in individual development. The damaging effects of malnutrition at this point are permanent since cells need nutrients for the development process itself. If undernourished during the critical fetal or early infancy years, a child's growth will remain stunted, and he can suffer deficient mental development as well.

Nutritional deficiencies are currently regarded as metabolic problems resulting from a lower than desirable availability of several nutrients whose functions are interrelated.[5] Rather than concentrating on the acute lack of specific nutrients, which can cause such diseases as scurvy or rickets, nutritionists presently consider nutritional deficiencies as an expression of several nutrient inadequacies. One particular nutrient cannot be utilized efficiently without adequate supplies of the other essential nutrients. For example, protein functions interdependently with riboflavin. An oral manifestation of angular cheilosis, which is usually related to riboflavin deficiency, will not improve when only riboflavin supplements are given if the patient is also deficient in protein. Both adequate protein intake and riboflavin are necessary to eliminate the angular cheilosis.

However, each nutrient, if sufficiently deficient, can also produce bodily manifestations.[6] Because each nutrient has a primary function, its deficiency can be characterized as occurring in specific areas. Thus, vitamin B complex deficiencies are associated with disorders of the oral mucous membranes and vitamin C deficiencies with vascular integrity.

Malnutrition may be caused by a dietary inadequacy in the case of a primary nutritional deficiency; or it may result from a systemic disorder or secondary nutritional deficiency which inhibits digestion, ingestion, absorption, transportation, or utilization of nutrients.[7] Malnutrition may also be caused by a combination of both primary and secondary nutritional deficiencies. Primary deficiencies appear when the diet fails to provide essential nutrients. Several factors may enter into this condition: (1) lack of knowledge of what comprises an adequate diet, (2) fad diets, (3) poor eating habits, (4) unavailability of good food, (5) poverty, (6) improper facilities to prepare food, (7) lack of desire to eat, (8) emotional or cultural prejudices making some good foods unacceptable, and (9) physical handicaps such as blindness.

Secondary deficiencies occur after food has been eaten and the body is not able to metabolize the essential nutrients. Conditioning factors that may result in secondary nutritional deficiencies include: (1) interference with food intake as occurs with anorexia, fever, infection, nausea, allergy, neurologic disorders, or poor dentition; (2) interference with digestion such as pancreatic insufficiency, which can cause deficiencies of calcium, fat-soluble vitamins, calories, or protein; (3) interference with absorption as occurs with diarrhea, celiac disease, or liver and gall bladder diseases; (4) interference with utilization of nutrients such as diabetes or alcoholism; (5) increases in nutritional requirements as caused by pregnancy, fever, growth, or physical exercise; and (6) excessive excretion as caused by sweating, dehydration, or Addison's disease.

When primary nutritional deficiencies are combined with systemic factors that interfere with nutrient utilization, a sequence of bodily events can occur which leads to eventual cell and tissue death.[8] The speed with which a deficiency syndrome develops and becomes manifest depends on (1) the relative severity of the dietary inadequacy, (2) the amount of nutrient stored in the body, and (3) the body's capacity to adapt to lower intakes of a nutrient.[9]

A deficiency begins by gradual depletion of tissue reserves of nutrients.[10] Researchers have biochemically measured this process by determining nutrient levels in a subject's blood, urine, or tissues. Reduced enzyme activity follows progressive tissue depletion of the nutrient. Physiological or functional disturbances then appear; these are reversible when the deficiency is treated. If the nutritional deficiency continues over a long period, anatomical lesions appear. At this point, cells are dying, and tissue has begun to break down. This damage is irreversible unless the dead cells are replaced with new cells.

Researchers are less informed about the progress of nutritional disease produced by an excess of calories or other nutrients.[11] It is believed that a stepwise progression also occurs, with body stores building up high nutrient levels, then the development of biochemical lesions, and, finally, the impairment of physiological function and/or the appearance of clinical signs and symptoms. Researchers are just beginning to discover methods to assess relative oversupplies of nutrients.

Related to this discussion is the effect of nutrition on infection. While adequate diets do not prevent infection, nutritional status has been shown consistently to affect the outcome.[12] Nutrition must be adequate to maintain the skin and internal membranes that are the first barriers to invading microorganisms. Also, nutrients are needed for the formation of antibodies. When an infection is established, those individuals who are well-nourished are more likely to survive the onset than those who are weakened by nutritional deficiencies or whose bodily nutrient reserves are not sufficient to support them during illness. For example, the individuals living in the tropics often have worm populations in the intestine but are able to cope with this condition as long as their diet remains adequate. However, when nutritional status declines or if an individual becomes stressed, the disease will manifest itself.

Infection can also condition nutritional deficiency.[13] Children with deficient diets may develop cases of marasmus or kwashiorkor as a result of contracting an ordinary childhood disease such as measles. Their bodily nutrient reserves are so depleted that they cannot tolerate any additional loss caused by a fever or nausea. Such children may die of malnutrition consequent to the infection.

Assessing a patient's nutritional status is usually accomplished by checking for common complaints, obtaining a medical and social history, obtaining and evaluating a dietary history, conducting a physical examination, and making various laboratory tests.[14] Of particular importance in the physical examination are oral manifestations of nutritional deficiencies.

ORAL MANIFESTATIONS OF NUTRITIONAL DEFICIENCIES

Color changes in the oral mucous membranes mirror systemic changes.[15] The redness or pallor of the membranes can be interpreted as the result of increased or decreased vascularity and/or increased or decreased keratinization of the overlying epithelium. The lips can signal angular cheilosis, a fairly common lesion with either a nutritional or nonnutritional etiology. Pallor of the labial commissures is the first symptom. This is followed by fissuring, ulceration, and bleeding. The lesions often have a crusty yellow appearance due to secondary bacterial infection, and there may be a sharp red line along the lip closure plus increased vertical fissuring. This disease has usually been associated with riboflavin deficiency, but it may also be related to deficiencies in iron, niacin, B_6, B_{12}, or folic acid.

Color changes and topographic differences in the dorsum, apex, and lateral margins of the tongue are also clinical evidence of nutritional deficiencies.[16] Color changes can range from pallor to strawberry red, dark red, or magenta. The tongue surface may be smooth, pebbled, furrowed, or hairy. In niacin deficiency or anemias, the filiform papillae, which are small and scattered over the dorsum and margin of the apical two thirds of the tongue, hypertrophy. They then atrophy and disappear, giving the tongue a smooth appearance. The fungiform papillae, located above the general epithelial surface of the tongue, are scattered over the dorsum and apex of the tongue and are generally large and deep red. With riboflavin deficiency these papillae hypertrophy, giving the tongue a granular, pebbly appearance. Sometimes the papillae turn a purplish color. If the deficiency continues, the fungiform flatten, fuse, and atrophy.

In pellagra, the tongue appears swollen, and the pressure of the teeth against the anterior and lateral margins produces indentations and a beefy, red color.[17] Tongue changes progress rapidly in this deficiency, and the tongue becomes dry, smooth, shiny, and atrophic.

Alterations in gingival health can also signal several vitamin deficiencies.[18] Scurvy is commonly associated with red, spongy, swollen interdental papillae and the hypertrophy of marginal gingiva. Usually, the local irritating effects of calculus and bacterial infection give rise to inflammatory changes with ascorbic acid deficiency functioning as the conditioning factor. A deficiency in B complex vitamins, especially niacin deficiency, can lower gingival resistance so the gingiva are secondarily infected with Vincent's disease. Gingival inflammation also frequently occurs in cases of pellegra.

Buccal and palatal mucosa may evidence hypochromic anemia with pallor and vesicular eruptions.[19] The mucosa can also appear red and swollen, with sensitivity to touch, as a result of the hyperemia associated with B complex deficiencies.

NUTRITION AND ORAL HEALTH

The above examples of oral manifestations of various nutritional deficiencies demonstrate the link between nutrition and oral health. In summary, good nutrition influences the development and maintenance of healthy, sound teeth and gum structures; healthy dental structures contribute to an individual's ability to consume an adequate diet.[20] Nutritionists early established that nutritional deficiencies influence the integrity of the tissues responsible for tooth development. Studies with experimental animals and humans have demonstrated that nutritional status during the period of tooth formation can affect the chemical composition and size of the teeth, the shape of cusps and fissures, the time of tooth eruption, and the susceptibility of the teeth to decay.

Nutrition is also related to oral health through dietary interactions at the surfaces of erupted teeth and the gingival margins.[21] Thus, food composition and dietary patterns contribute to creating the oral environment in which microbial agents live and function.

The choice and consumption of food are closely related to both dental caries and periodontal disease.[22] Each of these diseases has a complex etiology with interrelationships along the following parameters: (1) the agent, such as dental plaque; (2) the proneness of the host, such as the tooth and its supporting structures, to disease; and (3) the oral environment around the teeth and supporting structures, such as saliva. The proneness of the teeth and supporting structures to disease depends to varying degrees upon the sufficiency of an individual's diet to encourage adequate development and maintenance of these structures. The relationship of nutrition to oral destructive processes is of particular importance due to the nature of the dental tissues affected by caries and periodontal disease.[23] The accellular enamel and dentin of erupted teeth have no reparative ability, and the periodontal tissues have only limited ability to regenerate when the disease process has been halted.

The effect of severe and prolonged nutritional deficiencies

upon the development and maintenance of oral tissues is similar to the effect upon related tissues elsewhere in the body.[24] However, oral tissues may reflect nutritional deficiencies sooner because they are exposed to greater mechanical, chemical, and thermal stresses during chewing and swallowing.

NUTRITION AND PERIODONTAL DISEASE

As the specific relationship between nutrition and dental caries will be fully treated in a future chapter, this chapter will concentrate on defining the relationship between nutrition and periodontal disease, a much more elusive topic. Periodontal disease is a multifactorial disease.[25] Unlike the metabolically inert tooth, the periodontal tissues experience active interchange with the vascular nutrient supply and are more readily affected by systemic factors and old age.[26] The disease is predominantly inflammatory in origin.[27] This response is mostly caused by local irritating factors such as dental plaque. Other local irritants which can contribute to initiating periodontal disease are calculus, materia alba, food impaction, occlusal disharmonies, faulty restorations, and mechanical, chemical, and thermal extremes. Systemic factors such as age, nutrition, hormonal imbalances, and emotional or medical disabilities may also influence the inflammatory response to a lesser degree.

The pathogenesis of periodontal disease begins with local irritants which produce gingivitis.[28] If the gingivitis remains untreated, infection and toxins develop. These invade the supporting periodontal tissues which may have a lowered resistance. The products of inflammation in combination with lytic enzymes destroy the periodontal ligament and supporting bone, and the bone and connective tissue are replaced by inflammatory tissue. The tooth then becomes loose and detached from the bone as the bone is resorbed.

Effect of Food Consistency on Periodontal Disease

A soft diet tends to produce more bacterial plaque and, thus, contributes more to initiation of gingivitis than does a coarse diet.[29] In experimental animals, a soft diet has led to gingival inflammation with associated consequences such as downgrowth of the epithelial attachment and resorption of the crestal bone.[30-39] Krasse and Brille[35] observed that animals fed a soft, sticky diet produced plaque consisting of spirochetes and fusiform bacilli, but the animals had less plaque and a different kind of flora when fed a diet of firm consistency. Stahl and coworkers[40] evaluated histologically the periodontal health of rats on diets of dry whole milk, liquid whole milk, or diet pellets. Rats on the pellet diet evidenced extensive wear of teeth and food impaction, while those on the liquid diet exhibited little tooth wear or significant impaction. The powder-fed rats evidenced some impaction of soft debris but had less gingival inflammation than the pellet-fed animals.

Firm foods such as raw fruits and vegetables can benefit the gingiva by providing limited cleansing action and minimizing accumulation of food debris.[41] Such foods also improve gingival circulation as they increase the exchange of nutrients between blood and tissues.[31, 42] A firm diet that produces frictional rubbing on the gingiva will increase the degree of keratinization of the stratified squamous epithelium.[43] This hornified layer of epithelium provides protection against chemical and bacterial irritants which can cause inflammation.[44, 45] Also, firm foods may help maintain a balance between bone resorption and new bone formation; frequent consumption of soft foods leads to underutilization of the masticatory function and can produce atrophic bone changes.[46]

The mastication necessitated by foods of firm consistency also affects the periodontal ligament.[47] The mechanical action of chewing results in compression and expansion of the periodontal spaces around teeth. This stimulates the removal of waste products and introduction of nutrients into the periodontium. Evidence indicates firm foods aid the formation of a fibrous suspensory structure in the periodontal ligament by increasing circulation and fibroplastic activity.[48] A direct correlation between width of the periodontal ligament and the intensity of mastication has also been established.[49]

Systemic Effects of Nutrition on Periodontal Disease

The influence of nutrition on the development of periodontal disease is not yet well defined. Some investigators believe nutritional deficiencies affect the rate and severity of the disease rather than its initiation.[2, 27, 40, 50, 51] After reviewing many human epidemiological surveys relating to periodontal disease and malnutrition, Stahl concluded that periodontal disease is not a manifestation of a specific nutritional deficiency, but the process of deterioration may be hastened by nutritional deficiency or depletion in combination with other factors.[52] Nizel describes nutritional deficiencies as "secondary contributors or modifiers of the disease."[53] However, Mayer stresses that a number of nutrients, if absent from the diet or present in excess, can affect the onset and course of periodontal disease.[54] These nutrients will be reviewed below.

Carbohydrates

The role of carbohydrates in periodontal disease is related to the ability of soft carbohydrate foods and simple sugars to cling to tooth surfaces, increasing plaque formation and promoting dental decay. Because carbohydrates (granular sucrose mixed in a soft diet) have been found to be retained around rat molars, researchers concluded this nutrient could also be influential in the etiology of periodontal disease.[55] This observation has been confirmed by other investigators.[34, 56] In humans, the amount and/or composition of dental plaque can be changed by varying the amount of dietary sucrose.[57] Patients who eat diets higher in sucrose tend to demonstrate a higher plaque formation rate and greater plaque accumulation.[58, 59]

Protein

Protein-calorie deficiency can cause an increase in cornified cells among the buccal mucosal cells, but this may also result from infection and aging.[60] A deficiency in protein may reduce resistance to antibody production, toxins, leukocyte activity, and adrenocortical function. Hormonal activities in the endocrine system also need protein; their malfunctioning can adversely affect periodontal tissues. In addition, the body needs protein and vitamin D for effective metabolism of calcium, phosphorus, and magnesium.

Animal studies have illustrated that the periodontal tissues are more susceptible to inflammation and degeneration due to a local irritant if protein deficiency exists.[61] Protein deficiency has also been shown to slow the rate of wound healing and to retard repair of local tissue irritation.[62] Another investigation found high protein feedings reduced alveolar bone loss in mice.[63]

The literature provides many documented studies of humans experiencing protein deprivation. In a comparison of 100 healthy children and 100 children with kwashiorkor in Banglor, South India, researchers found the children with kwashiorkor had more cases of acute necrotizing gingivitis and significantly higher periodontal disease index scores.[64] Studies of Nigerians on protein-deficient diets indicate these people suffer severe periodontal disease; the acute necrotizing gingivitis often develops into acute oral necrosis in malnourished African children.[65–67] Malberger[67] has suggested a sequential relationship between systemic stresses, such as generalized infectious disease, and the occurrence of acute oral necrosis. The common state of malnutrition may also be somewhat responsible for the low resistance to disease evidenced by Gambian children, 50 percent of whom die before they are five years old.[68]

In a short-term study, protein versus placebo supplementation upon gingivitis was tested on forty-four dental students over a four-day period. Significant reduction in gingivitis occurred only in the group treated with protein. The researchers further observed that combining prophylaxis procedures with protein supplementation most improved host resistance. The effects of protein supplementation were also observed on tooth mobility. Researchers reported a decrease in tooth mobility when patients with periodontal disease were given diets supplemented by protein.[70] Investigators have claimed a twenty-one-day period of protein supplementation was responsible for decreased gingival inflammation but did not affect sulcus depth.[71]

Findings concerning the benefits of protein supplementation conflict, however. In one study, blood serum and parotid fluid was collected from 508 healthy males and analyzed for uric acid and protein content.[72] The subjects were divided into four periodontal index groups, and the researchers could find no significant differences between the groups in the rate of parotid gland function or in any chemical variables.

Ascorbic Acid

Most research relating nutritional deficiency to periodontal disease has dealt with the effect of ascorbic acid. Ever since it was discovered that vitamin C affected the gingiva (scorbutic gingivitis), many dentists have prescribed the vitamin for treatment of bleeding gingival margins, inflamed periodontal tissues, and loose teeth.[73] This practice seemed justified since researchers found vitamin C deficiency retards gingival healing, weakens the walls of small blood vessels, and reduces collagen formation, leading to increased tooth mobility and loss. To this evidence was added the fact that humans cannot synthesize their own vitamin C, while most animals, who generally experience a low incidence of periodontal disease, are able to synthesize the vitamin. However, there are now two schools of thought regarding the use of ascorbic acid supplementation.

As early as 1933, Hanke et al.[74] reported that gingivitis in children could be improved with daily intake of orange and lemon juice. If the juice intake was stopped, gingivitis recurred. Blockley and Barzinger[75] advocated ascorbic acid supplementation because they found no local treatment could eliminate inflammation in patients with low vitamin C levels until ascorbic acid therapy was added. Carvel and Halperin[76] gave gingivitis patients ascorbic acid and bioflavinoid supplements and found gingivitis bleeding stopped within two weeks of beginning supplementation. Another group[77] noted reduction in gingivitis in individuals receiving periodontal treatment and systemic therapy, consisting of vitamin C supplements with and without bioflavinoids. These same investigators[78] also reported reduction of sulcus depth after dietary supplements of vitamin C were combined with local periodontal treatment.

Other studies have related tooth mobility to vitamin C fluctuations. One study[79] established significant positive correlations between the lingual vitamin C tests and tooth mobility; with longer lingual tests, the vitamin C state was poorer and the tooth mobility was greater. Similar reduction in tooth mobility was reported after massive vitamin C supplements over a two-week period.[80]

Despite these positive findings, other investigators could establish only a marginal role for vitamin C in periodontal disease. "No one has ever demonstrated a relationship between levels of the vitamin and periodontal disease."[81] This area clearly calls for more investigation. In one study,[82] chronically ill mental patients, with low serum ascorbic acid and high incidence of gingivitis and bleeding from the gingival crevice, were given daily ascorbic acid supplements for six weeks. Although their plasma ascorbic acid level increased from 0.254 to 0.81 mg per 100 mg, their gingival condition did not improve. In his self-deprivation study,[83] Crandon experienced no gingival changes during five months on a diet deficient in vitamin C. He observed only slight changes at the gingival margin after six months.

Glickman[84] has shown that local irritants such as food debris must first initiate gingival inflammation, and then vitamin C deficiency will accentuate destruction of the periodontal membrane and alveolar bone. In a subsequent study, Glickman and Dines[85] found that daily ascorbic acid supplements did not affect the ascorbic acid level of the gingival tissues. Local treatment improved the gingivitis, and the patients with gingivitis had normal blood ascorbic acid levels. In a similar study,[86] blood ascorbic acid determinations were conducted on 341 healthy males before and after administration of ascorbic acid; urine recovery rates were also calculated. The researchers concluded that periodontal status did not correlate with ascorbic acid levels.

A study conducted by Linghorne et al.[87] again emphasizes the conflicting nature of studies of this type. In examinations of

Royal Canadian Air Force personnel, the investigators concluded gingival inflammation was common in healthy young adults, and large vitamin doses of vitamin C appeared to delay the recurrence of inflammation.

Vitamin B

Several oral changes can be attributed to deficiencies in components of the vitamin B complex group: glossitis, glossodymia, and cheilosis.[91] Investigators have further attributed herpetic-like oral vesicles to lack of thiamine.[92] Riboflavin deficiency can produce loss of crest in alveolar bone, with subsequent tooth mobility. Nicotinic acid has not been definitely established as a causative agent in gingivitis or ulcerative gingivitis, but there has been a correlation in dogs between vitamin B complex deficiencies and nonspecific gingivitis and periodontal lesions.[93] It is believed, as in other nutritional deficiencies, that gingivitis is caused by a local irritant, but is subject to the modifying effect of the systemic vitamin B deficiency.[94]

Vitamin D, Calcium and Phosphorus

Vitamin D determines the effectiveness of calcium, phosphorus, and magnesium metabolism in the body.[95] A diet with a high calcium : phosphorus ratio but deficient in vitamin D resulted in defective calcification of the cementum and alveolar bone.[96]

Researchers feeding young rats an experimental diet with a calcium : phosphorus ratio of approximately 1 : 20 found their rats' alveolar bone was more porotic than their long bones, and their cementum was reduced.[97] Mature rats on the same diet did not evidence this reaction; the researchers concluded that calcium deficiency produces osteoporosis mainly in young animals.

In another study,[98] adult beagle dogs were fed a diet with a 1 : 10 calcium : phosphorus ratio over a twelve-month period. The dogs suffered alveolar bone resorption due to osteolysis, leading the researchers to conclude that a dietary low-calcium : high-phosphorus ratio produces nutritional secondary hyperparathyroidism. They also postulated that an excess of phosphorus, even with adequate calcium intake, can cause hyperphosphatemia and hypocalcemia which eventually develops into a secondary hyperparathyroidism. The increased parathyroid level supposedly causes bone resorption because the body tries to achieve an equilibrium of calcium : phosphorus ratios by raising serum calcium levels and lowering serum phosphorus levels.

Lutwak et al.[99] and Krook et al.[100, 101] also contend that the primary morphologic feature of periodontal disease in humans is accentuated osteolysis caused by dietary calcium deficiency, a phosphorus excess, or both. Other investigators using similar experimental methods could not confirm these claims.[102]

Nizel notes that there is not adequate proof of such postulations, so there is no justification for reducing phosphorus intake or supplementing the diet with calcium pills to bring patients to a 1 : 1 calcium : phosphorus level.[103]

Fluoride

The role of fluoride in strengthening tooth resistance to decay has been well documented. Studies also indicate a possible correlation between increased fluoride intake and periodontal status in adults.[104] The effect may be due to retardation of osteoporosis by fluoride. Wade[105] has reported that when high levels of experimental fluoride are injected, extensive periosteal deposition occurs at the muscle sites where osteoporosis has already formed in the bone.

The above discussion emphasizes that while a dentist may not be able to eliminate periodontal disease and gingivitis through dietary manipulations, he can ensure good oral health for his patients by encouraging them to adopt patterns of adequate nutrition. Nutrition then becomes a valuable tool in preventive efforts.

As a conclusion to this chapter, the author will briefly discuss how individuals develop their present food habits and the processes involved in trying to attain desired eating behavior changes. Both areas are complex, but some understanding of how they relate to the counseling experience is necessary if counseling is to modify destructive eating patterns.

NUTRITION AND BEHAVIOR CHANGE

Eating is one of the fundamental activities of life. Like many other human activities, eating patterns are determined by cultural factors. Every society has developed its own traditional ways of growing or collecting, preparing, serving, and eating food according to adaptations the society makes to its physical and sociocultural environment.[106] Such practices are termed "foodways"; they are part of a society's cultural heritage and are taught to each succeeding generation as are other behaviors such as ethical norms or governing principles.

Those items used as food by a group are limited by availability, but no society ever regards all the potentially edible food in its environment as food.[107] Instead, through experience, a group develops a list of culturally acceptable foods and usually singles out particular foods as the mainstays of the diet. Americans tend to regard meat as the most important food, while the Japanese hold rice as being most essential.

Environmental changes tend to result in changes in a group's foodways.[108] Failure to adapt often ends in deterioration of individual well-being and may even lead to the destruction of a society. However, adaptations may also have an adverse effect upon a society. The effect of changes on a group's welfare is determined primarily by two factors: whether the diet's nutritional quality is improved or decreased by the change, and whether the change negatively or positively influences behavior patterns which are important in maintaining a society's strength. The changes in American eating patterns over the last fifty years demonstrate the interplay of these adaption variables. Many refined grains and cereal products are now enriched for better nourishment, but less popular whole grains are still better for people, from a nutritional viewpoint. Food industry technology has made it possible for today's cooks to prepare a meal in minutes rather than hours, but it is often at the expense of many food additives, some of which have harmful bodily effects. With the proliferation of restaurants and the tendency to provide meals for students and workers near their jobs, most families eat far fewer meals together at home, leading to some deterioration in family influence.

Individual food choice behaviors are termed "food habits," characteristic and repetitive acts that an individual performs to provide himself with nourishment and to fulfill a variety of social and emotional goals.[109] These habitual food choices become a way to satisfy needs such as security, comfort, status, pleasure, and ego enhancement.

A child learns food habits as part of the socialization process.[110] By the time a child is old enough to make his own decisions about what, where, when, and how much to eat, his habits and attitudes are already shaped by past experience, and he is resistant to change. The child's family is the predominant influence on his food habits and beliefs, as parents, consciously and unconsciously, teach their children how to behave in regard to food. In early childhood, the mother or whoever plans, prepares, and serves the food is the major influence upon what the child learns to eat. Personal experience with the sight, smell, and taste of food eventually leads a person to form food preferences. However, parental likes and dislikes may also provide the basis for food preferences.

As children grow up, other influences enter their development of food habits. The media, peer group members, and increased social encounters begin to increase an individual's awareness of the many roles of food.[111] For example, adolescent conflicts may generate disruptions in established food habits by the increase in snacking or the emotional disturbance caused by poor family relationships.

Any changes in food habits are difficult to bring about since these behaviors have emotional ties.[112] Resentment often occurs with attempts to enforce change. However, voluntary changes in food habits are possible and frequently accompany changes in the environment—physical, physiological, psychological, or social —when an individual understands the personal advantages of such modifications.

Basically, the goal of a nutrition educator is to help individuals evaluate their diets in light of desirable eating patterns and help them develop new, healthy eating behaviors. In the book, *Nutrition, Behavior and Change* by Gifft, Washbon, and Harrison, five phases in the process of change are identified:[113]

1. Awareness
2. Development of a receptive framework for learning
3. Trial
4. Reinforcement
5. Adaptation.

Awareness

No behavior change will occur until an individual is aware that he has a problem and that an alternative exists to his present behavior. At this stage, the educator may be involved in describing the essentials of good nutrition and helping the individual evaluate his own behavior in terms of these standards. Many individuals at this point are receptive to guidance on how to change their behavior, although most prefer to set the actual guidelines for themselves.

DEVELOPMENT OF RECEPTIVE FRAMEWORK FOR LEARNING

If an individual is to accept change, he must believe in the desirability of that change. For example, many teenagers can be motivated to practice better oral hygiene procedures when they appreciate the improvement this will make in their appearance. In this case, the educator draws upon natural teenage self-consciousness and extreme desire for peer acceptance to provide a meaningful reason for change.

Prior perceptions of an individual may also have to be dealt with before learning and behavior change can be initiated. An individual may be able to repeat dutifully the four basic food groups but may have no appreciation of the dynamic interplay of these groups in the diet, especially if previous nutrition instruction was dull or uninspired. Another individual may demonstrate erroneous concepts of nutrition that the educator must eliminate; false ideas about the calorie value of foods are common. However, the method of correction is again vital to the receptivity of the individual. If the erroneous belief is deeply rooted, forceful denigration might produce the opposite results. Gradual erosion of the belief as new information is explored is a more successful technique for changing habits and attitudes.

Lastly, how nutritional information is communicated can significantly affect listener receptivity. Nutrition is a personal matter, and an individual trying to change eating patterns needs someone who can help him without destroying his self-image and who also can empathize with his problems and individual situation. If an educator communicates the impression that his values are superior to those of the learner, no learning leading to behavior change will transpire. Instead, when an educator is caught up in his subject, when his interest and enthusiasm and his concern for the individual's needs are apparent, communication is facilitated and a learning environment is created. The learner grows to trust the educator; he knows the educator has faith in his personal ability to learn and change.

Trial

One step in the process of behavior change is experimenting with alternatives to present behavior. Again, the educator must be sensitive to the needs and flexibility levels of his audience. The trial may be to have the individual cook a meal based on guided planning or to experiment with new foods to vary the content of his diet. Any proposed trial must be feasible for the individual involved and produce tangible results, so the learner can see evidence of his efforts to improve.

Reinforcement

In this phase of the change process, the lessons learned during the trial period are strengthened by repetition, by transfer of the learning to similar situations and by encouragement and support from the educator. During this period, the learner tests his grasp of the basic principles by applying them on an ever-broader scale. For example, when an individual learns how to apply the basic four food groups to a single meal, the next logical step would be to plan and evaluate daily and weekly food intake until correct food choices become an assimilated behavior. Again, the educator's support is essential since criticism at this point can still discourage and turn away a learner.

Adoption

Adoption of a behavioral change occurs when the new pattern has become a functional part of an individual's actions.

SUMMARY

At every stage in the process of behavioral change, the educator must be especially sensitive to the needs and messages of the learner if fruitful communication is to take place. Individuals will learn to the extent that they are motivated to do so and to the degree that they perceive the information to be gained as beneficial or useful. This necessitates the educator's attention to a learner's interests and concerns, his prior beliefs and behaviors, his potential for learning, and the feasibility for a particular individual of any planned change.

When the educator has gained acceptability and credibility from the listener, he has set the stage to involve the individual actively in the learning process. Active participation of the patient is particularly important in nutritional counseling. When an individual realizes and accepts his personal responsibility for his food intake, behavior change then becomes personally desirable and meaningful. He becomes an active agent in promoting his own oral health.

REFERENCES

1. L. J. Bogert, G. M. Briggs, and D. H. Calloway, *Nutrition and Physical Fitness* (Philadelphia, Saunders, 1973), p. 8.
2. A. E. Nizel, *Nutrition in Preventive Dentistry: Science and Practice* (Philadelphia, Saunders, 1972), p. 4.
3. Bogert, et al., *Nutrition and Physical Fitness*, p. 8.
4. H. H. Gifft, M. B. Washbon, and G. G. Harrison, *Nutrition, Behavior, and Change* (Englewood Cliffs, P-H), p. 123.
5. Nizel, *Nutrition in Preventive Dentistry*, p. 316.
6. Nizel, p. 316.
7. Nizel, p. 317.

8. Nizel, p. 318.
9. Gifft, Washbon, and Harrison, *Nutrition, Behavior, and Change,* p. 213.
10. Nizel, *Nutrition in Preventive Dentistry,* p. 318.
11. Gifft, Washbon, and Harrison, *Nutrition, Behavior, and Change,* p. 214.
12. Bogert et al., *Nutrition and Physical Fitness,* p. 522.
13. Bogert et al., p. 522.
14. Nizel, *Nutrition in Preventive Dentistry,* p. 319.
15. S. Dreizen, R. E. Stone, and F. D. Spies, "Oral Manifestations of Nutritional Disorders," *Dent Clin North Am,* p. 429, 1958.
16. Nizel, *Nutrition in Preventive Dentistry,* p. 324.
17. Nizel, p. 324.
18. Nizel, p. 325.
19. Nizel, p. 326.
20. Bogert et al., *Nutrition and Physical Fitness,* p. 493.
21. J. H. Shaw, "New Knowledge of Nutrition and Dental Health," *Med Clin North Am,* 54:1556, 1970.
22. Shaw, p. 1555.
23. Shaw, p. 1556.
24. Shaw, p. 1556.
25. Nizel, *Nutrition in Preventive Dentistry,* p. 397.
26. L. D. McBean and E. W. Speckmann, "A Review: The Importance of Nutrition in Oral Health," *JADA,* 89:111, 1974.
27. A. E. Nizel, "Nutrition and Oral Problems," *World Rev Nutr Diet,* 16: 240, 1973.
28. Nizel, *Nutrition in Preventive Dentistry,* p. 400.
29. Nizel, *Nutrition in Preventive Dentistry,* p. 401.
30. P. Baer, "The Relation of the Physical Character of the Diet to the Periodontium and Periodontal Disease," *Oral Surg,* 9:839-44, 1956.
31. P. Burwasser and T. J. Hill, "The Effect of Hard and Soft Diets on the Gingival Tissues of Dogs," *J Dent Res,* 18:389-93, 1939.
32. J. Egelberg, "Local Effect of Diet on Plaque Formation and Development of Gingivitis in Dogs," *Odontol Rev,* 16:31-41, 1965.
33. A. D. Ivy, J. F. Morgan, and S. L. Farrell, "The Effects of Total Gastrectomy," *Surg Gynecol Obstet,* 53:612-16, 1931.
34. J. Klingsberg and E. O. Butcher, "Aging, Diet and Periodontal Lesions in the Hamster," *J Dent Res,* 38:421, 1959.
35. B. Krasse and N. Brill, "Effect of Consistency of Diet on Bacteria in Gingival Pockets in Dogs," *Odontol Rev,* 11:152-64, 1960.

36. D. F. Mitchell, "Periodontal Disease in the Syrian Hamster," *JADA*, 49:177-83, 1954.

37. P. Person, "Diet Consistency and Periodontal Disease in Old Albino Rats," *J Periodontol*, 32:308-11, 1961.

38. M. P. Ruben, J. McCoy, P. Person, and D. W. Cohen, "Effects of Soft Dietary Consistency and Protein Deprivation on the Periodontium of the Dog," *Oral Surg*, 15:1061-70, 1962.

39. S. S. Stahl, S. C. Miller, and E. D. Goldsmith, "Effects of Various Diets on the Periodontal Structures of Hamsters," *J Periodontol*, 29:7-14, 1958.

40. S. S. Stahl, "Nutritional Influences on Periodontal Disease," *World Rev Nutr Diet*, 13:279, 1971.

41. I. Glickman, "Nutrition in the Prevention and Treatment of Gingival and Periodontal Disease," *J Dent Med*, 19:181, 1964.

42. R. Pelzer, "A Study of the Local Oral Effects of Diet on the Periodontal Tissues and the Gingival Capillary Structure," *JADA*, 27:13-25, 1940.

43. Nizel, *Nutrition in Preventive Dentistry*, p. 403.

44. J. T. O'Rourke, "The Relation of the Physical Character of the Diet to the Health of the Periodontal Tissues," *Am J Ortho Oral Surg* 33:687, 1947.

45. J. Weinmann, "Keratinization of the Human Oral Mucosa," *J Dent Res*, 19:57, 1940.

46. Nizel, *Nutrition in Preventive Dentistry*, p. 403.

47. Nizel, *Nutrition in Preventive Dentistry*, p. 403.

48. P. J. Brekhus, W. D. Armstrong, and W. J. Simon, "Stimulation of Muscles of Mastication," *J Dent Res*, 20:87, 1941.

49. E. D. Coolidge, "The Thickness of the Human Periodontal Membrane," *JADA*, 24:1260, 1937.

50. L. N. Peterson, "Nutritional Influence on Periodontal Disease," *J Appl Nutr*, 24:87, 1972.

51. J. D. Suomi, "Prevention and Control of Periodontal Disease," *JADA*, 83:1271, 1971.

52. Stahl, "Nutritional Influences on Periodontal Disease," p. 286.

53. Nizel, *Nutrition in Preventive Dentistry*, p. 403.

54. J. Mayer, "Diet and Periodontal Disease," *Postgrad Med*, 49:250, 1971.

55. J. H. Shaw and D. Griffiths, "Relation of Protein, Carbohydrates and Fat Intake to the Periodontal Syndrome," *J Dent Res*, 40:614, 1961.

56. D. F. Mitchell and M. Johnson, "The Nature of the Gingival Plaque in Hamsters—Production, Prevention and Removal," *J Dent Res*, 35:651, 1956.

57. Nizel, *Nutrition in Preventive Dentistry*, p. 402.

58. J. Carlsson and J. Egelberg, "Effect of Diet on Early Plaque Formation in Man," *Odontol Rev*, 16:112, 1965.

59. J. Carlsson, "Effect of Diet on Presence of Streptococcus Salivarius in Dental Plaque and Saliva," *Odontal Rev*, 16:336, 1965.

60. Mayer, "Diet and Periodontal Disease," p. 250.

61. S. S. Stahl, H. C. Sandler, and L. R. Cahn, "The Effect of Protein Deprivation Upon the Oral Tissues of the Rat and Particularly Upon Periodontal Structures under Irritation," *Oral Surg Oral Med Oral Pathol*, 8:760, 1955.

62. S. S. Stahl, "The Influence of Prolonged Low Protein Feeding on Epithelized Gingival Wounds in Adult Rats," *J Dent Res*, 45:1448, 1966.

63. P. Baer and C. L. White, "Studies on Periodontal Diseases in the Mouse. IV. The Effects of a High Protein, Low Carbohydrate Diet," *J Periodontol*, 32:328-30, 1961.

64. J. J. Pindberg, M. Bhat, and B. Roed-Petersen, "Oral Changes in South Indian Children with Severe Protein Deficiency," *J Periodontol*, 38:218-21, 1967.

65. A. Sheehan, "The Prevalence and Severity of Periodontal Disease in Rural Nigerians," *Dent Pract Dent Rec*, 17:51, 1966.

66. R. D. Enslie, "Cancrum Oris," *Dent Pract*, 13:481-94, 1963.

67. E. Mahlberger, "Acute Infectious Oral Necrosis Among Young Children in Gambia, West Africa," *J Periodont Res*, 2:154, 1967.

68. I. A. McGregor, W. Z. Billewicz, and A. M. Thompson, "Growth and Mortality in Children in an African Village," *Brit Med J*, 2:1661-66, 1961.

69. W. M. Ringsdorf and E. Cheraskin, "Periodontal Pathosis in Man. IV. Effect of Protein vs. Placebo Supplementation Upon Gingivitis," *J Dent Med*, 18:92-4, 1963.

70. E. Cheraskin, W. M. Ringsdorf, A. T. S. H. Setyaadmadia, and D. W. Ray, "An Ecologic Analysis of Tooth Mobility: Effect of Prophylaxis and Protein Supplementation," *J Periodontol*, 38:227, 1967.

71. S. F. Dachi, H. M. Bohannan, and S. R. Saxe, "The Failure of Short Term Vitamin Supplementation to Reduce Sulcus Depth," *J Periodontol*, 37:221, 1966.

72. I. L. Shannon, J. M. Terry, and H. H. Chauncey, "Uric Acid and Total Serum in Parotid Fluid in Relation to Periodontal Status," *J Dent Res*, 45:1539-40, 1966.

73. G. J. Parfitt and D. M. Speirs, "Role of Nutrition in the Prevention and Treatment of Periodontal Disease," *J Can Dent Assoc*, 6:226, 1970.

74. M. T. Hanke, M. J. Needles, C. M. Marberg, W. H. Tucker, C. L.

Ghent, J. M. Williams, and M. D. Bartholomew, "Nutritional Studies on Children. The Effect upon Gingivitis of Adding Orange and Lemon Juice to the Diet," *Dent Cosmos*, 75:570, 1933.

75. C. H. Blockley and P. E. Baenziger, "An Investigation into the Connection Between the Vitamin C Content of the Blood and Periodontal Disturbances," *Brit Dent J*, 73:57, 1942.

76. R. L. Carvel and V. Halperin, "Therapeutic Effect of Water-Soluble Bioflavinoids in Gingival Inflammatory Conditions," *Oral Surg Oral Med Oral Pathol*, 14:847, 1961.

77. G. M. El-Ashiry, W. M. Ringsdorf, and E. Cheraskin, "Local and Systemic Influences in Periodontal Disease. II. Effect of Prophylaxis and Natural Versus Synthetic Vitamin C Upon Gingivitis," *J Periodontol*, 35:250-59, 1964.

78. G. M. El-Ashiry, W. M. Ringsdorf, and E. Cheraskin, "Local and Systemic Effects in Periodontal Disease. III. Effect of Prophylaxis and Natural Versus Synthetic Vitamin C Upon Sulcus Depth," *NY J Dent*, 34:254-62, 1964.

79. E. Cheraskin, W. M. Ringsdorf, D. W. Aspray, D. Michael and D. Preskitt, "A Lingual Vitamin C Test. X. Relationship to Tooth Mobility," *Int J Vitam Res*, 38:434-37, 1968.

80. F. A. Karlson, E. Cheraskin, and J. B. Dunbar, "Subclinical Scurvy and Subclinical Tooth Mobility," *J West Soc Periodontol*, 7:6-28, 1959.

81. Parfitt and Speirs, "Role of Nutrition in the Prevention and Treatment of Periodontal Disease," p. 226.

82. G. J. Parfitt and C. D. Hand, "Reduced Plasma Ascorbic Acid Levels and Gingival Health," *J Periodontol*, 34:347, 1963.

83. H. J. Crandon, C. D. Lund, and D. E. Dill, "Experimental Human Scurvy," *New Engl J Med*, 223:353, 1940.

84. I. Glickman, "Acute Vitamin C Deficiency and Periodontal Disease. I. The Periodontal Tissues of the Guinea Pig in Acute Vitamin C Deficiency," *J Dent Res*, 27:9, 1948.

85. I. Glickman and M. M. Dines, "Effect of Increased Ascorbic Acid Blood Levels on the Ascorbic Acid Level in Treated and Non-Treated Gingiva," *J Dent Res*, 42:1152, 1963.

86. I. L. Shannon and W. A. Gibson, "Intravenous Ascorbic Acid Loading in Subjects Classified as to Periodontal Status," *J Dent Res*, 44:355-61, 1965.

87. W. J. Linghorne, W. G. McIntosh, J. W. Tice, F. F. Tisdall, J. F. McCreary, T. G. H. Drake, A. V. Greaves, and W. M. Johnston, "The Relation of Ascorbic Acid Intake to Gingivitis," *Can Med Assoc J*, 54:106-19, 1946.

88. A. L. Russell, "International Nutritional Surveys: A Summary of Preliminary Dental Findings," *J Dent Res*, 42:233, 1963.

89. H. Mellanby, "Effect of Maternal Dietary Deficiency of Vitamin A on Dental Tissues in Rats," *J Dent Res, 20:*489, 1941.
90. I. Glickman and M. Stoller, "The Periodontal Tissues of the Albino Rat in Vitamin A Deficiency," *J Dent Res, 27:*758, 1948.
91. Glickman, "Nutrition in the Prevention and Treatment of Gingival and Periodontal Disease," p. 180.
92. Mayer, "Diet and Periodontal Disease," p. 250.
93. J. D. King, and N. E. Glover, "The Relative Effects of Dietary Constituents and other Factors Upon Calculus Formation and Gingival Disease in the Ferrets," *J Pathol, 57:*353, 1945.
94. Glickman, "Nutrition in the Prevention and Treatment of Gingival and Periodontal Disease," p. 180.
95. Mayer, "Diet and Periodontal Disease," p. 250.
96. H. W. Ferguson and R. L. Hartles, "The Effect of Vitamin D on the Bones of Young Rats Receiving Diets Low in Calcium or Phosphorus," *Arch Oral Biol, 8:*407, 1963.
97. H. W. Ferguson and R. L. Hartles, "The Effects of Diets Deficient in Calcium or Phosphorus in the Presence and Absence of Supplements of Vitamin D on the Secondary Cementum and Alveolar Bone of Young Rats," *Arch Oral Biol, 9:*647, 1964.
98. P. A. Henrikson, "Periodontal Disease and Calcium Deficiency," *Acta Odontol Scand, 26* (Suppl. 50), 1968.
99. Nizel, *Nutrition in Preventive Dentistry,* p. 406.
99. L. Lutwak et al., "Calcium Deficiency and Human Periodontal Disease," *Isr J Med Sci, 7:*504, 1971.
100. L. Krook et al., "Human Periodontal Disease and Osteoporosis," *Cornell Vet, 62:*371, 1972.
101. L. Krook et al., "Human Periodontal Disease. Morphology and Response to Calcium Therapy," *Cornell Vet, 62:*32, 1972.
102. G. Svanberg et al., "Effect of Nutritional Hyperparathyroidism on Experimental Periodontis in the Dog," *Scand J. Dent Res, 81:*155, No. 2, 1973.
103. Nizel, *Nutrition in Preventive Dentistry,* p. 406.
104. Mayer, "Diet and Periodontal Disease," p. 250.
105. A. B. Wade, *Basic Periodontology,* 2nd ed. (Bristol, John Wright & Sons, 1965).
106. Gifft et al., *Nutrition, Behavior, and Change,* p. 27.
107. Gifft et al., p. 28.
108. Gifft et al., p. 29.
109. Gifft et al., p. 30.
110. Gifft et al., p. 74.
111. Gifft et al., p. 79.
112. Gifft et al., p. 30.
113. Gifft et al., p. 258.

6

MICROBIOLOGICAL BASIS FOR CHANGES IN THE PERIODONTIUM

Russell Nisengard
Robert Genco

PERIODONTAL DISEASE
Relationship of Oral Hygiene to the Periodontal Lesion

ORAL HYGIENE PROCEDURES that control microbial dental plaque and gingival crevicular debris are directly related to prevention, initiation, and treatment of inflammatory periodontal disease. In fact, oral hygiene currently affords the only practical method for prevention of periodontal disease in large populations. The absence of oral hygiene or reduced efficiency of oral hygiene allows establishment of a complex microbial flora in close approximation to gingival tissues. This microbial accumulation is thought to be responsible for the periodontal lesion. Thus, in considering relationships between oral hygiene and periodontal disease, it is necessary to understand the crevicular microorganisms, their composition, establishment in plaque, pathogenic capabilities, and modes of control. These will be reviewed in this chapter.

Epidemiologic studies including several prevalence studies and longitudinal incidence studies have revealed a positive relationship between the severity of periodontal disease and degree of oral hygiene. Greene's report[1] of the prevalence of periodontal

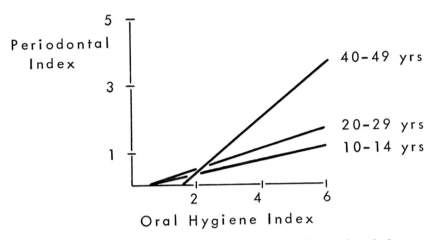

Figure 6-1. Relationship between oral hygiene and periodontal disease. Adapted from J. C. Greene, *Am J Pub Hlth,* 53:913, 1963.

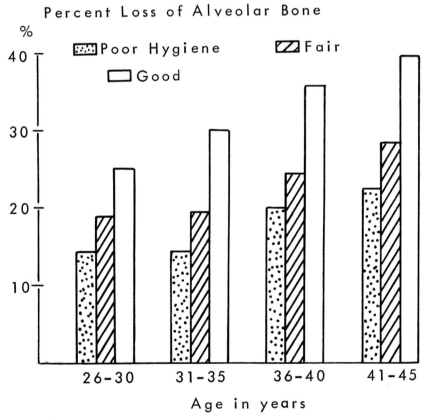

Figure 6-2. Alveolar bone loss as a function of oral hygiene. Adapted from Schei et al., *J Periodont,* 30:7, 1959.

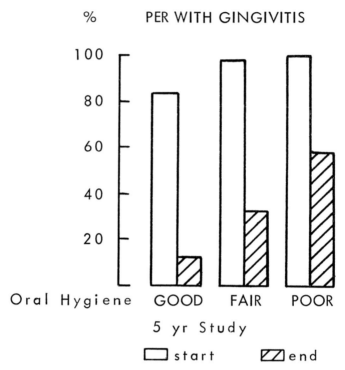

% PER WITH GINGIVITIS

Oral Hygiene   GOOD   FAIR   POOR

5 yr Study

☐ start   ▨ end

Figure 6-3. Gingivitis as a form of oral hygiene. Adapted from Loval et al., *Acta Odont Scand, 19:537,* 1961.

disease illustrates findings repeatedly demonstrated throughout the world. A combined population of 3,851 from Ecuador and Montana were examined for severity of periodontal disease using Russell's Periodontal Index[2] and for efficiency of oral hygiene using Greene's Simplified Oral Hygiene Index.[3] The results summarized in Figure 6-1 indicate a straight line relationship between severity of periodontal disease and degree of oral hygiene. The slope of this line increases with age so that for a given level of oral hygiene, there was more severe periodontal disease in older age groups. Greene has suggested this "age factor" may be related to increased time of bacterial exposure, or possibly to increased inflammatory response and decreased potential for repair with age.

Advanced periodontal disease measured in terms of alveolar

bone loss has also been correlated with efficiency of oral hygiene by Schie et al.[4] Figure 6-2 summarizes the alveolar bone loss observed around mandibular right central incisors which was similar to the bone loss observed around other teeth. In this study, bone loss was calculated from radiographs and expressed as a percentage change from the ideal, which was considered to be 1 mm below the cemento-enamel junction. These authors found that periodontal disease directly correlated with efficiency of oral hygiene. That is, reduced levels of oral hygiene were associated

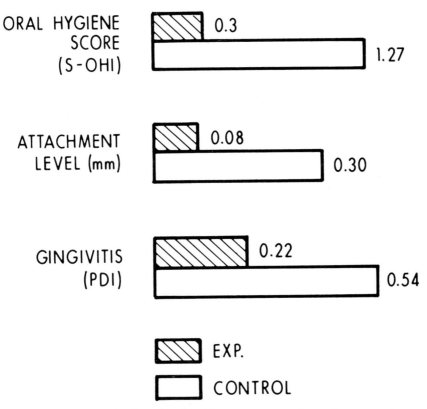

Figure 6-4. Longitudinal study of oral hygiene, gingival attachment, and gingivitis. Adapted from J. Suomi et al., *J Periodont,* 42:152, 1971.

with greater alveolar bone loss. In this study, age again was seen to modify the severity of bone loss accompanying a given degree of oral hygiene.

Longitudinal population studies have also revealed a direct relationship between oral hygiene and severity of periodontal disease. Lovdal et al.[5] reported results of a five-year study in which 808 subjects received a routine regimen of subgingival scaling and oral hygiene instruction. The severity of the measured interproximal gingivitis has been tabulated in Figure 6-3. During the five years when the subjects received routine scaling and reinforced oral hygiene instruction, the percentage of gingivitis decreased from 50 to 60 percent. This decrease was significantly greater in individuals exercising good oral hygiene compared to those with poor plaque control.

Studies reported by Suomi et al.[6,7] tested the hypothesis that the development and progression of periodontal disease could be retarded by high levels of oral hygiene. During the three-year test period, a large experimental group was given eleven routine prophylaxes in conjunction with oral hygiene instructions and dental health education. At the same time, a matched control group received no dental attention except for annual examinations. Changes that occurred in oral hygiene scores, gingivitis scores, and the level of gingival attachment are tabulated in Figure 6-4. Oral hygiene was measured by Greene's index, and gingivitis was measured by Ramfjord's Index.[8] In the experimental group with good oral hygiene there were relatively low levels of gingivitis and little change in the epithelial attachment. In comparison, the control group exhibited gingivitis and apical migration of the epithelial attachment. In addition (Table 6-I) there

TABLE 6-I

ALVEOLAR BONE LOSS IN A THREE-YEAR PERIOD*

Distance CEJ to Alveolar Crest (mm)	Alveolar Bone Loss	
	Control	Experimental
Initial	1.25	1.33
Final	1.44	1.34
Change	0.19	0.01

* Adapted from J. D. Suomi et al., *J Periodont*, 42:562, 1971.[7]

was relatively little radiographic evidence of alveolar bone loss in the experimental group. Thus, routine oral hygiene and scaling effectively controlled periodontal disease.

If effective oral hygiene could prevent periodontal disease, would the converse be true? That is, would elimination of oral hygiene lead to periodontal disease? This question was posed by Löe et al.[9, 10] and tested in a series of classic experiments. Dental students were given a dental prophylaxis followed by intensive oral hygiene practice until they had little or no measurable plaque or gingivitis. The participants were then instructed to stop all forms of oral hygiene. The rate of plaque accumulation and gingivitis that resulted are seen in Figure 6-5. Plaque began to accumulate rapidly; after nine to twenty-one days without oral hygiene, all students developed heavy plaque and generalized mild gingivitis. The development of gingivitis correlated well with the rate of plaque formation in each individual. Characteristic changes in the bacterial flora found at the gingival margin also correlated with development of gingivitis. Within one to two days after reinstitution of oral hygiene, the dental plaque was removed, and gingival inflammation subsequently disappeared. This experimental model provides direct evidence that the accumulation of dental plaque at the gingival margin causes gingivitis, and this gingivitis can be reversed by plaque removal. While the gingivitis model only relates to gingivitis and

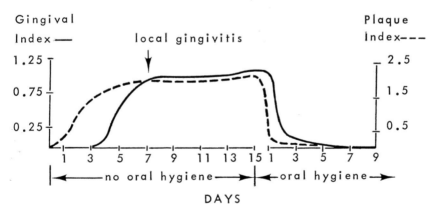

Figure 6-5. Experimental gingivitis. Adapted from E. Theilade et al., *J Periodont Res, 1:1*, 1966.

does not provide evidence relating oral hygiene to periodontitis, previously discussed research of Schei and Suomi provides evidence for this relationship.

The clinical development of experimental gingivitis as related to the rate of plaque formation is seen in Figures 6-6 to 6-13. Two subjects were observed for sixteen days during which time no oral hygiene was practiced. In the first subject (M.M.), plaque formed rapidly with heavy accumulation by sixteen days. Mild gingivitis was seen by seven days and was progressively more severe at sixteen days. In the second subject (N.B.), plaque formed relatively slowly, and little gingivitis was seen after sixteen days of no oral hygiene. Presumably, if plaque were allowed to accumulate for longer periods in this subject, more severe gingivitis would have occurred.

The lesson from the studies discussed in this section is clear; microbial dental plaque causes gingivitis and most likely is a major factor in periodontitis. Regular dispersal of dental plaque will markedly prevent the loss of the periodontal attachment apparatus. For most healthy individuals the so-called systemic factors play a *minor* role in the progression of periodontal disease.

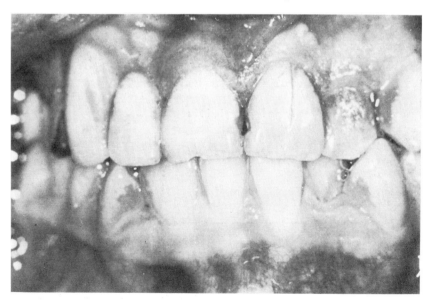

Figure 6-6. Two days after elimination of oral hygiene in subject M.M.

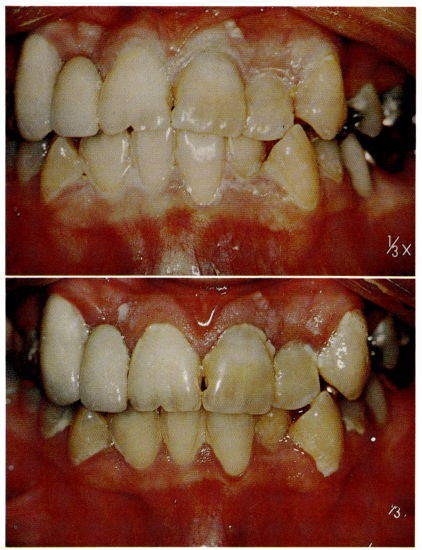

Plate 1. Two days after elimination of oral hygiene in subject M. M.
Plate 2. Sixteen days after elimination of oral hygiene in subject M. M.
Gingivitis is now seen in papillary and gingival margins of most teeth.

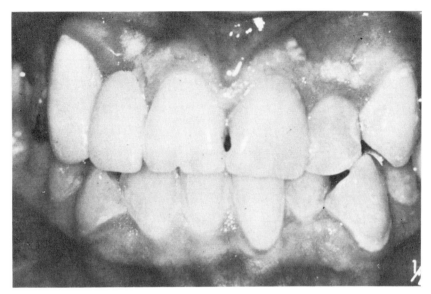

Figure 6-7. Seven days after elimination of oral hygiene in subject M.M. Gingivitis most noticeable mesial to mandibular cuspids.

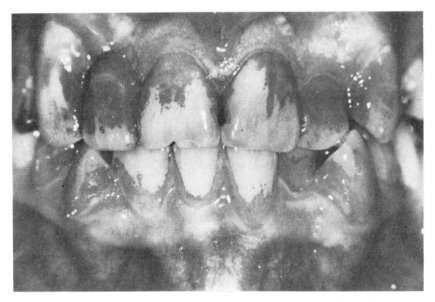

Figure 6-8. Plaque disclosed in subject M.M. seven days after elimination of oral hygiene. Plaque has progressed coronally from gingival margins.

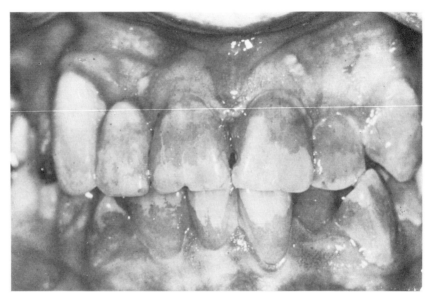

Figure 6-9. Plaque disclosed in subject M.M. sixteen days after elimination of oral hygiene.

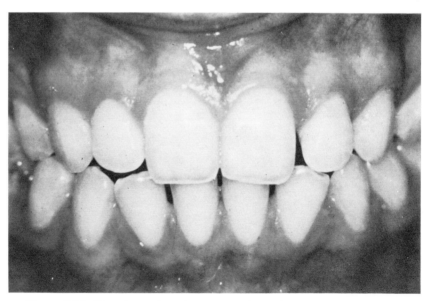

Figure 6-10. Two days after elimination of oral hygiene in subject N.B.

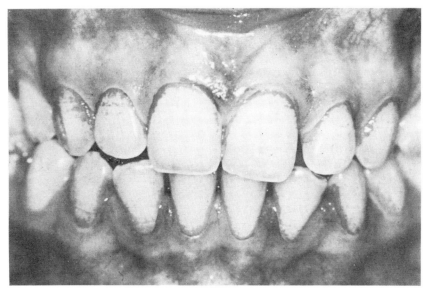

Figure 6-11. Plaque disclosed in subject N.B. two days after elimination of oral hygiene.

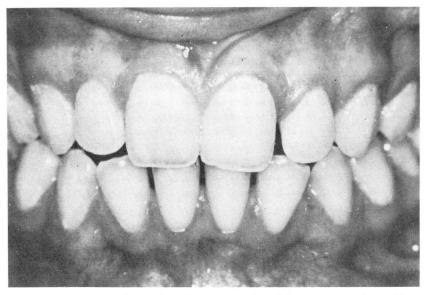

Figure 6-12. Sixteen days after elimination of oral hygiene in subject N.B. Minimal signs of gingivitis are seen compared to subject M.M. (see Plate 2).

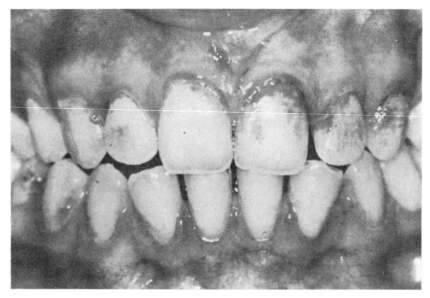

Figure 6-13. Plaque disclosed in subject N.B. sixteen days after elimination of oral hygiene. Rate of plaque formation is considerably slower than in subject M.M. (see Figure 6-9).

Microbial Flora of the Gingival Crevice

Because of the importance of microorganisms in periodontal disease, it is valuable to consider the organisms commonly found, dynamic changes in the flora with occurrence of periodontal disease, structure, composition, and development of microbial accumulations or aggregates, and the relationship of these aggregates to the hard and soft tissues.

Bacteria may be found free in the crevice or associated with teeth in various forms of aggregations. Differentiation must be made between aggregated deposits of food debris, materia alba, acquired salivary pellicle, bacterial dental plaque, and dental calculus.[11, 12] Food debris, as implied by its name, is retained food that frequently impacts interproximally. Materia alba, which in the earlier literature was sometimes considered synonomous with food debris, and at other times with plaque, actually consists of bacteria, some desquamated epithelial cells, and leukocytes. Materia alba loosely adheres to the gingiva, alveolar mucosa, teeth, plaque, and to restorations. It differs from plaque in that it has no definite structure and is easily removed from teeth by water spray or rinsing. Dental plaque is a dense microbial layer consisting of a variety of bacteria embedded in an intermicrobial matrix. The bacterial composition varies with the age of plaque. Plaque has a definite architecture and is found closely adherent to teeth or restorations. It is not removed by rinsing or by a moderate water spray. The acquired pellicle on which plaque forms is an amorphous material primarily of salivary origin; it varies from 0.1 μ to 0.8 μ in thickness and is composed of carbohydrates, mucopolysaccharides, and lipids. Pellicles form within minutes on pumiced tooth surfaces. Dental calculus in humans is mainly mineralized or calcified plaque. Mineralized deposits resembling calculus occur in germ-free animals, suggesting that bacterial plaque is not necessarily a precursory calculus. On the outer surface of the calculus, there is always a layer of unmineralized bacteria or plaque.

Subgingival deposits are thought to be pathogenic in periodontal disease since they are in close proximity to the site of initial lesions. Generally, plaque is the most important form of bacterial deposit because it allows the greatest numbers of viable bacteria to be maintained closely approximated to gingival tissue. Materia alba and calculus may also play a role in the disease since some bacterial pathogenic mechanisms do not require viable organisms or long exposure to the gingival tissue.

Many methods have been elaborated for examination of bacteria from the gingival area. The most common methods include average wet weight of samples, microscopic counts, and viable counts. Generally, the viable counts of culturable bacteria are considerably less than the microscopic counts. This results from problems of numbers, sizes, and dispersability of clumps, spontaneous reaggregation of bacteria in suspensions, loss of bacterial viability during specimen handling, and suitability of cultivation methods.[13] A common problem inherent in all techniques for identifying the gingival flora is one of sampling variability.

The resident gingival flora are dynamic, resulting in changes in numbers and possibly species of bacteria found in particular locations at different times of the day.[13] If changes in flora occur with time in one gingival crevice location, then greater microbial variability must occur in samples randomly removed from different areas of the mouth and in pooled samples. Thus, a "representative sample" of the flora around specific gingival areas cannot exist. What is actually seen is an average representation. In spite of these problems, considerable knowledge exists concerning the bacteria of the gingival area.

Microscopic and viable counts from normal gingival sulci and periodontal pockets reveal differences.[14] The microscopic counts in normal sulci were 1.3×10^{11} counts per gm wet weight, while counts in periodontal pockets averaged 2.1×10^{11}. This concentration assumes real significance when one realizes that these numbers are similar to pure cultures of streptococci packed by centrifugation.[15] The total viable anaerobic and aerobic counts in sulci were 3.5×10^{10} and 4.6×10^{10} while in pockets the counts were 2.0×10^{10} and 1.2×10^{10}, respectively.[16, 17] Microscopically, there was approximately a five-fold increase in counts of spirochetes in periodontal pockets compared to normal sulci. Viable counts of *Bacteriodes melaninogenicus* were twice as

TABLE 6-II

ORGANISMS OF THE HUMAN GINGIVAL CREVICE
AND DENTAL PLAQUE*

Group	Gingival Crevice	Dental Plaque
Gram-positive facultative cocci	29[†]	28
Gram-positive anaerobic cocci	7	13
Gram-positive facultative rods	15	24
Gram-positive anaerobic rods	20	18
Gram-negative facultative cocci	0.4	0.4
Gram-negative anaerobic cocci	11	6
Gram-negative facultative rods	1.2	0
Gram-negative anaerobic rods	16	10
Spirochetes	1-3	< 0.1

* Adapted from Gibbons et al., *Arch Oral Biol,* 8:281, 1963; *Arch Oral Biol,* 9:365, 1964.[16, 17]

† Approximate percentage of cultivable microbiota.

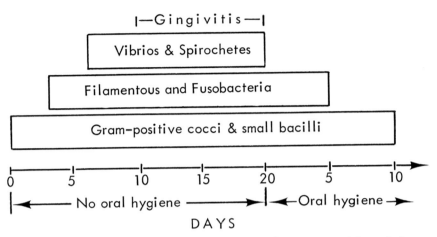

Figure 6-14. Bacterial changes in experimental gingivitis. Adapted from H. Löe, *J Periodont, 36:*177, 1965.

great, and fusobacteria were six times more numerous in periodontal disease.

A comparison of the predominant cultivable microbiota of the gingival crevice region in dental plaque has been summarized in Table 6-II. The flora in the crevicular debris and in plaque were similar. There were, however, some interesting differences. *B. melaninogenicus* was found in gingival debris but was not isolated from plaque; spirochetes, on the other hand, were not seen in plaque but were detected in gingival debris.

What dynamic changes occur in the microbiota during development of human "experimental gingivitis" resulting from a period of no oral hygiene? The flora at the gingival margin were identified microscopically by Löe et al.,[9] and changes in composition were followed during development of gingivitis. Results have been illustrated in Figure 6-14. Three phases in the development of the flora could be distinguished. Initially, from zero to two days during which time no oral hygiene was practiced, the flora were predominantly Gram-positive cocci and small bacilli. Gram-negative cocci and rods made up 30 percent of the microbial population at this time. From day one to four, there was significant increase in the numbers of filamentous bacteria and fusobacteria. The third phase from four to nine days was characterized by the appearance of vibrios and spirochetes. Population shifts in developing human plaque have been described by other authors. Plaque samples taken at one, three, five, seven, and nine days were assayed for their content of neisseria, nocardia, streptococcus, fusobacteria, veillonella, actinomyces, and corynebacteria. Early plaque had predominantly streptococci, neisseria, and nocardia; plaque nine days old had actinomyces, veillonella, and corynebacteria in addition to numerous streptococci. At least some of the changes can be related to changes in the oxygen tension of the local plaque environment, which in later stages promotes anaerobic growth.[18] Comparisons of supragingival plaque and subgingival plaque from periodontal pockets revealed that during forty-nine days of no oral hygiene, significant increases in vibrios and fusobacteria occurred.[19] These organisms were always present in greater proportions in subgingival plaque. Population shifts in microorganisms during periods of no oral hygiene do not allow conclusions as to which organisms cause inflammation, since it is likely that the increase in some organisms may result from the inflammation.

The potential pathogenicity of gingival bacteria has been well documented, but the potential importance of viruses, mycoplasma, and protozoa can only be surmised until they are studied further. Viruses, as will be discussed later, can cause severe alveolar bone loss in experimental animals. The protozoans, *Entamoeba gingivalis* and *Trichomonas tenax,* both occur four to eight times more frequently in individuals with periodontitis than in normal mouths.[2] *E. gingivalis* apparently do not invade gingiva but are limited to plaque or debris adjacent to gingival epithelium; they have been observed more frequently in advanced periodontitis than in moderate periodontitis.[21] Again, these increases in numbers with severity of inflammation may *result from rather than cause* periodontal disease.

The development, structure, and location of plaque with respect to the gingiva are also important in considering plaque pathogenesis.[22-26] The formation of plaque is controlled by the local environment. Supragingival plaque is under the influence of saliva, while subgingival plaque is mediated by crevicular fluid. In addition, the metabolic balance of bacteria in the gingival area is regulated by factors such as pH, the concentration of available carbohydrate, amino acids, minerals, host factors, and toxic products produced by microorganisms.

Plaque formation occurs rapidly. Within five minutes after pumicing, approximately one million organisms per square millimeter are deposited on an enamel surface.[27] Globules or aggregates of fifty to two hundred organisms can be seen by twenty minutes.[25] Because of the size of these aggregates, it is thought that rather than growing *in situ* from a single bacteria which adheres to the tooth, the aggregates may first form in the sulcus and then stick to the surface. The notion of this mode of adhesion or attachment is supported by current concepts of plaque formation. Microorganisms are thought to adhere to the tooth or pellicle by extracellular polysaccharides. Some of these adherent polysaccharides include dextran produced by *Streptococcus mutans* and levan produced by *Actinomyces viscosus*. Hillman, Gibbons, and van Houte have also postulated the existence of receptors on bacterial cells that are specific for tooth surface and pellicle.[28, 29] Once plaque begins to form, it rapidly enlarges by interbacterial agglutination.

As plaque develops, the bacterial flora change from a predominantly coccal form to a filamentous form. In older, thicker plaque, the basal portions consist mainly of closely packed, fine filamentous bacteria at right angles to the enamel surface.[30] The filaments closer to the periphery curve and are varied in size. In the outer layer, other morphological types are more commonly seen, including Gram-positive and Gram-negative cocci and bacilli.

The relationship of plaque to the hard and soft tissues has been studied by electron microscopy.[26] Several types of plaque structure have been differentiated. At the gingival margin, there is a loose accumulation of Gram-positive cocci. A second type of plaque occurs within the sulcus area; it is composed primarily of Gram-positive microorganisms in a dense microbial aggregation. The third type of plaque within the sulcus is divided into two distinct portions. The deep portion consists of cocci and rod-like microorganisms, while the superficial layer is predominantly filamentous. Plaque localized in the sulcus extends to within 0.1 mm of the bottom of the sulcus and is associated with migration of leukocytes through the junctional epithelium.

Chemically, plaque is approximately 80 percent water and 20 percent solids. The solids are inorganic salts and organic matrix. Dextran, which has been implicated in plaque formation, comprises 95 percent of the hexose-containing polysaccharide, while most of the remaining hexose is levan.

The pathogenicity of microorganisms will be considered later. For plaque to cause periodontal disease, however, either whole bacteria, bacterial fragments, bacterial enzymes, metabolic products, or endotoxins must enter the tissue to produce direct tissue damage or an indirect host immune response. This tissue infiltration must occur repeatedly to produce the chronic lesion characteristic of periodontal disease. While the only real evidence for direct tissue invasion is found in acute necrotizing ulcerative gingivitis, a variety of experiments point to routine passive bacterial infiltration of the periodontium.

Bacteremias detected by culture of venous blood occur following physical manipulation of gingival tissues. Bacteremias following these activities imply bacteria must enter the gingival tissue and vasculature in order to be isolated from the systemic circulation. Routine activities such as brushing teeth and chewing hard substances set up transient bacteremias in about one fifth of individuals studied.[31, 32] These bacteremias were reported as frequently in individuals with periodontitis as in those with clinically normal gingivae. The incidence of bacteremias following subgingival scaling, however, was directly related to severity of periodontal disease.[33] For example, bacteremias following subgingival scaling and root planing occurred in 22 percent of patients with normal gingiva, in 29 percent with gingivitis and in 51 percent with periodontitis.

Other techniques have demonstrated that intact bacteria as well as bacterial fragments and metabolic products enter the tissue. *Bacteroides melaninogenicus* antigens have been demonstrated by immunofluorescence in tissues taken from patients with periodontitis.[34] From half of the cultured strips of human gingiva, Gram-positive filamentous bacteria have been identified.[35]

Histologic localization of bacteria in gingiva has been equivocal; conflicting reports probably result from the insensitivity of the histologic method and inherent problems of contamination during sectioning.[36, 37] However, as few as one bacterium per oil immersion field ($\times 1,000$) in a 6μ section would be equivalent to 10^7 bacteria/ml.[38] Passive infiltration both inward and outward through the gingiva has been demonstrated utilizing carbon particles with a size similar to bacteria.[39, 40] Carbon particles gently applied to the crest of the free gingiva and allowed to flow into the gingival crevice were consistently found in the underlying connective tissue of clinically normal and periodontally involved humans. Similarly, intravenous injection of India ink resulted in histological localization of carbon particles not only in the connective tissue and basement membrane area, but also intercellularly throughout the epithelium and within the gingival sulcus. Evidence also indicates the importance of an intact gingival sulcus epithelial barrier.[41] When this barrier breaks down, relatively low concentrations of antigens produce pathologic changes in tissues.

Thus, in periodontal disease microbial products seem to be constantly entering the tissues. As the disease progresses with further tissue degeneration, the infiltration and pathology increase.

The Pathogenicity of Microorganisms in Periodontal Disease

Of primary importance is whether bacteria associated with calcified deposits can act as the primary etiologic agent in periodontal disease. Convincing experimental evidence has been provided by Rovin et al.[42] They produced gingival irritation by placing 000 silk ligature at the cervical margins of molars in germ-free and conventional rats. Histologic examination revealed that the local irritation did not produce periodontal inflammation in the absence of microorganisms. Inflammation was only produced by the combination of a local irritant (ligature) and a microbial flora. The ligature, it appears, acted as a nidus for bacterial accumulation near the tissue, and this increased bacterial concentration led to the inflammation.

Bacteria can play two basic roles in the pathogenicity of periodontal disease. This has been demonstrated by intraperitoneal injection of sterile, autoclaved calculus, and by injection of non-sterile calculus into guinea pigs.[43] Initially, the response to both types of calculus was suppuration and proliferation. Subsequently, the sterile calculus with nonviable bacteria evoked a granulomatous "foreign body" type response, while the non-sterile calculus continued to evoke suppuration. By eliciting host responses, bacteria may induce direct effects requiring viable multiplying organisms and indirect effects in which viability is not necessary.

The identification of specific microorganisms responsible for periodontal disease has been approached primarily by two methods. One approach involves obtaining pure cultures of punitive pathogens and introducing these into experimental animals, either by injection into the tissues or by inoculation into the oral cavity of germ-free animals. The second approach has been to study bacterial interactions in naturally occurring periodontal disease of animals. Animals used in both of these types of studies have included mice, rats, hamsters, rabbits, dogs, and monkeys.

One of the earliest experimental models has been the transmissible mixed infection produced by subcutaneous injection into the guinea pig or rabbit of bacterial debris from the gingival crevice. Following serial transmission, the supportive, inflammatory lesion was found to be populated by *Treponema microdentium*, Fusobacterium, vibrios, spirella, bacteroides, anaerobic streptococci and anaerobic diphtheroids.[44] While pure cultures inoculated singly were unable to produce the disease, recombinations with four organisms sufficed. The four organisms consisted of *Bacteroides melaninogenicus*, a second strain of bacteroides, a motile, Gram-negative anaerobic bacillus, and a facultative diphtheroid. Deletion of *B. melaninogenicus* from the mixture of organisms resulted in a minor, atypical nontransmissible lesion, indicating the importance of *B. melaninogenicus* to this particular mixed anaerobic infection.[45] The possible importance of *B. melaninogenicus* in the pathogenesis of human periodontal disease is further emphasized by the demonstration of tissue-destroying factors such as collagenase, fibrolysin, endotoxin, deoxyribonuclease, hydrogen sulfide, indole, ammonia, and various organic acids.[46] Although *B. melaninogenicus* may not initiate human periodontal disease, its wide spectrum of toxic products may play a role in the progression of the disease after the gingiva becomes permeable to these substrates.

Introduction of certain human oral bacteria as monocontaminants in gnotobiotic animals frequently leads to periodontal disease characterized by alveolar bone loss. Organisms shown to elicit this response include *Streptococcus mutans, Actinomyces viscosus, Actinomyces naeslundii,* and a strain of Bacillus.[46-49]

The etiology of naturally occurring periodontal disease in hamsters has been extensively studied.[50] Pure cultures of a filamentous bacteria, initially isolated from hamster plaque and later identified as *Actinomyces viscosus,* induced periodontal disease and cervical caries when inoculated orally into uninfected hamsters in which the disease did not occur spontaneously. Similar periodontal pathology was seen in gnotobiotic rats infected with *A. viscosus.* Other plaque organisms including streptococci, sarcina, Gram-negative rods, and Gram-negative oval-shaped cells failed to produce similar pathology. The circle of evidence implicating filamentous organisms in periodontal disease and root surface caries is now nearly complete with the demonstration that filamentous isolates from the carious dentin of human teeth with root surface caries and from humans with periodontal disease can induce the periodontal syndrome as well as cervical caries in the hamster.[51, 52] Filaments isolated include *Rothia dentocariosa,* strains of Actinomyces resembling *A. naeslundii, A. viscosus* (serotypes 1 and 2), and *A. odontolyticus.*

Natural periodontal disease in mice appears to be a continuous process of gradual alveolar bone loss somewhat independent of the presence of microorganisms. The process however, is greatly accelerated by the presence of large numbers of bacteria in the gingival crevice area. It has been suggested that an analogous situation occurs in man, although it is clear that in most individuals bacterial accumulation at the gingival crevice is by far the most important factor in alveolar bone loss.

The rice rat exhibits a spontaneous periodontal syndrome consisting of gingival distortion, periodontal pockets, alveolar resorption, and tooth mobility. The bacterial etiology of this disease has been demonstrated by a dramatic improvement in the disease state upon administration of antibiotics. The disease can be transmitted by transferring plaque from rice rats with the disease to normal rice rats.[53] It has also been demonstrated that periodontal disease in rice rats occurs as a result of oral inoculations with a pooled culture containing four microorganisms: a Gram-negative, thin filamentous rod, a thick pleomorphic coccus or rod; and two types of Gram-positive thick rods.[54] The etiologic agents in the periodontal syndrome of rice rats apparently include Gram-positive rods.

The role of viruses in periodontal disease has received little attention. Infection with viruses has led to experimental periodontal disease, which includes apical migration of the epithelial attachment, periodontal pocket formation with purulent exudate, and extensive resorption of alveolar bone. The viruses used include the polyoma virus from mice and a virus from a rat.[55, 56]

Thus, evidence indicates bacteria can experimentally duplicate many aspects of human periodontal disease. Present evidence suggests that a multiplicity of organisms may be involved in the etiology of periodontal disease. Further animal studies will undoubtedly reveal additional organisms capable of producing periodontal pathology.

Is Human Periodontal Disease Contagious?

The possibility that human periodontal disease might be contagious is not completely established. The available evidence to date, however, indicates human periodontal disease is not highly contagious. The possibility exists that periodontal disease has a low level of transmissibility, requiring multiple challenges by new bacteria until they can colonize the recipient. This is supported by studies of animal periodontal disease, which can be transmitted from animal to animal by specific bacteria. However, human studies have demonstrated the difficulties of upsetting the natural ecological balance between organisms found in the mouth to allow implantation of new bacteria. Frequently, gross changes in diet are necessary for successful implantation.

The study of transmissibility of human periodontal disease will require more sophisticated indicators. Rather than studying the species of bacteria present in the gingival area, the identification of serotypes of species may be necessary, assuming that some serotypes are more virulent than others.

In any bacterial infection there are several potential mechanisms by which bacteria can cause pathogenesis. Where infection is caused by one genus of bacteria, only a few mechanisms may be operative. In periodontal disease, however, a variety of bacteria may be involved, so all possible mechanisms must be evaluated. Table 6-III summarizes both the direct and indirect mechanisms possibly active in human periodontal disease. Those mechanisms most likely participating in periodontal disease or about which most is known will be discussed later in greater detail.

Table 6–III

POTENTIAL BACTERIAL MECHANISMS
IN PERIODONTAL DISEASE

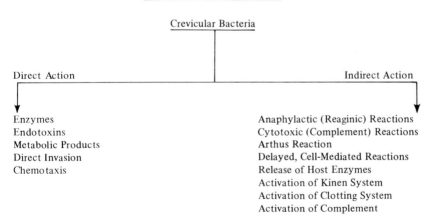

Crevicular Bacteria

Direct Action

Indirect Action

Direct Action	Indirect Action
Enzymes	Anaphylactic (Reaginic) Reactions
Endotoxins	Cytotoxic (Complement) Reactions
Metabolic Products	Arthus Reaction
Direct Invasion	Delayed, Cell-Mediated Reactions
Chemotaxis	Release of Host Enzymes
	Activation of Kinen System
	Activation of Clotting System
	Activation of Complement

Immunologic Mechanisms: Potential Pathogenic Agents in Periodontal Disease

Although immune mechanisms are thought to be protective responses of the host to the presence of foreign substances such as bacteria and viruses, they may also result in local tissue destruction. That is, the host, in its efforts to eliminate the bacteria, may overreact in the form of a hypersensitivity reaction characterized by a greater inflammatory response than the bacteria could elicit by direct attack. Such a situation most likely occurs in inflammatory periodontal disease as a response to the antigens of crevicular microorganisms.

Tissue damage (or immunopathology) may occur in a sensitized host upon subsequent exposure to the sensitizing antigen or allergen.[57-59] The four types of hypersensitivity reactions described by Gell and Coombs[56] are (1) anaphylactic, (2) cytotoxic, (3) Arthus, and (4) delayed or cell-mediated hypersensitivity.

(1) Anaphylactic or Reagin-Dependent Reactions

In these reactions, a unique immunoglobulin, called reagin or IgE, is produced by plasma cells and fixes to or sensitizes mast cells and basophilic leukocytes. Subsequent antigenic challenge releases the biochemical mediators of the anaphylactic reaction: histamine, a slow-reacting substance of anaphylaxis (SRS-A), bradykinin, prostaglandins, and eosinophil chemotactic factor. These mediators bring about smooth muscle constriction, edema resulting from increased vascular permeability, constriction of small venules, and mobilization of phagocytes. Complement does not appear to play a role in anaphylactic reactions since IgE does not bind complement.

(2) Cytotoxic Reactions

Cytotoxic reactions occur when antigens intimately associated with cell or other tissue components react with antibodies of the IgG or IgM class. Complement fixation by these immune complexes is usually necessary for subsequent cell damage. Tissue cells become susceptible to the damage or lytic effects of antibody when bacterial antigens temporarily absorb cells. Pharmacological mediators such as histamines or SRS-A are not important for cytotoxic reactions.

(3) Arthus (Toxic Complexes) Reactions

Arthus reactions result when antigen reacts in tissue spaces or in blood vessels with precipitating antibody of the IgG or IgM class. Microprecipitates, which form in moderate antigen excess, activate the complement system and lead to hormonal, vascular, and cytotoxic actions or effects, depending on the location where the antigen-antibody complexes lodge. Pharmacological mediators such as histamines do not play an important role in the pathogenesis, and antihistamines, therefore, are ineffective in this reaction. Rather, there is marked leukocytic infiltration, possibly in response to complement-activated chemotactic factors. These infiltrating leukocytes are thought to lead to the thrombosis, hemorrhage, edema, endothelial destruction, and local necrosis which characterize Arthus reactions.

(4) Delayed or Cell-Mediated Reactions

These reactions differ from the other hypersensitivity reactions in that sensitized lymphocytes rather than humoral antibodies mediate the hypersensitivity. In fact, transfer of delayed hypersensitivity occurs only with the transfer of cells or cell extracts and not with sera (antibodies), while the other three forms of hypersensitivity can be transferred with sera containing specific antibodies. In a sensitized animal, minute amounts of antigen cause localization of mononuclear cells and exudation. Stimulation of sensitized lymphocytes by antigen produces many factors or mediators which are important in the pathogenesis of delayed reactions. Some of the factors demonstrated are migration inhibition factor (MIF) which inhibits migration of normal macrophages, a chemotactic factor for macrophages, and cytotoxic factors such as lymphotoxin.

The antigen-antibody complexes formed in cytotoxic reactions and Arthus reactions fix complement. Complement, once activated, acts as an effector system for these immune complexes.[60, 61]

The nine components of complement are activated in this order: C1, C4, C2, C3, C5, C6, C7, C8, and C9. During this sequential activation, biologically active products form. Activation of C3 allows immune adherence which enhances phagocytosis. Anaphylatoxin formed by activation of C3 and C5 releases histamine from mast cells. Chemotactic factors for polymorphonuclear leukocytes are also released by activation of C3 and C5. Death and lysis of cells occur after activation of C8 and C9. Recently,[61] endotoxins have been shown to activate complement, probably starting with the C3 component. Thus, endotoxins, acting through the complement effector system with or without antibodies, may cause leukocyte chemotaxis changes in vascular permeability and cell lysis.

The immune mechanisms described above can all contribute to soft tissue inflammatory lesions as seen in periodontal disease. Some recent evidence indicates complement-dependent immunopathology also includes bone resorption.[62, 63] The *in vitro* models studied have demonstrated that a complement-dependent antigen-antibody reaction can lead to resorption of bone.

If periodontal disease is a manifestation of the immunopa-

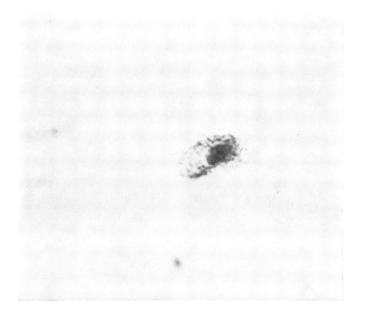

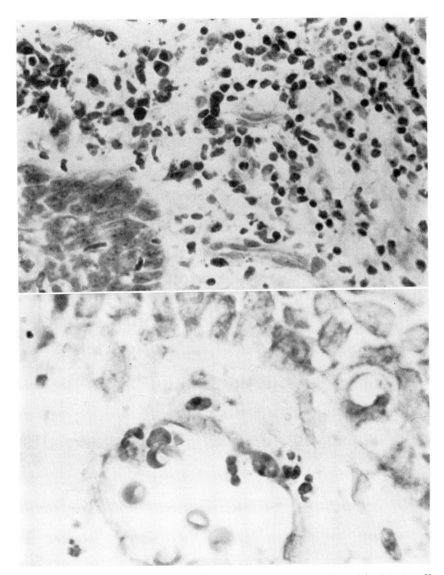

Figure 6-15. Connective tissue of inflamed human gingiva. (a): Mast cell stained with methyl green-thionin stain (×1000). (b): Accumulation of plasma cells and lymphocytes beneath the crevicular epithelium (×100). (c): Perivascular migration of polymorphonuclear leukocytes in gingival vessel (×500).

thology that occurs when microorganisms challenge a sensitized host, one would expect to see evidence of this immune response in the gingival tissue. Indeed, diseased gingival tissue is infiltrated with plasma cells which produce immunoglobulins, lymphocytes which are active in delayed or cell-mediated reactions, mast cells, and polymorphonuclear leukocytes (Fig. 6-15a, b, c).

Specifically, what is the localization of inflammatory cells in human periodontal disease? Plasma cells and lymphocytes have been observed in the connective tissue of the gingiva; polymorphonuclear leukocytes have been isolated in the gingival sulcus, junctional epithelium, and the connective tissue underlying the junctional epithelium.[23, 26] Lymphocytes have been reported to be within the gingival connective tissue and the basal cell layer of the epithelium,[65] while proliferating plasma cells frequently are found clustered around the capillaries of the inflamed gingiva.[66, 67] Examination of gingival specimens from fifty patients with gingivitis to determine the relative proportions of lymphocytes and plasma cells indicated a predominance of plasma cells. Plasma cells were found in 96 percent of the biopsies and comprised over 80 percent of the inflammatory cells in 78 percent of the biopsies.[68] The number of lymphocytes may have been underestimated, however, since they are difficult to demonstrate in tissue sections. Mast cell numbers are inversely related to the extent of gingival inflammation.[69] Normal gingiva contains more mast cells per area than moderately inflamed tissue. Severely inflamed gingiva contains the fewest mast cells. This strongly suggests that mast cells degranulate in the development of periodontal disease. In support of the role of mast cells in periodontal disease, it has been reported that mast cell counts decrease during periodontitis and increase following successful periodontal therapy.[70] Ultrastructural features of mast cells from periodontitis specimens characteristically include predominant granules with a granular matrix of varying density.[71] Similar features have occurred in mast cell granules following elicitation of immediate hypersensitivity reactions.[72] Mast cells also contain heparin. Goldhaber[73] has found that heparin potentiates the effect of parathyroid hormone in stimulating bone resorption. He feels that heparin release from gingival mast cells could lead to local alveolar bone resorption, even with physiologic levels of parathyroid hormone.

Although several types of antibody-mediated reactions may occur separately or in various combinations in the gingiva, some of the reactions may be of less consequence than others. The relative importance of different hypersensitivity reactions and other bacterial pathogenic mechanisms in periodontal disease has not yet been ascertained, but it is likely that the importance varies from individual to individual since persons with agammaglobulinemia have a form of periodontal disease.[74] In cases where particular immune mechanisms are inactive, other pathogenic mechanisms may assume greater importance in the etiology of periodontal disease.

Several approaches have been followed in examining the role of immune mechanisms in periodontal disease. Animal models were utilized to elicit hypersensitivity and to compare the resultant immunopathology with human periodontal disease. Studies in humans have attempted to demonstrate the potential for hypersensitivity responses and antibody formation to oral bacteria.

As anticipated, hypersensitivity reactions in the oral cavity can be elicited. Immediate and delayed-type reactions have been elicited in the oral mucosa of rabbits and guinea pigs.[75, 76] Delayed hypersensitivity has been passively transferred by sensitized lymphoid cells.[77] Arthus reactions have also been produced in gingiva and oral mucosa.[78, 79]

Gingival histopathology resulting from experimental hypersensitivity has revealed many similarities to human periodontal disease. Gingival immune reactions in the early phase frequently exhibit edema, venule congestion, venous thrombosis, extravascular fibrinoid, and a cellular exudate characterized by polymorphonuclear leukocytes. By the fifth day after challenge, the reaction sites mainly have a plasma cell infiltrate.[80] The histopathology reported in some studies also includes osteoclastic activity.[81] Placement of antigen directly into the gingival crevice permitted sensitization of an animal to the antigen and later acted as a challenging stimulus to evoke an immune response.[82] In addition to local histopathology within the gingiva, there is a systemic immune response characterized by serum antibodies. Multiple challenges of sensitized animals cause periodontal pocket formation and proliferation of epithelium into the gingival connective tissues.[83] Many characteristics of human periodontal disease are therefore duplicated experimentally by hypersensitivity reactions in the gingiva.

Do immune reactions to bacterial stimulation develop in the gingiva? Does this response correlate with periodontal disease? Immunofluorescent studies have revealed immunoglobulins in gingival plasma cells. Most plasma cells found in clinically normal tissue contain IgG, very few cells contain IgA, and only rare cells contain IgM.[84] Some gingival plasma cells contain IgE, and their numbers increase in more severely inflamed tissue.[85] Immu-

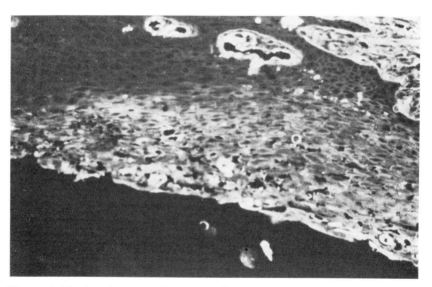

Figure 6-16. Localization of immunoglobulin G in epithelium lining the crevice of normal human gingiva. This is an area of junctional epithelium (JE) and oral epithelium (OE) treated with fluorscein-labelled antibodies to human IgG. The immunoglobulin is localized mainly in the junctional epithelium and connective tissue (CT); no immunoglobulin is detectable in the oral epithelium which lines part of the gingival crevice (GC) in health (×100).

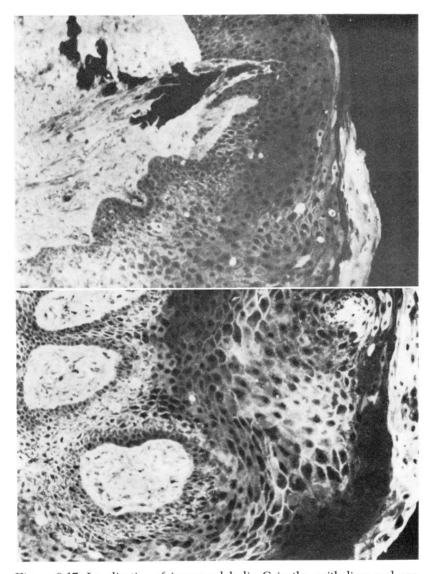

Figure 6-17. Localization of immunoglobulin G in the epithelium and connective tissue of inflamed human gingiva. Figure 6-17a shows the keratinized, free marginal gingiva (FM) blending into the crevicular epithelium,
and Figure 6-17b shows the inflammed crevicular epithelium lining the
periodontal pocket. Both photographs show localization of immunoglobulin
G between the cells of the inflamed crevicular epithelium and in the connective tissue. There is little or no immunoglobulin G detectable in the
keratinized epithelium at the margin of the gingiva (×100).

noglobulins also have been reported in the cytoplasm of gingival and crevicular epithelium.[86] In clinically normal gingiva, IgG immunoglobulins have been localized between junctional epithelial cells within the crevice, but few or no immunoglobulins have been detected in oral epithelium which borders part of the crevice.[87] (See Figures 6-16, 6-17, 6-18.)

Many of the immunoglobulins in gingival tissue have been shown to be antibodies to bacteria. In one study, the morphology of bacteria adhering to gingival tissue in areas of globulin concentration included bacilli, cocci, and filaments, suggesting a multiplicity of antibodies to many bacterial antigens.[87] This adherence of bacteria to areas of globulins was thought to be related to the specificity of the antibodies. More direct evidence has demonstrated that bacterial antigens from *E. Coli,* Veillonella and Fusobacterium form immune complexes with gingival immunoglobulins obtained from thin slices of gingival tissues or from spent media of gingival organ cultures.[88] These immune complexes were also observed to activate the complement system.

The possibility also exists that hypersensitivity reactions oc-

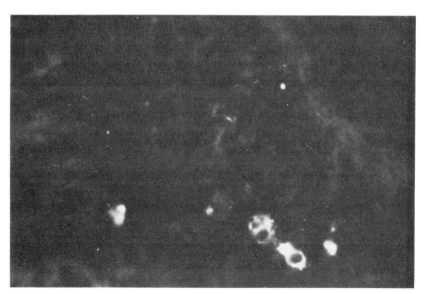

Figure 6-18. IgE-containing plasma cells in connective tissue of inflamed human gingiva as detected by direct immunofluorescence (×500).

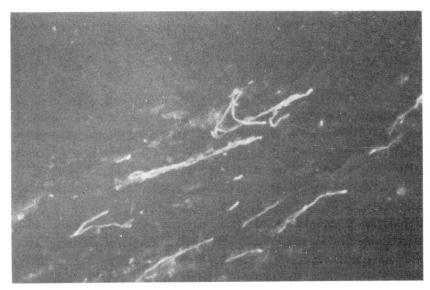

Figure 6-19. IgE coating of filamentous bacteria from subgingival debris.

cur within the gingival crevice. Complement, IgG, and IgM have been detected in gingival crevicular fluid.[89, 90] Quantitative studies of the concentrations of IgG, IgA, and IgM in crevicular fluid indicated their concentrations are similar to serum.[91] The relative concentration of EgG and C3 are lower, however, than those of IgM and IgA.[92] Because the flow rate of crevicular fluid increases with severity of inflammation, the absolute amounts of immunoglobulins would actually increase in periodontal disease. The presence of these components in crevicular fluid makes it possible for cytotoxic reactions to occur. The antigenic specificities for immunoglobulins in crevicular fluid are suggested by the finding (Figure 6-19) that some crevicular bacteria, particularly filamentous forms, have been coated *in vivo* with IgE.[85] This reaction of crevicular bacteria with IgE also makes possible reaginic reactions in the crevice.

Animal experiments have demonstrated the importance of the dose or size of antigenic stimulation.[93] Results suggest that low doses of antigen administered intramucosally stimulate an immune response not only in the local nodes, but also systemically.

Such experiments may relate to humans where serum antibody titers poorly correlate with the amount of local antibodies.[88] Serum antibodies have been described for *Leptotrichia buccalis, Fusobacterium polymorphum, Veillonella alcalescens, Escherichia coli, Treponema microdentium, Actinomyces naeslundii, Actinomyces israelii,* and *Bacterionema matruchotti.*[94-99]

The antibodies in human gingival tissue, gingival fluid, and sera could function protectively by eliminating and controlling antigen entrance into the gingiva, or they could be responsible for the disease in the form of reaginic reactions, cytotoxic reactions, and Arthus reactions. A third possibility is that immunoglobulins react with gingival tissue rather than reacting with bacteria, causing periodontal disease by an autoimmune response similar to that seen in some types of thyroiditis. In a careful study of seventy-six humans with periodontal disease, no such autoantibodies to gingival tissue occurred.[90] Such negative findings in a population of this size make this theory highly doubtful.

Anaphylactic-type reactions to oral bacteria have also correlated with severity of periodontal disease. Skin test reagents prepared from an extract of Actinomyces have provided an *in vivo* test demonstrating that humans have both immediate and delayed reactions to this oral filamentous bacteria.[100] A statistically significant correlation was found between the incidence of immediate hypersensitivity and severity of periodontal disease. Patients with generalized gingivitis evidenced a significantly depressed incidence of immediate hypersensitivity compared to patients with normal gingiva, localized gingivitis, or periodontitis. Preliminary evidence demonstrating an inverse relationship between immediate hypersensitivity and humoral antibody titers suggests a blocking antibody active in generalized gingivitis.

Delayed hypersensitivity has also been detected by an *in vitro* test, lymphocyte transformation, which demonstrated that patients with gingivitis or mild or moderate periodontitis had lymphocytes stimulated by *Actinomyces viscosus, Veillonella alcalescens, Bacteroides melaninogenicus,* and *Fusobacterium fusiforme.*[101] Lymphocyte transformation, however, was significantly depressed in severe periodontitis compared to transformation in mild or moderate periodontitis. A more recent study demonstrated a direct correlation between severity of periodontal disease and lymphocyte transformation in response to plaque antigens.[102] The correlation between severity of periodontal disease and degree of delayed hypersensitivity as measured by lymphocyte transformation is striking. An additional factor which will inhibit lymphocyte transformation has been found in the serum of patients with severe periodontitis. It is possible that severe periodontal disease is associated with the appearance of serum-blocking factors which act to limit the disease.[103]

Thus, it appears that several types of immunopathologic reactions, both antibody mediated and cell mediated, may occur in human periodontal disease. The precise role of these reactions and their interaction with other pathogenic factors in determining the severity of the acute or chronic phases of periodontal disease has yet to be established.

Endotoxin: Potential Pathologic Agent in Periodontal Disease

Endotoxins, lipopolysaccharide cell wall components of Gram-negative bacteria, have a multitude of pathogenic activities.[104-106] Many effects may result from activation of complement, clotting, and the kinin systems. By rendering blood hypercoagulable, endotoxin leads to slow deposition of fibrin aggregates and the formation of small thrombi which interfere with blood flow to tissues.

In addition, endotoxin interferes with removal of fibrin from the blood by the reticuloendothelial system. Endotoxin also causes platelet aggregation with release of serotonin and accumulation of polymorphonuclear leukocytes, followed by accumulation of small lymphocytes and mononuclear leukocytes. Endotoxin increases permeability of cell lysozymes, leading to the release of hydrolases which are normally contained in lysozymes in the inert form. Potentially injurious enzymes are thus released into the surrounding fluid. Bacterial endotoxins may also enhance or inhibit the pathogenicity of infection, depending upon the infecting organism, dose, route of endotoxin injection, and the interval between administration of endotoxin and initiation of infection. A transient increase in susceptibility to infection occurs when endotoxin is injected immediately preceding or shortly before initiation of infection. Such a situation could be found in a gingival pocket. Cellular and subcellular metabolic alterations are also consequences of endotoxin. Changes include increased aerobic glycolysis, hyperglycemia or hypoglycemia, and inhibition of protein synthesis. Endotoxin injection, on the other hand, increases the activity of histidine decarboxylase. This has been interpreted to mean that an increased rate of histamine synthesis occurs, resulting in a disturbance in the homeostatic relationship between histamine and the catecholamines. Several physiological effects of endotoxin such as clotting system activation, anaphylatoxin generation, and chemotaxis appear to occur indirectly through the activation of complement.

The effects of endotoxins isolated from oral bacteria have also been studied. Since endotoxins from all bacteria behave similarly, effects observed with nonoral bacteria should apply to endotoxins from oral bacteria and vice versa. Fusobacteria endotoxin influences infection to oral streptococci.[107] Pretreatment with this endotoxin increases susceptibility to infection during the first six to eight hours, followed by increased resistance after twenty-four hours. Associated with this resistance is an accelerated inflammatory response.[108] Similar influences on local defense mechanisms may occur in periodontal tissues, leading to a disturbance in host-parasite equilibrium.

Since human periodontal disease probably is a response to multiple bacterial challenges, the effects of single and multiple applications of endotoxin have also been studied.[109] Small multiple applications resulted in a similar, but more prolonged leukocytic response than that seen with single larger applications of endotoxins.

In addition to soft tissue effects, endotoxin also causes bone responses. Endotoxins from several bacterial strains including *Bacteroides melaninogenicus* were found to be effective in stimulating bone resorption *in vitro*.[110] This resorption, similar in

TABLE 6-IV

ORAL MICROORGANISMS HAVING ENDOTOXIN ACTIVITY

Actinomyces	(113)
Bacteroides melaninogenicus	(115)
Borrelia buccalis	(115)
Borrelia vincentii	(115)
Fusobacterium nucleatum	(115)
Fusobacterium polymorphum	(112)
Leptotrichia buccalis	(114)
Selenomia sputegena	(115)
Treponema microdentium	(115)
Veillonella	(112, 115)

many respects to that seen with parathyroid hormone, occurs as a result of proliferation of osteoclasts. Recent studies have shown that (1) endotoxin, in addition to stimulating bone resorption on its own, can also potentiate the effects of parathyroid hormone; and (2) heparin, which alone cannot stimulate bone resorption, will potentiate the effects of endotoxin, thus stimulating bone resorption.[111]

The multiplicity of these tissue responses to endotoxin could assume real importance in periodontal disease when one considers the variety of oral microorganisms with demonstrable endotoxin activity which are found in the gingival crevice.[112-115] Some of these microorganisms are listed in Table 6-IV. Not only do crevicular bacteria have endotoxins, but crevicular exudate from periodontitis patients has demonstrable endotoxin activity, suggesting that free endotoxin is present in effective concentrations in the gingival crevice.[116] A correlation was found between quantity of endotoxin in gingival exudate and degree of clinical inflammation.[117] Examination of some endotoxin preparations from oral bacteria suggests that they not only have different potencies (Table 6-V), but are frequently serologically distinct.[118-121] Thus, not all bacteria with endotoxin may be equally important in periodontal disease when one considers the direct actions of endotoxins and their indirect effects as antigens.

Experimentally, the histopathologic effects of endotoxin on rabbit mucosa and gingiva have been examined.[122, 123] A single

TABLE 6-V

RELATIVE POTENCIES IN LOCAL SHWARTZMAN REACTIONS*

Oral Bacteria	Relative Potency
Veillonella alcalescens	1
Leptotrichia buccalis	1
Selenomonas sputigena	1/4
Fusobacterium polymorphum	1/25
Bacteroides melaninogenicus	1/100
Small treponeme	1/100

* Adapted from S. E. Mergenhagen, "Nature and Significance of Somatic Antigens of Oral Bacteria," *J Dent Res, 46:*46, 1967.[120]

injection into a palatogingival site resulted in gross abscesses evident for up to ten days with involvement of lamina propria, bone, and epithelium. A neutrophilic infiltrate occurred early, followed later by increased numbers of macrophages, and still later by increased numbers of lymphocytes. Fibrinoid thrombi were found in the blood vessels. By eighteen hours, increased numbers of osteoclasts and well-developed resorption lacunae were found on bone underlying the site of injection.

It is not yet clear at what stage endotoxin plays a role in periodontal disease. It is reasonable to expect that in the later stages of gingivitis and in periodontitis, during which the crevicular epithelium is ulcerated and very permeable, that endotoxin has easy entrance to the periodontal tissues and plays a major role in soft tissue and bone destruction.

Enzymes: Potential Pathogenic Agents in Periodontal Disease

Many crevicular microorganisms elaborate enzymes which are capable of hydrolyzing gingival tissue substrates. If these enzymes accumulate in sufficient quantity within the gingival crevice and enter the tissue, periodontal pathology may occur. Some of the bacterial enzymes which could assume importance in periodontal disease are listed in Table 6-VI. This list includes enzymes active against connective tissue matrix, ground substance, epithelial intercellular matrix, cellular components of blood, and cell components of the tissue.[124-133]

TABLE 6-VI

BACTERIAL ENZYMES POTENTIALLY ACTIVE IN
PERIODONTAL DISEASES

Enzyme	Source of Enzyme
Chondroitin sulfatase	Microaerophilic diphtheroids[124]
Coagulase	Staphylococci[125]
Collagenase	*Bacteroides melaninogenicus*[126]
Deoxyribonuclease	Diphtheroids, bacteroides[126]
Fibrinolysin	*Bacteroides melaninogenicus*[126]
Gelatinase	Unfiltered gingival debris[127]
Glucuronidase	*Streptococcus mitis, Streptococcus salivarius,* staphylococci diphtheroids[128]
Hyaluronidase	Peptostreptococci, staphylococci diphtheroids, enterococci, B-hemolytic streptococci, *Streptococcus mitis, Streptococcus salivarius*[128, 129]
Kinase	Group A hemolytic streptococci, some staphylococci[125]
Neuraminidase	Subgingival bacteria, Gram-positive cocci and rods, Gram-negative cocci and rods, some strains *S. mitis* and *S. sanguis*[130, 131]
Protease	Unfiltered gingival debris[127, 132, 133]
Ribonuclease	Diphtheroids, bacteroides[126]

If bacterial enzymes are important in the pathogenesis of periodontal disease, some quantitative increase in the amount of enzyme or in the number of bacteria producing these enzymes would be expected in periodontal pockets. Schultz-Haudt and Scherp[124] have studied this question; results of their experiments

TABLE 6-VII

PRODUCTION OF HYALURONIDASE AND BETA-GLUCURONIDASE
BY SUBGINGIVAL STREPTOCOCCI*

	Hyaluronidase		Beta-Glucuronidase	
	Subjects (N = 17)†	Strains (N = 121)‡	Subjects (N = 17)	Strains (N = 121)
Gingival Condition	%	%	%	%
Normal	29	6	0	0
Gingivitis	100	47	60	23

* Adapted from S. D. Schultz-Haudt and H. W. Scherp, *J Dent Res*, 34:924, 1955.[128]

† Percentage of subjects with bacterial strains producing hyaluronidase or beta-glucuronidase.

‡ Percentage of isolated strains producing enzyme.

are illustrated in Table 6-VII. They examined individuals with gingivitis and normal gingiva to detect bacterial strains from the gingival crevice that produce hyaluronidase or beta-glucuronidase, and in each individual they determined the number of bacterial strains that produce these enzymes. Results indicated that a significantly greater percentage of individuals with gingivitis had strains of subgingival bacteria producing these enzymes. In gingivitis there was also a significantly greater percentage of the gingival flora capable of producing these enzymes. Thus, in gingivitis an alteration in bacterial flora led to potentially greater amounts of enzymes. Similar studies of chondroitin sulfatase did not reveal clear-cut differences between normal and gingivitis subjects.[124] Levels of neuraminidase in saliva also did not correlate with periodontal disease severity.[134]

In vivo evidence of the tissue-destroying capacity of bacterial enzymes comes from studies in which hyaluronidase was injected into monkey gingival tissue and found to duplicate some of the histopathology seen in human periodontal disease.[135] Changes included disruption of connective tissue and subsequent downgrowth of epithelium with periodontal pocket formation.

In addition to bacterial enzymes in the gingival environment, there is evidence for the production of tissue or endogenous (nonbacterial) enzymes in the periodontium during periodontal disease. Because of the extensive connective tissue breakdown observed in periodontal disease, much effort has gone into studying collagenase. Endogenous collagenase activity was found in gingival explants from patients with periodontitis but not in explants from normal human gingiva.[136] This collaganese activity appeared to be associated with inflammatory foci and accumulation of immunoglobulins. Recent evidence has demonstrated collagenase production by both epithelial and connective tissue cells of human gingiva.[137] The mechanism responsible for release of endogenous collagenase remains elusive. One theory suggests that a hypersensitivity reaction to the microbial antigens is at least partially responsible.

MICROBIOLOGY OF ACUTE NECROTIZING ULCERATIVE GINGIVITIS

Acute necrotizing ulcerative gingivitis (ANUG) is considered separately from gingivitis and periodontitis. This separation is based on differences in clinical signs, symptoms, epidemiology, and bacteriology between ANUG and the gingivitis-periodontitis form of periodontal disease.

Originally ANUG was considered a fusospirochetal infection. This concept developed from examination of direct smears taken superficially from areas of necrosis in which *Borellia vincentii* and *Fusobacterium fusiformis* were identified. Examination of biopsy specimens by electron microscopy, however, allows a different interpretation. Tissue specimens from an ulcerated lesion could arbitrarily be divided into four main zones.[138] Starting with the most superficial layer, these zones were the bacterial zone, the neutrophile-rich zone, the necrotic zone, and the zone of spirochetal infiltration.

Within the outer *bacterial zone,* many bacterial forms were seen; however, it was only possible to identify spirochetes with certainty because of their characteristic morphology as seen in thin sections. The spirochetes were small, intermediate, and large types. The *neutrophile-rich zone,* consisting mainly of neutrophiles, was infiltrated with a variety of bacteria including spirochetes. In the *necrotic zone* overlying the ulcerated lesions, spirochetes were found in large numbers with few other bacteria present. The zone of *spirochetal infiltration,* the deepest site of bacterial penetration, occurred approximately 250μ beneath the ulcerated surface within normal-appearing tissue. There were, however, areas of lysis containing clumps of spirochetes. These spirochetes included primarily the intermediate and large variety with very few small spirochetes present. Spirochetes were also observed within the intercellular spaces of the epithelium adjacent to the ulcer.

Attempts to identify the predominant spirochetes within the lesion revealed their difference from *Treponema microdentium* and *Borrelia vincentii* in the size and/or number of axial fibrils.[139] The spirochetes seen in tissue from patients with ANUG could not be detected in samples of dental plaque from periodontally normal individuals or in plaque or tissue from individuals with acute periocoronitis or severe gingivitis.

Because of conflicting evidence about the numbers of small-size spirochetes seen deep in ANUG tissue and difficulties in identification of spirochetes in ultrathin sections of tissue, scrapings of lesions have also been studied.[140, 141] In pooled scrapings from lesions, median values for small, intermediate, and large spirochetes were 28 percent, 72 percent, and 3 percent, respectively. If spirochetes with six or fewer fibrils are identical to *Borrelia vincentii*, the results indicate that spirochetes with seven or more fibrils tend to outnumber *Borrelia vincentii* in pooled scrapings of ANUG lesions and appear in larger percentages in deeper portions of the lesions.

The main issue is whether spirochetes have actually caused the lesion seen in ANUG or are simply saprophytic organisms taking advantage of cultural conditions within the tissue. Some evidence suggests that spirochetes do cause tissue lesions. Certainly the best example would be syphilitic lesions caused by *Treponema pallidum*, in which the spirochete is the only organism implicated. Oral spirochetes including a small oral treponema (possibly *Treponema microdentium*), *Borrelia vincentii*, and *Borrelia buccalis* injected subcutaneously as monocontaminants into animals cause localized infections terminating in abscesses.[142] These abscesses reach maximum intensity in five to seven days and persist up to one month. Similar lesions occurring with heat-killed or fragmented cells suggest the importance of a spirochete endotoxin. Injection of a cell-free filtrate from a culture of an oral microaerophilic diphtheroid containing hyaluronidase and chondroitinase or injection of the diphtheroid itself led to enhancement and extension of the lesion without abscess formation. Frequently, clusters of spirochetes were located in the normal surrounding tissue. Human ANUG presents a similar possibility for potentiation of response by tissue-destroying enzymes. Intracutaneous injection of pure cultures of *Fusobacterium nucleatum* or *Fusobacterium polymorphum* led to abscesses similar to those observed with spirochetes.[143] Fusobacteria also have been shown to have endotoxins.[144] When fusobacteria and spirochetes were injected together there was a synergistic effect with formation of fulminating abscesses and invasion of both organisms into the surrounding tissues. These studies of experimentally induced spirochetal, fusobacterial, and fusospirochetal infections lend support to the potential pathogenicity of oral fusobacteria and oral spirochetes.

Immunologic studies of ANUG have attempted to clarify the specific organisms implicated in ANUG and determine if any changes in immune responses occur during the disease.[145, 146] No significant differences in serum antibody titers to *B. vincentii, F. fusiformis, B. melaninogenicus Candida albicans, Actinomyces viscosus,* or *Veillonella alcalescens* were observed in ANUG patients, normal patients, or in those with recurrent ulcerative gingivitis. Where studied, no rise in antibody titers took place during the convalescent phase of the disease as is usually found when there is an etiologic relationship between an organism and a disease. Cell-mediated immunity as measured by the Lymphocyte Transformation Test showed significantly greater responses to *O. viscosus, V. alcalescens, B. melaninogenicus,* and *F. fusiforme* in ANUG patients as compared to controls. Except for responses to *F. fusiforme,* which were significantly greater in ANUG, similarly high responses were also seen in patients with chronic marginal gingivitis. Similarities in cell-mediated immunity observed in ANUG and gingivitis patients suggests that ANUG may have been superimposed on a preexisting gingivitis. The significantly greater cell-mediated immunity to *F. fusiforme* in ANUG suggests that this organism might be involved in the change to ANUG from gingivitis.

Current evidence permits the theory that specific spirochetes and possibly other bacteria cause ANUG by an invasion of periodontal tissue, a process which may be facilitated by tissue-destroying enzymes from other bacteria. As the number of spirochetes increase, the endotoxin levels in tissue increase, causing necrotic tissue changes. In addition, changes in host immune responses occurring before, concurrently, or after tissue invasion may be protective or destructive.

ANUG was once thought to be communicable. Experimental

attempts to transmit the disease have been uniformly unsuccessful. ANUG may be a transmissible disease, although as yet conditions for transmission have not been found. It is clearly not a highly contagious disease as was once thought.

ANUG tends to recur.[147] These authors analyzed the factors involved in recurrence of sixty-one cases of ANUG and found that recurrence is most frequently associated with persistence of gingival deformity leading to difficulty in eliminating local factors such as plaque. These findings emphasize the role of extrameticulous plaque control in individuals who have had ANUG. It is reasonable to treat these patients surgically to eliminate the gingival defects if they otherwise cannot maintain plaque control. Recurrence of ANUG should be avoided since it can lead to extensive interproximal bone loss, a condition which might then be referred to as acute necrotizing, ulcerative periodontitis (ANUP).

HOST RESISTANCE TO PERIODONTAL DISEASE

Even though the prevalence of inflammatory periodontal disease is almost universal, some host resistance can be postulated. Certainly, most dentists are familiar with traumatic periodontal injuries and surgical periodontal procedures where not only soft tissue, but also alveolar bone is exposed to the highly septic oral environment for periods ranging from minutes to days. Generally, even without antibiotic coverage, these lesions heal rapidly. This suggests that during the time in which the lesion has not healed sufficiently to isolate the tissues from oral microorganisms, the host tissue must be able to control and prevent a bacterial infection. In addition, in periodontal disease it is known that a reduction in bacteria through scaling decreases periodontal inflammation, and inflammation can be entirely prevented by decreasing bacterial plaque formation.

While several explanations are conceivable, it is possible that periodontal disease occurs only after an overload of the host defense mechanisms or when a critical threshold is reached. That is to say, the host has a weak defense against crevicular bacteria or products entering crevicular tissue and only limited control on plaque formation by bacteria. Once some critical number of bacteria, which varies for each individual, is reached, the host defenses are inadequate and periodontal disease ensues. Obviously, an alternate or concomitant possibility is that the host over-reacts in a hypersensitivity response which is seen as periodontal disease. This situation will be discussed elsewhere.

What host factors may play a role in modifying, preventing, or controlling periodontal disease? These factors include physical, biochemical, and immunologic activities, some of which could be effective in the gingiva and some effective within the tissue.

Present evidence suggests several possible defenses in the gingival crevice. The gingival fluid bathing this area contains immunoglobulins (IgG, IgA, IgM, and IgE) and complement. Reaction of antibodies with bacteria may enhance phagocytosis, or subsequent complement activation may lead to cell lysis. Many polymorphonuclear leukocytes are found in the gingival crevice where there is inflammation. These cells may function in the phagocytosis of bacteria or in the release of lysozyme. Lysozyme, which has been reported in pocket fluid in higher concentrations than serum,[148] could also contribute to lysis of bacteria. One study has demonstrated at least two antibacterial mechanisms in the rabbit gingival sulcus *in situ* killing and mechanical removal.[149] The viability of *Serratia marcescens* placed in the sulcus rapidly decreased from 67 percent after one minute to 0 percent after sixty minutes. At the same time bacteria were quickly mechanically removed. Only a small percentage of inoculated bacteria could be recovered by ten minutes, and virtually complete elimination had occurred by one hundred twenty minutes.

Within the gingival tissues, all normal body defense mechanisms may be operative. Such defenses include phagocytosis, complement-mediated immune lysis, and lysozyme release. In fact, disruption of these defense mechanisms, which occurs in cyclic neutropenia and agranulocytosis, may account for the severe periodontal disease seen in individuals with these diseases.

CONTROL OF PERIODONTAL DISEASE BY
NONMECHANICAL MEASURES

Since gingivitis and periodontitis are primarily bacterial diseases, these diseases are controlled by preventing the subgingival bacteria from either colonizing the tooth as plaque or growing free in the crevice. The dental profession currently can offer the public mechanical prevention measures, which are very effective if routinely followed. This approach, however, has not been as successful as expected. To be more effective and reach a greater proportion of the population, measures amenable to use with large populations, i.e. public health measures, may be necessary. This permits a passive, more effortless patient participation compared to current mechanical plaque disposal methods which usually require concentrated instruction, close supervision, regular monitoring, and reinforcement.

Plaque control through chemical or biological procedures may provide modes of periodontal disease prevention in the future. Biological procedures are presently only theoretical with little experimental data demonstrating their application. These biological procedures include (1) immunization against specific bacteria or groups of bacteria, (2) interference with the important biochemical or cellular mediation of periodontal inflammation, and (3) increasing the resistance of alveolar bone to resorption as is projected with fluoride.

Chemical methods of disease control are nearer at hand. Included in this group are enzymes, antibiotics, and disinfectants in the form of mouthwashes and toothpastes or gum which could inhibit plaque or calculus and thereby control periodontal disease. These agents have met with considerable success in periodontal disease control, and it is worthwhile considering the possible characteristics of an ideal antiperiodontal disease agent. Although these agents generally have been considered as either "antiplaque" or "anticalculus" agents, this terminology is too limited. As newer agents are introduced, clinicians hope to avoid a shotgun approach which disrupts the entire local bacterial ecology in preventing plaque and calculus. Instead, agents may be employed that affect only those portions of plaque or calculus which are important in the pathogenesis of periodontal disease. The primary goal of any agent is not plaque or calculus control but control of periodontal disease.

Two activities of an antiperiodontal disease agent may be considered: the effects on bacteria and the effects on the host. Bacteriologically, the chemotherapeutic agent should alter sufficiently the microbial character of plaque and calculus to prevent periodontal disease. It is currently thought that rendering plaque nonpathogenic may be sufficient. Secondly, the agent must not lead to superinfection of the mouth or other areas of the body. Superinfection may be prevented by modifying the microbial spectrum of the agent to include possible superinfecting organisms or by using agent delivery methods that localize its effects to the gingival area. Lastly, the agent should not adversely disrupt the gastrointestinal flora.

The possible unfavorable biological effects of an antiperiodontal disease agent on the host must also be evaluated. Any agent must be hypoallergenic. Because of the extended long-term exposure, allergic manifestations must be carefully studied in experimental animals. The agent must be noncarcinogenic; long-term tissue contact makes this of considerable importance. Lastly, there should be no adverse direct effects on the periodontium, tooth structure, and other oral areas in contact with the agent. Specific evaluation of the periodontium must include epithelial detachment, epithelial attachment, and collagen metabolism. Important changes in tooth structure would include staining and loss of tooth structure. Other undesirable changes to be evaluated in the oral cavity include loss of taste, paresthesia, and hyperkeratosis.

Several approaches utilizing chemical agents have been attempted to control periodontal disease clinically. These include agents that affect attachment of bacteria and organic matrices to teeth, alter the nature of plaque and affect the salts of calculus.[150]

One promising area of interest is the prevention of bacterial attachment and/or organic matrices to the teeth. Oral bacteria are known to adhere selectively to different oral surfaces.[28, 29] As an example, *Streptoccus salivarius* and *S. sanguis,* which are commonly found in significant numbers on epithelial surfaces, show a definite capacity to adhere to epithelial cells and not to enamel. In contrast, *S. mutans,* which are commonly found in large numbers on enamel surfaces and not on epithelial surfaces, selectively adhere to enamel powder. An attempt to duplicate pellicle on enamel by treating enamel powder with saliva frequently increased the percentage of adsorbed bacteria as is seen with *Actinomyces visosus.* On the other hand, saliva treatment of enamel sometimes decreased adsorption as occurs with some strains of *S. sanguis.* This decreased adherence may be explained by some salivary factor. Identification and exploitation of this factor may provide a preventive measure.

Another mechanism of bacterial adhesion to the tooth and to other bacteria involves the adhesive, bacterial polysaccharide dextran. Two approaches to studying this mechanism have been utilized. One is the use of the enzyme dextranase. Initial studies with dextranase in hamsters revealed its effectiveness in plaque reduction and suggested a reduction in alveolar bone loss.[151] Subsequent human studies utilizing dextranase as a mouthwash have met with only limited success.[152] A partial explanation may be that other mechanisms of bacterial adherence to teeth are important in humans or that a mouthwash is ineffective in getting adequate amounts of active enzyme to the gingival area for sufficient lengths of time. Many other enzyme preparations in the form of dentifrices or chewing gums have been tested, including proteolytic enzymes and carbohydrate-hydrolyzing enzymes. These have been clinically ineffective.

A second approach to controlling dextran-mediated adherence is competitive inhibition of the enzymatic synthesis of insoluble, high-molecular weight dextran.[153] In animal experiments, addition of 16 percent low-molecular weight dextran to the diet effectively prevents formation of gelatinous plaque. This low-molecular weight dextran does not prevent colonization by the organism, but it does inhibit the organism's ability to form gelatinous deposits on tooth surfaces. There is apparently a receptor site on *S. mutans,* possibly dextransucrase, which agglutinates with high-molecular weight dextran.[154] A competitive inhibition occurs with low-molecular weight dextran which is not large enough to bridge the space between two bacteria. Additions of dextrans to food products containing sucrose could attenuate the plaque-forming potential of the streptococci; however, many clinical experiments with low-molecular weight dextran have been disappointing.[155]

Several antimicrobial agents have been tested for their ability to control plaque. These include both antibiotics and disinfectants. Some antibiotic studies suggest systemic antibiotics such as penicillin, erythromycin, lincomycin, and tetracycline may be partially effective in plaque control.[156, 157] Because of their frequent systemic usage, however, there is a danger of sensitization and subsequent anaphylaxis by the topical oral route. Penicillin in particular frequently leads to allergy when applied topically as in the oral cavity. Researchers have also tested other antibiotics with low allergenicity on topical application such as vancomycin, spiramycin, kanamycin sulfate, CC 10232, polymyxin B, neomycin, bacitracin, and thiostrepton.[158-160] Some antibiotics such as bacitracin, neomycin, and thiostrepton had no effect on plaque formation. Other topical antibiotics had varying success in controlling plaque. Most studies to date have examined only short-term effects. Long-term administration of antibiotics not only leads to allergies, but also alters the basic flora of plaque[160] and/or allows emergence of resistant strains of bacteria. For example, vancomycin initially appeared useful in a short-term eight-day study for controlling plaque.[158] However, during a three-week period of no oral hygiene utilizing the experimental gingivitis model, the flora changed, but plaque accumulation and gingivitis developed at the same rate as in controls not taking vancomycin.[160] Similar initial improvements in gingivitis scores resulted from kanamycin treatment; but by the fourth to eighth week after antibiotic treatment, no differences in gingivitis were seen between the subjects and controls.[162] At present, research indicates that no antibiotic tested is proven for routine clinical usage as a plaque control agent. Future research in this area may prove fruitful.

Other antimicrobial agents have been tested for plaque control. These include fluoride compounds, laurylsulfates, chlorophyll derivates, hexachlorophene, polyvinylpyrrolidone-iodine complex (Betadine®), benzethonium chloride, cetylpyridinium chloride, chlormethyl analogue of victamine C, chlorhexidine, alcohols, iodophores, quaternary ammonium bases, and guanadines.[159, 161, 163–165] Only the fluorides, benzethonium chloride, cetylpyridinium chloride, chlormethyl analogue of vitamine C, and chlorhexidine reduced plaque formation. As with the antibiotic studies, many of these agents were only tested on a short-term basis. Long-term results must await further experiments. Chlorhexidine has been tested for up to four weeks during which plaque did not form, and gingivitis did not develop. Part of the success of chlorhexidine may result from its adsorption to tooth surfaces, pellicle, plaque, and mucous membranes with release when the concentration in the environment is low.[166] Its undesirable side effects include disturbed taste sensation, brown staining of teeth, and occasionally oral ulceration. Some of these side effects may be eliminated by varying the concentration or the mode of application, or by modifying the molecule.

The last agents of interest in control of periodontal disease are those which affect the salts of calculus. These agents would be expected to inhibit most calculus formation if they prevent plaque formation. For example, both erythromycin and CC 10232, antibiotics which decrease plaque formation, also reduce calculus deposition.[167, 168] One agent of particular interest is disodium etidronate, a crystal-growth inhibitor.[169] Over a six-month study there was a significant protection against new calculus formation and no adverse changes in the oral tissues. Anticalculus agents that act by dissolving calculus have also been studied. These agents may ultimately prove to be of little value since they frequently dissolve dentin and enamel as well.[170]

None of the agents currently being considered for periodontal disease protection have been studied beyond initial observations of their effects on periodontal disease. Before these agents become available clinically, their effects on bacteria, plaque, and calculus must be evaluated and their effects on the host must be studied.

SUMMARY AND CONCLUSIONS

1. Gingivitis and periodontitis are bacterial diseases. These diseases are, therefore, a result of poor oral hygiene which allows plaque development near the gingival tissues. At the present time, regular removal of microbial dental plaque affords the best method for periodontal disease prevention.

2. Bacteria from the gingiva have a multitude of pathogenic capabilities and are capable of producing periodontal disease experimentally. Several modes of bacterial action probably play a role in disease. The etiologic bacteria and mechanisms of action in gingivitis and periodontitis may vary from individual to individual. The etiologic bacteria and operative bacterial mechanisms in disease may differ for gingivitis and periodontitis.

3. Acute necrotizing ulcerative gingivitis probably differs from gingivitis and periodontitis in causative bacteria and pathogenesis.

4. Plaque control by mechanical methods currently affords the best method for control. Future prospects for control of periodontal disease include procedures based on the mechanisms of plaque attachment to teeth, host responses to the bacteria, and actions of bacterial products.

REFERENCES

1. J. C. Greene, "Oral Hygiene and Periodontal Diseases," *Am J Public Health*, 53:913, 1963.
2. A. L. Russell, "A System of Classification and Scoring for the Prevalence Surveys of Periodontal Diseases," *J Dent Res*, 35:350, 1956.
3. J. C. Greene and J. R. Vermillion, "The Simplified Oral Hygiene Index," *JADA*, 68:7, 1964.
4. O. Schei, J. Waerhaug, A. Lovdal, and A. Arno, "Alveolar Bone Loss as Related to Oral Hygiene and Age," *J Periodontol*, 30:7, 1959.
5. A. Lovdal, A. Arno, O. Schei, and J. Waerhaug, "Combined Effect of Subgingival Scaling and Controlled Oral Hygiene on the Incidence of Gingivitis," *Acta Odontol Scand*, 19:537, 1961.
6. J. D. Suomi, J. C. Greene, J. R. Vermillion, J. Doyle, J. L. Chang, and E. C. Leatherwood, "The Effect of Controlled Oral Hygiene Procedures on the Progression of Periodontal Disease in Adults: Results after Third and Final Year," *J Periodontol*, 42:152, 1971.
7. J. D. Suomi, T. D. West, J. J. Change, and B. J. McClendon, "The Effect of Controlled Oral Hygiene Procedures on the Progression of

Periodontal Disease in Adults: Radiographic Findings," *J Periodontol, 42*:562, 1971.

8. S. P. Ramfjord, "Indices for Prevalence and Incidence of Periodontal Disease," *J Periodontol, 30*:51, 1959.

9. H. Löe, E. Theilade, and S. B. Jensen, "Experimental Gingivitis in Man," *J Periodontol, 36*:177, 1965.

10. E. Theilade, W. H. Wright, S. B. Jensen, and H. Löe, "Experimental Gingivitis in Man. II. A Longitudinal Clinical and Bacteriological Investigation," *J Periodont Res, 1*:1, 1966.

11. I. D. Mandel, "Dental Plaque: Nature, Formation and Effects," *J Periodontol, 37*:357, 1966.

12. R. S. Schwartz and M. Massler, "Tooth Accumulated Materials: A Review and Classification," *J Periodontol, 40*:407, 1969.

13. A. E. Poole and M. N. Gilmour, "The Variability of Unstandardized Plaques Obtained from Single or Multiple Subjects," *Arch Oral Biol, 16*:681, 1971.

14. S. S. Socransky, R. J. Gibbons, A. C. Dale, L. Bortnick, E. Rosenthal, and J. B. MacDonald, "The Microbiota of the Gingival Crevice Area of Man: I. Total Microscope and Viable Counts and Counts of Specific Organisms," *Arch Oral Biol, 8*:275, 1963.

15. A. Strailfor, "Investigations into the Bacterial Chemistry of Dental Plaques," *Odontol T, 58*:155, 1950.

16. R. J. Gibbons, S. S. Socransky, S. Sawyer, B. Kapsimalis, and J. B. MacDonald, "The Microbiota of the Gingival Crevice of Man. II. The Predominant Cultivable Microbiota of Dental Plaque," *Arch Oral Biol, 8*:281, 1963.

17. R. J. Gibbons, S. S. Socransky, W. C. deAraujo, and J. van Houte, "Studies of the Predominant Cultivable Microbiota of Dental Plaque," *Arch Oral Biol, 9*:365, 1964.

18. H. L. Ritz, "Microbial Population Shifts in Developing Human Dental Plaque," *Arch Oral Biol, 12*:1561, 1967.

19. A. Salkind, H. Oshrain, and I. D. Mandel, "Bacterial Aspects of Developing Supragingival and Subgingival Plaque," *J Periodontol, 42*:706, 1971.

20. W. W. Wantland and E. M. Wantland, "Incidence, Ecology and Reproduction of Oral Protozoa," *J Dent Res, 39*:863, 1960.

21. D. S. Gottlieb and L. H. Miller, "Entamoeba Gingivalis in Periodontal Disease," *J Periodontol, 42*:412, 1971.

22. C. Dawes, "The Nature of Dental Plaque, Films and Calcareous Deposits," *Ann NY Acad Sci, 153*:102, 1968.

23. I. D. Mandel, "Plaque and Calculus," *Ala J Med Sci, 5*:313, 1968.

24. S. S. Socransky, "Relationship of Bacteria to the Etiology of Periodontal Disease," *J Dent Res, 49*:203, 1970.

25. P. Critchley and C. A. Saxton, "The Metabolism of Gingival Plaque," *Int Dent J, 20:*408, 1970.
26. H. E. Schroeder, "The Structure and Relationship of Plaque to the Hard and Soft Tissues: Electron Microscopic Interpretation," *Int Dent J, 20:*353, 1970.
27. S. S. Socransky, A. D. Manganiello, J. V. Oram, D. Propas, I. L. Dogan, and J. van Houte, "Development of Early Dental Plaque," *IADR Abstracts,* March 1971.
28. J. D. Hillman, J. van Houte, and R. J. Gibbons, "Sorption of Bacteria to Human Enamel Powder," *Arch Oral Biol, 15:*899, 1970.
29. R. J. Gibbons and J. van Houte, "Selective Bacterial Adherence to Oral Epithelial Surfaces and its Role as an Ecological Determinant," *Infection and Immunity, 3:*567, 1971.
30. W. A. McDougall, "Studies on the Dental Plaque. I. The Histology of the Dental Plaque and its Attachment," *Aust Dent J, 8:*261, 1963.
31. H. M. Colbe, "Transitory Bacteremia," *Oral Surg Oral Med Oral Pathol, 7:*609, 1954.
32. M. Murray and F. Moosnick, "Incidence of Bacteremia in Patients with Dental Disease," *J Lab Clin Med, 26:*801, 1941.
33. H. D. Corner, S. Hamberman, C. K. Collings, and T. E. Winford, "Bacteremias Following Periodontal Scaling in Patients with Healthy Appearing Gingiva," *J Periodontol, 38:*466, 1967.
34. P. R. Courant and H. Bader, "Bacteroides melaninogenicus and its Products in the Gingiva of Man," *Periodontics, 4:*131, 1966.
35. T. E. Winford and S. Haberman, "Isolation of Aerobic Gram-positive Filamentous Rods from Diseased Gingiva," *J Dent Res, 45:*1159, 1966.
36. F. W. Wertheimer, "A Histologic Study of Microorganisms and Human Periodontal Tissues," *J Periodontol, 35:*406, 1964.
37. S. Haberman, "Inflammatory and Non-inflammatory Responses to Gingival Invasion by Microorganisms," *J Periodontol, 30:*190, 1959.
38. G. W. Burnett and H. W. Scherp, *Oral Microbiology and Infectious Disease,* 3rd ed. (Baltimore, Williams & Wilkins, 1968).
39. D. H. Fine, J. L. Perchersky and D. H. McKibben, "The Penetration of Human Gingival Sulcular Tissue by Carbon Particles," *Arch Oral Biol, 14:*1117, 1969.
40. P. A. Patcliff, "Permeability of Healthy Gingival Epithelium of Microscopically Observable Particles," *J Periodontol, 37:*291, 1966.
41. A. A. Rizzo, "Histologic and Immunologic Evaluation of Antigen Penetration into Oral Tissues After Topical Application," *J Periodontol, 41:*210, 1970.
42. S. Rovin, E. R. Costich, and H. A. Gordon, "The Influence of Bacteria and Irritation in the Initiation of Periodontal Disease in Germfree and Conventional Rats," *J Periodont Res, 1:*193, 1966.

43. D. L. Allen and D. A. Kerr, "Tissue Response in the Guinea Pig to Sterile and Non-Sterile Calculus," *J Periodontol, 36:*121, 1965.

44. J. B. MacDonald, R. J. Gibbons, and S. S. Socransky, "Bacterial Mechanisms in Periodontal Disease," *Ann NY Acad Sci, 85:*467, 1960.

45. J. B. MacDonald, S. S. Socransky and R. J. Gibbons, "Aspects of the Pathogenesis of Mixed Anaerobic Infections of Mucous Membranes," *J Dent Res, 42:*529, 1963.

46. S. S. Socransky, "Relationship of Bacteria to the Etiology of Periodontal Disease," *J Dent Res, 49:*203, 1970.

47. H. V. Jordan, R. J. Fitzgerald, and H. R. Stanley, "Plaque Formation and Periodontal Pathology in Gnotobiotic Rats Infected with an Oral Actinomycete," *Am J Pathol, 47:*1158, 1965.

48. P. J. Gibbons, K. S. Berman, P. Knoettner and B. Kapsimalis, "Dental Caries and Alveolar Bone Loss in Gnotobiotic Rats Infected with Capsule Forming Streptococci of Human Origin," *Arch Oral Biol, 11:*549, 1966.

49. S. S. Socransky, C. Hubersak, and D. Propas, "Induction of Periodontal Destruction in Gnotobiotic Rats by a Human Oral Strain of *Actinomyces naeslundii,*" *Arch Oral Biol, 15:*993, 1970.

50. H. V. Jordan and P. H. Keyes, "Aerobic, Gram-positive, Filamentous Bacteria as Etiologic Agents of Experimental Periodontal Disease in Hamsters," *Arch Oral Biol, 9:*401, 1964.

51. H. V. Jordan and B. F. Hammond, "Filamentous Bacteria Isolated from Human Root Surface Caries, *Arch Oral Biol, 17:*1333, 1972.

52. H. V. Jordan, P. H. Keyes, and S. Bellock, "Periodontal Lesions in Hamsters and Gnotobiotic Rats Infected with Actinomyces of Human Origin," *J Periodont Res, 7:*21, 1972.

53. D. S. Dick and J. R. Shaw, "The Infectious and Transmissible Nature of the Periodontal Syndrome of the Rice Rat," *Arch Oral Biol, 11* 1095, 1966.

54. D. S. Dick, J. H. Shaw, and S. S. Socransky, "Further Studies on the Microbial Agent or Agents Responsible for the Periodontal Syndrome in the Rice Rat," *Arch Oral Biol, 13:*215, 1968.

55. G. Shklar and M. M. Cohen, "The Development of Periodontal Disease in Experimental Animals Infected with Polyoma Virus," *Periodontics, 3:*281, 1965.

56. P. N. Baer and L. Kilham, "Rat Virus and Periodontal Disease. III. The Histopathology of the Early Lesion in the First Molar," *Oral Surg Oral Med Oral Pathol, 17:*116, 1964.

57. P. G. H. Gell and R. R. A. Coombs (Eds.), *Clinical Aspects of Immunology,* 2nd ed. (Philadelphia, Davis, 1968).

58. J. R. David, "The Elusive Humors of the Lymphocyte Mediators of Delayed Hypersensitivity," *J Allergy Clin Immunol, 47:*237, 1971.

59. C. G. Craddock, R. Longmire, and R. McMillan, "Lymphocytes and the Immune Response (Second of Two Parts)," *N Engl J Med,* 285:378, 1971.

60. H. J. Muller-Eberhard, "Complement," *Ann Rev Biochem,* 38:389, 1969.

61. S. E. Mergenhagen, T. R. Tempel, and R. Snyderman, "Immunologic Reactions and Periodontal Inflammation," *J Dent Res,* 49:256, 1970.

62. H. B. Fell, "Role of Biological Membranes in Some Skeletal Reactions," *Ann Rheum Dis,* 28:213, 1969.

63. R. Sacco, E. Hausmann, and R. Genco, "Immunologically Activated Factors: Stimulation of Bone Resorption in Tissue Culture," *IADR Abstracts,* 1972.

64. D. A. Grant and B. Orban, "Leukocytes in the Epithelial Attachment," *J Periodontol,* 31:87, 1960.

65. M. Cattoni, "Lymphocytes in the Epithelium of Healthy Gingiva," *J. Dent Res,* 30:627, 1951.

66. P. D. Toto, "Plasma Cells in Inflamed Oral Mucosa," *Dent Prog, 1:* 199, 1961.

67. P. D. Toto, R. J. Pollock, and A. W. Gargiulo, "Pathogenesis of Periodontitis," *Periodontics,* 2:197, 1964.

68. J. W. Wittmer, E. H. Dickler, and P. D. Toto, "Comparative Frequencies of Plasma Cells and Lymphocytes in Gingivitis," *J Periodontol,* 40:274, 1969.

69. B. U. Zachrisson, "Mast Cells of the Human Gingiva. II. Metachromatic Cells at Low pH in Healthy and Inflamed Tissue," *J Periodont Res,* 2:87, 1967.

70. L. E. Shelton and W. B. Hall, "Human Gingival Mast Cells," *J Periodont Res,* 2:214, 1968.

71. H. L. Freedman, M. A. Listgarten, and N. S. Taichman, "Electron Microscopic Features of Chronically Inflamed Human Gingiva,"

72. R. L. Nelson, H. I. Katz, and A. S. Aelickson, "An Electron Microscope Study of the Immediate Type Hypersensitivity Reaction," *Ann Allergy,* 26:281, 1968.

73. P. Goldhaber, "Tissue Culture Studies of Bone as a Model System for Periodontal Research," *J Dent Res,* 50:278, 1971.

74. R. Barrickman, M. Callerame, and J. Candemi, "Gingivitis in Hypogammaglobulinemic Patients," *IADR Abstracts,* No. 329, 1971.

75. S. E. Mergenhagen and A. A. Rizzo, "Allergic Response of Oral Mucosa to Foreign Protein," *J Dent Res,* 40:695, 1961.

76. J. D. Spouge and B. S. Cutler, "Hypersensitivity Reactions in Mucous Membranes. II. An Investigation into Induced Hypersensitivity Lesions in the Mucous Membranes of Laboratory Animals," *Oral Surg Oral Med Oral Pathol,* 16:539, 1963.

77. D. Adams, J. J. Williamson, and A. E. Dolby, "Delayed Hypersensitivity Response in Guinea Pig Oral Mucosa," *J Pathol, 97*:495, 1969.

78. H. M. Hyman and B. J. Zeldow, "A Comparison of the Cutaneous and Mucosal Arthus Reaction in the Guinea Pig and Hamster," *J Immunol, 91*:701, 1963.

79. C. Terner, "Arthus Reaction in the Oral Cavity of Laboratory Animals," *Periodontics, 3*:18, 1965.

80. A. A. Rizzo and S. E. Mergenhagen, "Studies on the Significance of Local Hypersensitivity in Periodontal Disease," *Periodontics, 3*: 271, 1965.

81. E. H. Beutner, C. Triftshauser, R. J. Nisengard, and A. J. Drinnan, "Gingival Hypersensitivity Reactions. An Experimental Model for Studies of Periodontal Disease," *IADR Abstracts,* No. 327, 1966.

82. A. A. Rizzo and C. T. Mitchell, "Chronic Allergic Inflammation Induced by Repeated Deposition of Antigen in Rabbit Gingival Pockets," *Periodontics, 6*:65, 1968.

83. R. R. Ranney and H. A. Zander, "Allergic Periodontal Disease in Sensitized Squirrel Monkeys," *J Periodontol, 41*:12, 1970.

84. P. Brandtzaeg and F. Kraus, "Autoimmunity and Periodontal Disease," *Odontol Tid, 73*:281, 1965.

85. R. J. Nisengard, E. H. Beutner, and M. S. Gauto, "Immunofluorescent Studies of IgE in Periodontal Disease," *Ann NY Acad Sci, 177*:39, 1971.

86. G. C. Cowley, "Fluorescence Studies of Crevicular Fluid," *J Dent Res, 45*:655, 1966.

87. T. F. Schneider, P. G. Toto, A. W. Gargiulo, and R. J. Pollock, "Specific Bacterial Antibodies in Inflamed Human Gingiva," *Periodontics, 4*:53, 1966.

88. S. E. Berglund, "Immunoglobulins in Human Gingiva with Specificity Oral Bacteria," *J Periodontol, 42*:546, 1971.

89. P. Brandtzaeg, "Immunochemical Comparison of Proteins in Human Gingival Pocket Fluid, Serum and Saliva," *Arch Oral Biol, 10*:795, 1965.

90. P. Brandtzaeg and F. Kraus, "Autoimmunity and Periodontal Disease," *Odontol Tid, 73*:285, 1965.

91. K. Holmberg and J. Killander, "Quantitative Determination of Immunoglobulin (IgG, IgA and IgM) and Identification of IgA-type in the Gingival Fluid," *J Periodont Res, 6*:1, 1971.

92. E. J. Shilletoe and T. Lehner, "Immunoglobulins and Complement in Crevicular Fluid, Serum and Saliva in Man," *Arch Oral Biol, 71*: 241, 1972.

93. S. E. Berglund, A. A. Rizzo, and S. E. Mergenhagen, "The Immune

Response in Rabbits to Bacterial Somatic Antigen Administered via the Oral Mucosa," *Arch Oral Biol, 14:*7, 1969.

94. S. E. Mergenhagen, W. C. deAranjo, and E. Varah, "Antibody to *Leptotrichia buccalis* in Human Sera," *Arch Oral Biol, 10:*29, 1965.

95. R. T. Evans, S. Spaeth, and S. E. Mergenhagen, "Bactericidal Antibody in Mammalian Serum to Obligatorily Anaerobic Gram-Negative Bacteria," *J Immunol, 97:*112, 1966.

96. A. E. Steinberg, S. S. Socransky, S. N. Gershoff, and A. Weinstock, "Use of Tanned-Cell Hemagglutination to Demonstrate Circulating Antibody Against an Oral Spirochete," *J Bacteriol, 91:*2114, 1966.

97. C. R. Ghosh and K. M. Stevens, "Complement-fixing and Hemagglutinating Antibodies to *Treponema microdentium,*" *Proc Soc Expt Biol Med, 124:*559, 1967.

98. R. J. Nisengard and E. H. Beutner, "Immunologic Studies of Periodontal Disease. V. IgG-type Antibodies and Skin Test Responses to Actinomyces and Mixed Oral Flora," *J Periodontol, 41:*149, 1970.

99. T. Kristoffersen, "Immunochemical Studies of Oral Fusobacteria," *Acta Pathol Microbiol Scand, 77:*717, 1969.

100. R. J. Nisengard, E. H. Beutner, and S. P. Hazen, "Immunologic Studies of Periodontal Disease. IV. Bacterial Hypersensitivity and Periodontal Disease," *J Periodontol, 39:*329, 1968.

101. L. Ivanyi and T. Lehner, "Stimulation of Lymphocyte Transformation by Bacterial Antigens in Patients with Periodontal Disease," *Arch Oral Biol, 15:*1089, 1970.

102. J. E. Horton, G. Gordon, S. Lecken, and J. J. Oppenheim, "Lymphocyte Transformation by Human Saliva and Periodontal Deposits," *IADR Abstracts,* No. 334, 1971.

103. L. Ivanyi and T. Lehner, "The Significance of Serum Factors in Stimulating Lymphocytes from Patients with Periodontal Disease by *Veillonella alcalescens,*" *Int Arch Allergy Appl Immunol, 41:*622, 1971.

104. L. E. Cluff, "Effects of Endotoxins on Susceptibility to Infections," *J Infect Dis, 122:*205, 1970.

105. B. W. Zweifach and A, Janoff, "Bacterial Endotoxemia," *Ann Rev Med, 16:*201, 1965.

106. S. E. Mergenhagen, R. Snyderman, H. Gerwurz, and H. S. Shin, "Significance of Complement to the Mechanism of Action of Endotoxin," *Curr Top Microbiol Immunol, 50:*37, 1969.

107. S. Börglum Jensen and S. E. Mergenhagen, "Influence of Endotoxin on Resistance of Mice to Intraperitoneal Infection with Human Oral Bacteria," *Arch Oral Biol, 9:*229, 1964.

108. S. Börglum Jensen and S. E. Mergenhagen, "Influence of Endotoxin on the Dermal Response of Rabbits to Human Oral Bacteria," *Arch Oral Biol, 9:*241, 1964.

109. S. Börglum Jensen, E. Theilade, and J. Smidt Jensen, "Influence of Oral Bacterial Endotoxin on Cell Migration and Phagocytic Activity," *J Periodont Res, 1:*129, 1966.

110. E. Hausmann, L. G. Raisz, and W. A. Miller, "Endotoxin: Stimulation of Bone Resorption in Tissue Culture," *Science, 168:*862, 1970.

111. E. Hausmann, N. Weinfeld, and W. A. Miller, "Effects of Lipopolysaccharides on Bone Resorption in Tissue Sections," *Calcif Tissue Res, 9:*272, 1972.

112. S. E. Mergenhagen, "Endotoxic Properties of Oral Bacteria as Revealed by the Local Schwartzman Reaction," *J Dent Res, 39:*267, 1960.

113. R. J. Nisengard and E. H. Beutner, "Relation of Immediate Hypersensitivity to Periodontitis in Animals and Man," *J Periodontol, 41:* 223, 1970.

114. R. L. Gustafson, A. V. Kroeger, J. L. Gustafson, and E. M. K. Vaichulis, "The Biologic Activity of *Leptotrichia buccalis* Endotoxin," *Arch Oral Biol, 11:*1149, 1966.

115. S. E. Mergenhagen, E. G. Hampp, and H. W. Scherp, "Preparation and Biological Activities of Endotoxins from Oral Bacteria," *J Infect Dis, 108:*304, 1961.

116. B. I. Simon, H. M. Goldman, M. P. Ruben, and E. Baker, "The Role of Endotoxin in Periodontal Disease," *J Periodontol, 40:*695, 1969.

117. B. I. Simon, H. M. Goldman, M. P. Ruben, and E. Baker, "The Role of Endotoxin in Periodontal Disease. II. Correlation of the Quantity of Endotoxin in Human Gingival Exudate with the Clinical Degree of Inflammation," *J Periodontol, 41:*81, 1970.

118. W. C. deAraujo, E. Varah, and S. E. Mergenhagen, "Immunochemical Analysis of Human Oral Strains of *Fusobacterium* and *Leptotrichia,*" *J Bacteriol, 86:*837, 1963.

119. S. E. Mergenhagen and E. Varah, "Serologically Specific Lipopolysaccharides from Oral *Veillonella,*" *Arch Oral Biol, 8:*31, 1963.

120. S. E. Mergenhagen, "Nature and Significance of Somatic Antigens of Oral Bacteria," *J Dent Res, 46:*46, 1967.

121. T. Hofstad, "Biological Activities of Endotoxin from *Bacteroides melaninogenicus,*" *Arch Oral Biol, 15:*343, 1970.

122. A. A. Rizzo and S. E. Mergenhagen, "Histopathologic Effects of Endotoxin Injected into Rabbit Oral Mucosa," *Arch Oral Biol, 9:*659, 1964.

123. A. A. Rizzo, "Absorption of Bacterial Endotoxin into Rabbit Gingival Pocket Tissue," *Periodontics*, 6:65, 1965.
124. S. D. Schultz-Haudt and H. W. Scherp, "The Production of Chondro-sulfatase by Microorganisms Isolated from Human Gingival Crevices," *J Dent Res*, 35:299, 1956.
125. B. D. Davis, R. Dubecco, H. N. Eisen, H. S. Ginsberg, and W. B. Wood, *Microbiology* (New York, Har-Row, 1968).
126. J. B. MacDonald, S. S. Socransky, and R. J. Gibbons, "Aspects of the Pathogenesis of Mixed Anaerobic Infections of Mucous Membranes," *J Dent Res*, 42:529, 1963.
127. M. R. Deward, "Bacterial Enzymes and Periodontal Disease," *J Dent Res*, 37:100, 1958.
128. S. D. Schultz-Haudt and H. W. Scherp, "Production of Hyaluronidase and Beta-Glucuronidase by Veridans Streptococci Isolated from Gingival Crevices," *J Dent Res*, 34:924, 1935.
129. B. Rosan and N. B. Williams, "Hyaluronidase Production by Oral Streptococci," *Arch Oral Biol*, 9:291, 1964.
130. S. A. Leach and M. L. Hayes, "Isolation in Pure Culture of Human Oral Organisms Capable of Producing Neuraminidase," *Nature*, 216:599, 1967.
131. K. Fukui, Y. Fukui, and T. Moriyama, "Neuraminidase Activity in Some Bacteria from the Human Mouth," *Arch Oral Biol*, 16:1361, 1971.
132. P. O. Söder and G. Frostell, "Proteolytic Activity of Dental Material. I. Action of Dental Plaque Material on Azocoll, Casein and Gelatin," *Acta Odontol Scand*, 24:501, 1966.
133. P. O. Söder, "Proteolytic Activity of Dental Plaque Material. II. Action on Gelatin of Proteolytic Enzymes from Dental Plaque Material," *Odontol Tid*, 75:50, 1967.
134. M. J. Perlitsh and I. Glickman, "Salivary Neuraminidase: III. Its Relation to Oral Disease," *J Periodontol*, 38:189, 1967.
135. M. S. Aisenberg and A. D. Aisenberg, "Hyaluronidase and Periodontal Disease," *Oral Surg*, 4:317, 1951.
136. E. H. Beutner, C. Triftshauser, and S. P. Hazen, "Collagenase Activity of Gingival Tissue from Patients with Periodontal Disease," *Proc Soc Exp Biol Med*, 121:1082, 1966.
137. H. M. Fullmer, W. A. Gibson, G. S. Lazarus, H. A. Bladen, and K. A. Whedon, "The Origin of Collagenase in Periodontal Tissues of Man," *J Dent Res*, 48:646, 1969.
138. M. A. Listgarten, "Electron Microscopic Observations on the Bacterial Flora of Acute Necrotizing Ulcerative Gingivitis," *J Periodontol*, 36:328, 1965.
139. M. A. Listgarten and S. S. Socransky, "Ultrastructural Characteristics

of a Spirochete in the Lesion of Acute Necrotizing Ulcerative Gingivostomatitis (Vincent's Infection)," *Arch Oral Biol,* 9:95, 1964.

140. R. T. Haylings, "Electron Microscopy of Acute Ulcerative Gingivitis (Vincent's Type)," *Brit Dent J, 122:*51, 1967.

141. M. A. Listgarten and D. W. Lewis, "The Distribution of Spirochetes in the Lesion of Acute Necrotizing Ulcerative Gingivitis: An Electron Microscopic and Statistical Survey," *J Periodontol,* 38:379, 1967.

142. E. G. Hampp and S. E. Mergenhagen, "Experimental Infections with Oral Spirochetes," *J Infect Dis, 109:*43, 1961.

143. E. G. Hampp and S. E. Mergenhagen, "Experimental Intracutaneous Fusobacterial and Fusospirochetal Infections," *J Infect Dis, 112:* 84, 1963.

144. S. E. Mergenhagen, E. G. Hampp, and H. W. Schert, "Preparation and Biological Activities of Endotoxins from Oral Bacteria," *J Infect Dis, 108:*304, 1961.

145. T. Lehner and E. D. Clarry, "Acute Ulcerative Gingivitis: An Immunofluorescent Investigation," *Brit Dent J, 121:*366, 1966.

146. J. M. Wilton, L. Ivanyi, and T. Lehner, "Cell-Mediated Immunity and Humoral Antibodies in Acute Necrotizing Ulcerative Gingivitis," *J Periodont Res,* 6:9, 1971.

147. J. D. Manson and H. Rand, "Recurrent Vincent's Disease," *Brit Dent J, 110:*386, 1961.

148. P. Brandtzaeg, "Local Factors of Resistance in the Gingival Area," *J Periodont Res,* 1:19, 1966.

149. L. H. Green and E. H. Kass, "Quantitative Determination of Antibacterial Activity in the Rabbit Gingival Sulcus," *Arch Oral Biol, 15:* 491, 1970.

150. E. Weinstein and I. D. Mandel, "The Present Status of Anti-calculus Agents," *J Oral Therap and Pharm,* 1:327, 1964.

151. R. J. Fitzgerald, P. H. Keyes, T. H. Stoudt, and D. M. Spinell, "The Effects of a Dextranase Preparation on Plaque and Caries in Hamsters, a Preliminary Report," *JADA,* 76:301, 1968.

152. P. H. Keyes, M. A. Kicks, B. M. Goldman, R. M. McCabe, and R. J. Fitzgerald, "Dispersion of Dextranous Bacterial Plaques on Human Teeth with Dextranase," *JADA,* 82:136, 1971.

153. R. J. Gibbons and P. H. Keyes, "Inhibition of Insoluble Dextran Synthesis, Plaque Formation and Dental Caries in Hamsters by Low Molecular Weight Dextran," *ArchOralBiol,14:*721,1969.

154. R. J. Gibbons and R. J. Fitzgerald, "Dextran-induced Agglutination of *Streptococcus mutans* and Its Potential Role in the Formation of Microbial Dental Plaques," *J Bacteriol,* 98:341, 1969.

155. R. R. Lobene, "A Clinical Study of the Effect of Dextranase on Human Dental Plaque," *JADA,* 82:132, 1971.

156. N. W. Littleton and C. L. White, "Dental Findings from a Preliminary Study of Children Receiving Extended Antibiotic Therapy," *JADA, 68:*520, 1964.

157. R. R. Lobene, M. Brion, and S. S. Socransky, "Effect of Erythromycin on Dental Plaque Forming Microorganisms of Man," *J Periodontol, 40:*287, 1969.

158. D. F. Mitchell and L. A. Holmes, "Topical Control of Dentogingival Plaque," *J Periodontol, 36:*202, 1965.

159. P. H. Keyes, S. A. Rowberry, H. R. Englander, and R. J. Fitzgerald, "Bio-Assays of Medicaments for the Control of Dentobacterial Plaque, Dental Caries and Periodontal Lesions in Syrian Hamsters," *J Oral Therap and Pharm, 3:*157, 1966.

160. S. Börglum Jensen, H. Löe, C. Pundom Schiött, and E. Theilade, "Experimental Gingivitis in Man. IV. Vancomycin Induced Changes in Bacterial Plaque Composition as Related to Development of Gingival Inflammation," *J Periodont Res, 3:*284, 1966.

161. A. R. Volpe, L. J. Kupczak, J. H. Brant, W. J. King, R. C. Kestenbaum, and H. J. Schlissel, "Antimicrobial Control of Bacterial Plaque and Calculus and the Effects of These Agents on Oral Flora," *J Dent Res, 48:*832, 1969.

162. W. J. Loesche, E. Green, E. B. Kenney, and D. Nafe, "Effect of Topical Kanamycin Sulfate on Plaque Accumulation," *JADA, 83:*1063, 1971.

163. S. Turesky, N. D. Gilmore, and I. Glickman, "Reduced Plaque Formation by the Chloromethyl Analogue of Victamine C," *J Periodontol, 41:*41, 1970.

164. H. Löe and C. Pundom Schiött, "The Effect of Mouthrinses and Topical Application of Chlorhexidine on the Development of Dental Plaque and Gingivitis in Man," *J Periodont Res, 5:*79, 1970.

165. P. Gjermo, K. L. Baastad, and G. Rolla, "The Plaque-Inhibiting Capacity of 11 Antibacterial Compounds," *J Periodont Res, 5:*102, 1970.

166. G. Rölla, H. Löe, and C. Pundom Schiött, "Retention of Chlorohexidine in the Human Oral Cavity," *Arch Oral Biol, 16:*1109, 1971.

167. J. Theilade and R. J. Fitzgerald, "Dental Calculus in the Rat: Effect of Diet and Erythromycin," *Acta Odontol Scand, 21:*271, 1963.

168. A. R. Volpe, S. M. Schulman, E. Goldman, W. J. King, and L. J. Kupczak, "The Long Term Effect of an Antimicrobial Formulation on Dental Calculus Formation," *J Periodontol, 41:*463, 1970.

169. O. P. Sturzenberger, J. R. Swancar, and G. Reiter, "Reduction of Dental Calculus in Humans Through the Use of a Dentifrice Containing a Crystal-Growth Inhibitor," *J Periodontol, 42:*416, 1971.

170. S. Mukhenjee, "An *In Vitro* Study of Anti-calculus Agents," *J Periodont Res, 4:*26, 1969.

RELATIONSHIP OF
ORAL HYGIENE
TO DENTAL CARIES

7

THE NATURE OF THE CARIOUS LESION

Louis W. Ripa

IN THIS CHAPTER the effects of caries on tooth tissue are described. Particular emphasis is placed on the alterations associated with the early lesion and on those changes considered reparative in nature. In succeeding chapters, the influence of oral hygiene procedures, topical fluoride applications and other methods of controlling or limiting the decay process will be described.

HISTORICAL OVERVIEW

Dental decay is an extremely ancient disease. Its effects are evident in the remains of Rhodesian man who existed one million years ago.[1] As civilization advanced, the incidence and prevalence of dental caries also increased. Spurred by man's attempt to ascribe causal relationships to events around him, numerous theories of dental decay have been advanced. Miller[2] cited several theories held in earlier times, including such diverse concepts as initiation by worms, electrolytic decomposition, and inflammation. The latter theory described dental caries as an inflammatory process originating independently in the dentin of the tooth; it probably was an attempt to equate caries with soft tissue pathology in which inflammation is a characteristic feature. Caries, however, is unique in that the initial lesion most commonly occurs in the highly mineralized enamel layer which is devoid of viable cellular elements and consequently lacks the ability to mobilize an inflammatory response.

In 1890, W. D. Miller[2] enunciated the chemicoparasitic theory of dental caries. Miller based his theory upon the observations of other investigators, such as Magitot,[3] Wedl,[4] and Tomes,[5] as well as his own. He showed that oral bacteria will ferment carbohydrates, producing lactic and other acids that are capable of destroying tooth enamel. Miller stated:

> Dental decay is a chemicoparasitical process consisting of two distinctly marked stages: decalcification, or softening of the tissue, and dissolution of the softened residue.

Since 1890, the theory of Miller has been modified but never abandoned.

GROSS APPEARANCE OF CARIES

Gross changes in the appearance of the tooth are detected by visual examination aided by proper illumination, by probing with a sharp instrument and by clinical radiographic analysis. Radiographs have been shown to increase the number of carious lesions detected.[6-8] Dunning and DeWilde[6] found an average increase of 4.91 carious surfaces per patient when bite-wing radiographs were included in the dental examination of twelve to twenty-three-year olds. All age groups, however, did not benefit equally. The greatest increase of detectable lesions was in seventeen-year olds. Other reports[7, 8] have indicated radiographs are of least value in eleven-year olds when primary molars are exfoliating and bicuspids are in an active state of eruption. Radiographs are especially important for the detection of proximal lesions because poor accessibility makes clinical diagnosis diffi-

TABLE 7-I

CARIES INCIDENCE (DMFS) OF CHILDREN IN A NONFLUORIDE COMMUNITY EVALUATED WITH AND WITHOUT RADIOGRAPHS*

Type of Surface	Examiner A Visual Exam	Examiner B Visual Exam	Visual + X-Ray Exam
Occlusal	4.09	4.14	4.14
Proximal	2.10	1.63	4.35
Buccolingual	2.11	2.00	2.00
Total	8.30	7.77	10.49

DMF surface rates for eleven and twelve-year-old children in a nonfluoride community. Note that the use of radiographs increases the DMFS score for proximal surfaces but not for occlusal or buccolingual surfaces.

* Adopted from H. S. Horowitz and J. K. Peterson, *Arch Oral Biol*, 1966.[10]

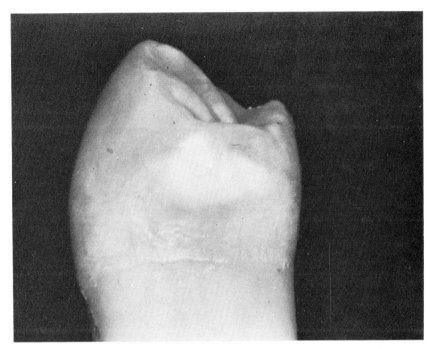

Figure 7-1. Clinical appearance of a "white spot" or early carious lesion on the proximal surface of a bicuspid tooth. Refractive changes associated with loss of mineral at the affected site cause the opaque appearance. The color change can best be discerned when the tooth is dried.

cult.[9] Table 7-I indicates the value of radiographs in the detection of caries on occlusal, proximal, and buccal or lingual surfaces.[10] Radiographs did not increase the incidence of clinically detectable occlusal, buccal, or lingual lesions above that recorded by visual (and probe) examination. The number of detectable lesions on proximal surfaces, however, was increased by approximately 50 to 60 percent.

Caries initiating in the enamel may be divided into two types: pit and fissure lesions and smooth surface lesions. The first macroscopic evidence of a smooth surface lesion is the appearance of a "white spot" (Figure 7-1). Because the affected area is less mineralized than the surrounding enamel, refractive differences cause it to appear opaque and white in contrast to the translucence of the surrounding normal enamel. The surface of the lesion is hard and resists penetration of an explorer tip. Although clinically and radiographically the lesion can go undetected,[11] there is histologic evidence that, at this early stage, dentin can be involved. As the lesion progresses, the surface becomes soft and chalky, and cavitation results. Before cavitation, it may be possible to reverse the advancement of the lesion by removing all tenacious plaque and debris from the surface and applying topical fluoride.[12] Lesions can also spontaneously arrest, in which case they may appear as "brown spots" due to the acquisition of protein material.[13] The greater uptake of fluoride in de-

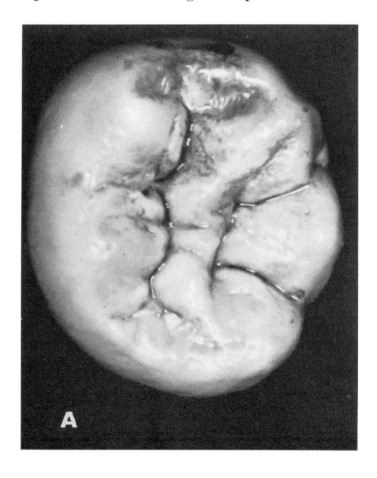

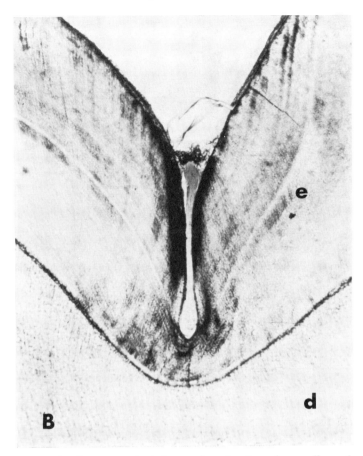

Figure 7-2. (A) The anatomical form of occlusal surfaces allows bacteria and food debris to be retained. (B) Histologic section through an occlusal fissure. The depth and configuration of the fissure prevent adequate cleaning with a toothbrush. Note the trapped debris. (e = enamel; d = dentin) Compliments of Doctor M. Buonocore.

mineralized enamel than in unaffected enamel[14, 15] may contribute to the spontaneous arrestment of the lesion.

Whereas smooth surface lesions develop beneath a plaque, pit and fissure lesions require a less specific dietobacterial environment.[16] The deep fissures and sloping cusps provide a shelter for food and bacteria to collect (Figure 7-2). It is generally impossible for toothbrush bristles to clean this area, and in spite of fluoride therapy, pit and fissure occlusal surfaces, especially on permanent molars, are the most caries-susceptible sites.[17] The initial pit and fissure lesion may also begin as a "white spot." However, because of the collection of debris, etc., in this area, the color change may go unnoticed so that the first evidence of caries is a clinically "sticky fissure" or frank cavitation.

Cavitation is an indication for restorative procedures, although even at this stage it is possible for the lesion to spontaneously arrest, e.g. eburnated caries. Massler[18] has described the gross appearance of actively progressing lesions and arrested lesions together with accompanying subjective symptomology (Table 7-II). This distinction is of practical importance to the clinician. The dentin of the arrested lesion is less permeable due to sclerosis of the tubules, and, therefore, the pulp is less likely to be traumatized by chemical and bacterial irritants diffusing through the tooth.[18]

Unlike the hard tissues of the tooth, the pulp, which contains nerves, blood vessels, and connective tissue, can undergo an inflammatory response. This response can be initiated when the dentin is invaded but before the pulp is actually penetrated by

TABLE 7-II

CLINICAL DIFFERENTIATION OF ACTIVE AND ARRESTED CARIOUS LESIONS*

	Active Lesion	*Arrested Lesion*
1. Pain	Elicited by (a) sudden change in temperature (b) intake of concentrated sugars (c) impaction of foods (d) probing the lesion	Absent
2. Color of surface layer	Light brown	Dark brown or black
3. Consistency of surface layer	Soft and friable	Firm and leathery; often eburnated

* From M. Massler, *Int Dent J*, 1967.[18] (Courtesy of Doctor M. Massler and *Int Dent J*)

bacteria.[18] The pulpal inflammation can be acute or chronic. If proper treatment is not instituted, necrosis is generally the terminal stage of pulpal involvement, although an exaggerated viable response, e.g. hyperplastic pulpitis or pulp polyp, may occur infrequently.

In older patients where gingival recession has exposed the root surface to the oral environment, caries may initiate in the root cementum, penetrate the dentin and invade the pulp. These lesions are diagnosed by their brownish discoloration and softening and, because they occur in older individuals, have been referred to as "senile caries."

HISTOLOGIC APPEARANCE OF CARIES

Microradiography (radiographs of microscopic sections) and polarized light microscopy are two methods that have been frequently employed to assess histologically demineralization within the early carious lesion. Microradiographic technics employ the same principles used in the interpretation of clinical radiographs; differences in mineralization are represented as variations in intensity of an image on a photographic emulsion. Polarized light studies measure the degree of mineralization either qualitatively or quantitatively based upon the retardation of plane polarized light as it passes through a thin ground section of a tooth.

These methods have demonstrated conclusively that the early carious or "white spot" lesion is a *subsurface* enamel lesion with the surface layer relatively intact.[19-21] Figure 7-3a, a low-power microradiograph of a longitudinal ground section prepared through a "white spot" lesion, exhibits the typical, intact radiopaque surface layer. The surface layer is continuous with adjacent, unaffected surface enamel and covers a radiolucent area of subsurface demineralization. Densitometric tracings of microradiographs[22] have demonstrated that although the outer layer is intact, it is less mineralized than normal enamel, indicating some acid dissolution has occurred. The persistence of this relatively intact, slightly demineralized surface layer has been variously attributed to the greater resistance of this layer to acid demineralization, to the physicochemical phenomenon of acid dissolution beneath the dental plaque and to a reprecipitation of previously dissolved calcium salts.

At higher magnification (Figure 7-3b), alternate fine lines of radiolucency and radiopacity have been observed within the area of subsurface demineralization. Two sets of these lines have been noted; they correspond to the direction of the enamel prisms as they traverse the enamel from the surface to the dentin-enamel junction and to the striae of Retzius, which run in a gingivoocclusal direction. Since outlines of these histologic details are not visible in microradiographs of normal enamel, it has been hypothesized that enamel demineralization progresses

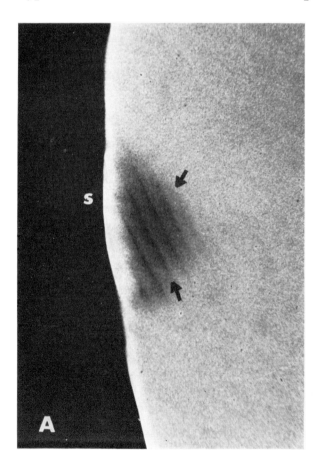

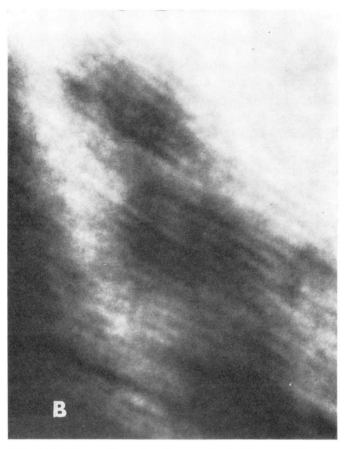

Figure 7-3. (A) Microradiograph of an early "white spot" lesion on the proximal surface of a permanent tooth. Note the subsurface radiolucent area (arrows) and the relatively intact radiopaque surface layer(s). (orig. mag. ×80) (B) At higher magnification, prism outlines, running diagonally from left to right, and outlines of the striae of Retzius running from top to bottom, are visible within the radiolucent lesion. These histologic details do not appear in the surrounding unaffected enamel. (orig. mag. ×450)

along two pathways: (1) inward, following the enamel prisms; and (2) laterally, along the striae of Retzius.[20, 23, 24]

On the basis of its appearance under polarized light, the "white spot" or early carious lesion has been divided into zones[19,]

[21, 25] that are believed to represent successive stages in the attack of enamel (Figure 7-4). Progressing inward from the relatively intact surface layer, the first identifiable zone is the *body of the lesion*. This zone constitutes the area of greatest demineralization and appears highly radiolucent in microradiographs (see Figure 7-3a). Lying deep to the body of the lesion is the *dark or positive zone*,[21, 25, 26] beneath which lies the *translucent zone*. The distinct appearance of these zones is believed to be related to the size and number of spaces (or micropores) they contain. The size and number of these micropores are associated with the acid dissolution and possible reprecipitation of calcium salts that have occurred as the lesion developed. Alterations of the birefringent qualities and radiodensity of these zones have been caused by immersing prepared longitudinal ground sections

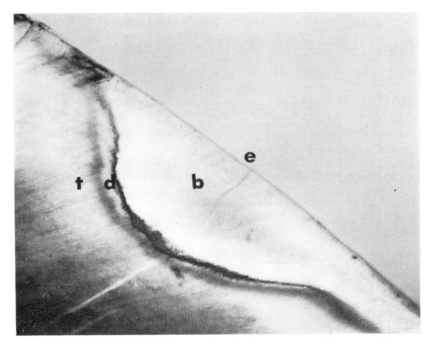

Figure 7-4. Histologic appearance of an early carious or "white spot" lesion viewed under polarized light. The body of the lesion (b) represents the principal area of mineral loss. Lying deep to this is the dark zone (d) and the translucent zone (t). (e = enamel surface) (quinoline; orig. mag. ×80)

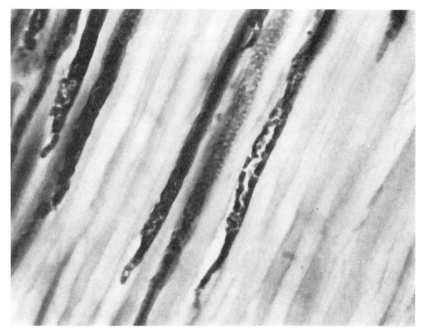

Figure 7-5. Decalcified section of carious human dentin showing the presence of bacteria within the tubules. (H. & E.; orig. mag. ×500) Compliments of Doctor O. Sarda.

through "white spot" lesions in either whole saliva or a solution of a calcium phosphate dihydrate.[27] The immersed sections were changed by deposition of mineral from the solutions into the demineralized early carious sites. Although no extrapolation to the clinical situation should be attempted from such *in vitro* investigation, these observations demonstrate that alterations of a "repair-like" nature can occur at the histologic level in lesions that clinically are known to arrest.

The histologic picture in the enamel of lesions exhibiting clinical cavitation is similar to that already described. However, the surface layer has been lost, there is greater internal destruction, and bacterial invasion is evident.

Microradiographs of carious lesions in the dentin also reveal the presence of several zones. The most superficial zone shows the greatest demineralization; next is an intermediate zone of variable radiodensity and an internal hypermineralized zone.[28] The hypermineralized zone is the result of the deposition of calcium salts into the dentinal tubules, producing a *sclerotic layer* of dentin. New *secondary dentin* is produced adjacent to the pulp as it recedes from the carious site. The sclerotic and secondary dentin are the tooth's defensive response to the noxious (physical, chemical, bacterial) agents of the carious attack.

As caries progresses, destruction of the peritubular and intertubular dentin occurs. Decalcified sections demonstrate the presence of bacteria in the dentinal tubules[29] (Figure 7-5). Nevertheless, it is believed that the advancing front of the lesion is one of acid dissolution of mineral salts rather than bacterial invasion. The organic matrix of the dentin is secondarily involved as it comes in intimate contact with the bacteria.[30]

In early dentinal caries, the pulp response is confined to the ends of the cariously involved tubules and is characterized by the presence of inflammatory cells and a reduced number of odontoblasts. The initial pulp response is stimulated by the destruction products of the carious lesion rather than the invading bacteria that have not yet reached the pulp.[31] As the dentinal lesion enlarges, the severity of the pulpal reaction increases. There is a dilatation of blood vessels and an increased number of lymphocytes and macrophages. An abscess develops in the adjacent odontoblastic layer as the pulp is invaded. A chronic inflammatory reaction occurs, and if the tooth goes untreated, there is eventual necrosis of the pulp.

Ultrastructural Changes Associated With Caries

Electron microscopy has permitted enlargement of such magnitude to allow visualization of the apatite crystallites that constitute the individual mineral components of the tooth and the organic framework. Because of the difficulty of sectioning hard dental enamel, and other technical problems, early electron microscopic studies were conducted on replicas prepared from fractured or etched surfaces rather than directly observing the enamel itself.[32-36] With technical advances such as the development of ultrathin sectioning equipment,[37] increased experience, and delineation of preparation artifacts, it has been possible to interpret carious destruction based on direct visualization of the damaged enamel crystallites.[38–40]

Electron microscopic studies of early carious lesions with clinically intact surfaces have demonstrated both preferential dissolution channels and areas of gross destruction within the "white spots."[39, 40] Surface penetration and advancement through the enamel followed the prism direction, confirming the polarized light and microradiographic investigations. By direct visualization of the defect at the ultrastructural level, it was found that the dissolution pathways could involve either the prism centers or the interprismatic enamel located between the prisms. Areas of abrupt change in crystallite orientation, which are located at prism boundaries,[41] were found to be especially susceptible sites to acid dissolution. *In vitro* demineralization of enamel with procian dye-formic acid mixtures has produced similar results.[42] Figure 7-6 is an electron micrograph of partially demineralized enamel prisms in which the prism centers are more demineralized than the peripheries.

The enlarged intercrystallite spaces created by acid dissolution were found to contain amorphous organic material[39] and, *in vivo*, may also contain water and possibly air. Since these materials have a different refractive index than crystalline apatite, they contribute to the birefringement changes (described when sections of carious enamel are examined with polarized light) and to the clinical appearance of the lesion as a "white spot."

Individual crystallites within the lesion are altered in both size and configuration. Selective dissolution of the crystallite centers has been reported by several investigators.[28, 38, 40] In longitudinal view, these elongate crystallites appear as hollow rods, and in cross section they look like hollow rectangles or hexagons (Figure 7-7). Crystallites measuring up to 1500 Å in width, which are larger than those in normal enamel, have been found at prism borders within the caries site.[40, 43] The nature of these large crystallites in demineralized enamel has been speculated about. It has been proposed that these larger crystallites result from re-

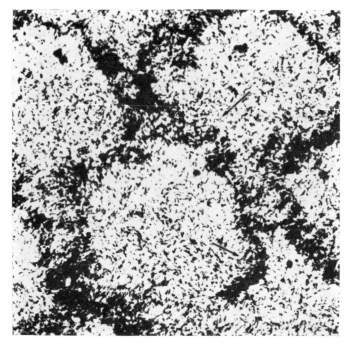

Figure 7-6. Electron micrograph of cross section of enamel prisms partially demineralized with procian dye-formic acid. The prism periphery (arrows) is less demineralized than the prism centers. (orig. mag. ×6500) Compliments of Doctors E. L. Smith and J. M. Shackleford, and *The Alabama Journal of Medical Sciences.*

crystallization occurring at the margins of dissolution channels within the lesion.

In the early stages of the development of the lesion in dentin, intact collagen fibrils are found associated with a sparse distribution of crystallites.[28, 38] The loss of mineral without corresponding alteration of the organic matrix is an indication that demineralization, rather than proteolysis, is the first stage of dentinal disintegration. At this early stage, bacteria cannot be demonstrated within the lesion, but acids, enzymes, debris, etc., diffusing ahead of the carious front, can stimulate intratubular mineralization. The sclerotic reaction, in which mineral crystallites are precipitated within the dentinal tubules, decreases the per-

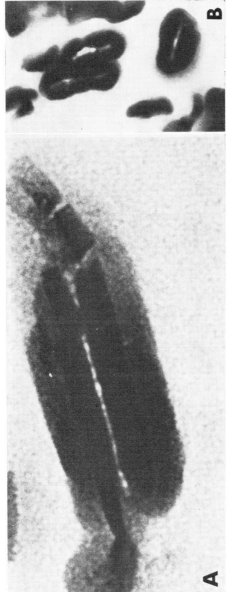

Figure 7-7. (A) Electron micrograph of a longitudinal view of a partially demineralized enamel crystallite. The crystallite appears to be composed of two halves with an intervening space. (orig. mag. ×416,000) (B) In cross section the partially demineralized enamel crystallites appear to have hollowed-out centers. (orig. mag. ×165,000) Compliments of Doctors E. L. Smith and J. M. Shackleford, and *The Alabama Journal of Medical Sciences.*

Oral Hygiene in Oral Health

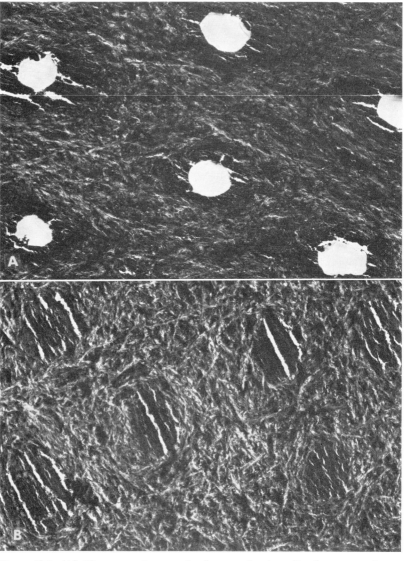

Figure 7-8. (A) Electron micrograph of an undemineralized section of normal (noncarious) deciduous dentin. Note the patent dentin tubules. (orig. mag. ×5000) (B) A section from the translucent zone of a carious lesion showing the tubules filled with material indistinguishable from peritubular dentin. (orig. mag. ×5000) Compliments of Doctors N. W. Johnson, B. R. Taylor, and D. S. Berman, and of *Caries Research*.

meability of the dentin lying pulpally to the advancing lesion and ameliorates the effects of irritants on the pulp.[18]

In the more advanced dentinal lesion, zones which can be correlated with those detected with the light or polarizing microscope have been described at the ultrastructural level.[44, 45] The most superficial zone is the *zone of destruction* in which structural details have been lost. There is little or no remaining mineral; collagen dissolution has occurred; and masses of both viable and degenerating bacteria are present. The next zone, the *zone of penetration,* is partially demineralized and also contains bacteria. The third zone, called the *translucent zone,* is at the internal periphery of the dentinal lesion closest to the pulp. It is characterized by an area of hypermineralization.

The ultrastructural appearance of the zone of penetration is one of both demineralization and mineralization. The areas of demineralization are characterized by enlarged dentinal tubules. Conversely, there are areas of mineralization that have tubules occluded by large needle-shaped crystals. Large rhombohedral crystals have also been found within the dentinal tubules, causing investigators to speculate that these morphologically unique crystals are associated with remineralization occurring within this zone.

The most internal zone, the zone of translucence, is hypermineralized due largely to the occlusion of the lumen of the tubules by crystals resembling those found in normal peritubular dentin (Figure 7-8). This zone appears radiopaque on clinical radiographs or microradiographs of ground sections. The occlusion of the tubule lumens by crystal precipitation appears to be a physiologic response of the tooth to confine the advancing lesion. If the caries attack is relatively mild, presumably sclerosis and secondary dentin deposition can protect the viable pulpal elements, and arrest of the lesion may even occur. If the attack is rapid, pulpal involvement will produce the pathologic response already described.

CHEMICAL CHANGES ASSOCIATED WITH CARIES

There is approximately 52 to 63 percent calcium and 53 to 63 percent phosphorus (by volume) in "white spot" lesions compared to sound enamel.[46] This reflects the fact that the initial carious attack is principally a demineralization phenomenon. There are other alterations in the chemical composition of enamel effected by early caries. There is a decrease in carbonate[28, 46, 47] and magnesium[28] and an increase in a number of trace elements, especially lead, zinc, and copper.[15] Of particular interest is the three to five-fold increase of fluoride found in "white spot" enamel[15, 28, 48] (Table 7-III). The increased concentration of fluoride indicates that there may be a preferential dissolution of crystals as the lesion develops (the fluoride-containing crystals being spared), and/or that the demineralized enamel is absorbing fluoride to a greater extent than sound enamel. Either explanation is tenable. Preferential dissolution of enamel crystallites has been reported, as described in the previous section, and *in vitro* studies have demonstrated that acid-etched enamel can absorb more fluoride than unaltered control samples.[49] Other chemical changes reported in the early lesion are an increase in water content[28, 46] and an increase in organic matter[28, 46] as reflected by higher nitrogen levels found within the lesion.[50]

Chemical investigations on carious dentin have also indicated that 50 percent or more of the mineral is lost; there is an increase in water content; and there is an alteration in trace element concentrations.[28, 51] There is also an increase in fluoride concentration. Ashed samples of sound dentin evidenced 175 ppm fluoride compared to an eight-fold increase (1,400 ppm) in ashed carious dentin.[28]

TABLE 7-III

FLUORIDE CONTENT OF EARLY CARIOUS ("WHITE SPOT")
ENAMEL AND SOUND ENAMEL (ppm Dry Weight)

Investigators	Age of Tooth Sample	ppm F Sound	ppm F Carious
Johansen (1962)		120	580
Little, Posen, Singer (1962)	< 30	190	528
	> 30	230	604
Little, Steadman (1966)	< 30	190	560

SUMMARY

Alterations of tooth tissue have been described in association with the advancement of the carious lesion through enamel, dentin, and pulp. Changes in the gross appearance of the tooth have been correlated with histologic, ultrastructural, and chemical changes. In order to diagnose and treat caries successfully, the practicing dentist need only be cognizant of the gross changes. Knowledge of the microscopic and chemical alterations, however, is important in order to assess present and future technics of caries prevention and tooth restoration.

It is believed that within the carious lesion both demineralization and remineralization are occurring.[52] In addition to destructive change, there are processes of repair and defense that operate concurrently. Caries arrestment, remineralization, sclerosis, secondary dentin deposition, and preferential uptake of fluoride and organic materials by the carious lesion all contribute to the defense mechanism of the tooth. As indicated in Fig-

FATE OF BUCCAL ENAMEL AREAS DURING A PERIOD OF SEVEN YEARS

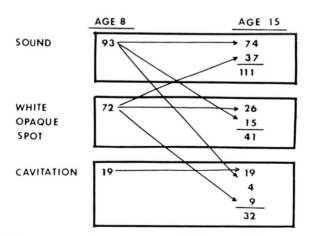

Figure 7-9. Seven years after seventy-two "white spot" lesions were diagnosed in eight-year-old children, only nine had progressed to the stage of cavitation, while thirty-seven were diagnosed as clinically sound. Adapted from O. Backer-Dirks, *J Dent Res*, 1966.[53]

ure 7-9, not all early carious lesions necessarily need to progress to the cavitation stage.[53] By an alteration of the external or internal environment of the tooth, it is possible to affect the advancement of the carious lesion or to prevent its inception. The following chapters will present the technics and rationale of caries control procedures that a dentist employs in his private dental office.

REFERENCES

1. M. F. A. Montagu, *An Introduction to Physical Anthropology*, 2nd ed. Springfield, Thomas, 1951, p. 159.
2. W. D. Miller, *Micro-organisms of the Human Mouth*. Philadelphia, S. S. White Dental Mfg. Co., 1890.
3. E. Magitot, *Recherches Experimentales et Therapeutiques de la Carie Dentaire*. Paris, J. B. Bailliere et Fils, 1866.
4. C. Wedl, *The Pathology of the Teeth*. Philadelphia, Lindsay and Blakiston, 1872.
5. J. Tomes, *Dental Surgery*. Philadelphia, Lindsay and Blakiston, 1859.
6. J. M. Dunning and M. D. DeWilde, "Variations in the Efficiency of Bite-wing Roentgenograms as Related to Age of Patient," *JADA*, 52:138-148, 1956.
7. N. W. Chilton and L. E. Greenwald, "Studies in Dental Public Health Administration. II. Role of Roentgenograms in Public Health Dental Surveys," *J Dent Res*, 26:129-141, 1947.
8. J. R. Blayney and J. F. Greco, "Evanston Dental Caries Study. IX. Value of Roentgenological vs. Clinical Procedures for the Recognition of Early Carious Lesions on Proximal Surfaces of the Teeth," *J Dent Res*, 31:341-345, 1952.
9. J. Van Aken, "Limitations in Clinical Diagnosis of Dental Caries of Approximal Surfaces," *Adv Fluorine Res Dent Caries Prev*, 4:89-92, 1966.
10. H. S. Horowitz and J. K. Peterson, "Evaluation of Examiner Variability and the Use of Radiographs in Determining the Efficacy of Community Fluoridation," *Arch Oral Biol*, 11:867-875, 1966.
11. T. M. Marthaler and M. Germann, "Radiographic and Visual Appearance of Small Smooth Surface Caries Lesions Studied on Extracted Teeth," *Caries Res*, 4:224-242, 1970.
12. V. H. Mercer and J. C. Muhler, "The Clinical Demonstration of Caries Arrestment Following Topical Stannous Fluoride Treatment," *J Dent Child*, 32:65-72, 1965.
13. B. R. Bhussry, "Chemical and Physical Studies of Enamel from Human Teeth. II. Specific Gravity, Nitrogen Content, and Hardness Rating of Discolored Enamel," *J Dent Res*, 37:1045-1053, 1958.

14. A. S. Hallsworth and J. A. Weatherell, "The Microdistribution, Uptake and Loss of Fluoride in Human Enamel," *Caries Res, 3*:109-118, 1969.

15. M. G. Little and L. T. Steadman, "Chemical and Physical Properties of Altered and Sound Enamel. IV. Trace Element Composition," *Arch Oral Biol, 11*:273-278, 1966.

16. P. H. Keyes, "Research in Dental Caries," *JADA, 76*:1357-1373, 1968.

17. O. Backer-Dirks, "The Distribution of Caries Resistance in Relation to Tooth Surfaces," G. E. W. Wolstenholme and M. O'Conner (Eds.) In *Ciba Foundation Symposium: Caries Resistant Teeth.* Boston, Little, 1965, pp. 66-83 and "Discussion."

18. M. Massler, "Pulpal Reactions to Dental Caries," *Int Dent J, 17*:441-460, 1967.

19. G. Gustafson, "The Histopathology of Caries of Human Dental Enamel with Special Reference of the Division of the Carious Lesion into Zones," *Acta Odontol Scand, 15*:13-55, 1957.

20. C. I. Guzman, F. Brudevold, and H. Mermagen, "A Soft Roentgen Ray Study of Early Carious Lesions," *JADA, 55*:509-515, 1957.

21. A. I. Darling, "Studies on the Early Carious Lesion of Enamel with Transmitted Light, Polarized Light and Radiography," *Brit Dent J, 101*:289-297, 329-341, 1956.

22. N. Soni and F. Brudevold, "A Microradiographic and Polarizing Microscope Study of Sound Enamel," *J Dent Res, 38*:1181-1186, 1959.

23. A. I. Darling, "The Pathology and Prevention of Caries," *Brit Dent J, 107*:287-302, 1959.

24. K. V. Mortimer, "The Pattern of Demineralization of the Enamel of Dental Caries," *Caries Res, 2*:180-192, 1968.

25. A. I. Darling, "Studies of the Early Lesion of Enamel Caries, Its Nature, Mode of Spread and Points of Entry," *Brit Dent J, 105*:119-135, 1958.

26. A. I. Darling, K. V. Mortimer, D. F. G. Poole, and W. D. Ollis, "Molecular Sieve Behavior of Normal and Carious Human Dental Enamel," *Arch Oral Biol, 5*:251-271, 1961.

27. L. M. Silverstone and D. F. G. Poole, "The Effect of Saliva and Calcifying Solutions Upon the Histological Appearance of Enamel Caries," *Caries Res, 2*:87-96, 1968.

28. E. Johansen, "The Nature of the Carious Lesion," *Dent Clin North Am, July*:305-320, 1962.

29. N. W. Johnson, B. R. Taylor, and D. S. Berman, "The Response of Deciduous Dentine to Caries Studied by Correlated Light and Electron Microscopy," *Caries Res, 3*:348-368, 1969.

30. R. M. Frank, "The Ultrastructure of the Tooth from the Point of View

of Mineralization, Demineralization and Remineralization," *Int Dent J, 17*:661-683, 1967.

31. K. Langeland, "Biologic Considerations in Operative Dentistry," *Dent Clin North Am, March*:125-146, 1967.

32. S. Takuma, "The Electron Microscopy of the Enamel Surfaces of Teeth Under Various Abnormal Conditions," *J Dent Res, 34*:152-163, 1955.

33. J. G. Helmcke, "Elektronenmikroskopishe Strukturuntersuchungen an Gesunden und Pathologischen Zahnen," *Schweiz Monats schr Zahnheilkd, 65*:629-635, 1955.

34. Y. Awazawa, "Electron Microscopy of Carious Dental Enamel. I. With Particular Reference to Development Behavior of Initial Dental Caries," *J Nihon Univ Sch Dent, 3*:79-82, 1960.

35. Y. Awazawa, "Electron Microscopy of Carious Dental Enamel. II. With Reference to Incipient Caries," *J Nihon Univ Sch Dent, 4*:25-39, 1961.

36. Y. Awazawa, "Electron Microscopy of Carious Dental Enamel. III. With Special Regard to Development and Progress Behaviours of Caries," *J Nihon Univ Sch Dent, 5*:99-115, 1962.

37. A. P. Murphy and G. McNeil, "Precision Ultramicrotome of Simplified Design," *Rev Sci Instrum, 35*:132-134, 1964.

38. R. M. Frank, "The Ultrastructure of Caries-Resistant Teeth," G. E. W. Wolstenholme and M. O'Connor (Eds.) In *Ciba Symposium: Caries Resistant Teeth.* Boston, Little, 1965, pp. 169-184 and "Discussion."

39. R. M. Frank and A. Brendel, "Ultrastructure of the Approximal Dental Plaque and the Underlying Normal Carious Enamel," *Arch Oral Biol, 11*:883-912, 1966.

40. N. W. Johnson, "Some Aspects of the Ultrastructure of Early Human Enamel Caries Seen with the Electron Microscope," *Arch Oral Biol, 12*:1505-1521, 1967.

41. A. H. Meckel, W. J. Griebstein, and R. J. Neil, "Structure of Mature Human Dental Enamel as Observed by Electron Microscopy," *Arch Oral Biol, 10*:775-783, 1965.

42. E. L. Smith and J. M. Shackleford, "Microradiographic, Transmitted Light and Electron Microscopic Studies of Human Tooth Enamel Demineralized in Procian Dye-Formic Acid Mixtures," *Ala J Med Sci, 5*:80-88, 1968.

43. J. E. Glas, M. W. Nylen and M. F. Little, "A Microradiographic and Electron Microscopic Study of Carious Enamel," *IADR Abstracts,* No. 121, 1965.

44. S. Takuman and Y. Kurahashi, "Electron Microscopy of Various Zones in a Carious Lesion in Human Dentine," *Arch Oral Biol, 7*:439-453, 1962.

45. N. W. Johnson, B. R. Taylor, and D. S. Berman, "The Response of Deciduous Dentine to Caries Studied by Correlated Light and Electron Microscopy," *Caries Res, 3:*348-368, 1969.

46. M. F. Little, E. S. Cueto, and J. Rowley, "Chemical and Physical Properties of Altered and Sound Enamel. I. Ash, Ca, P, CO_2, N, Water, Microradiolucency and Density," *Arch Oral Biol, 7:*173-184, 1962.

47. T. B. Coolidge and M. H. Jacobs, "Enamel Carbonate in Caries," *J Dent Res, 36:*765-768, 1957.

48. M. F. Little, J. Posen, and L. Singer, "Chemical and Physical Properties of Altered and Sound Enamel. III. Fluoride and Sodium Content," *J Dent Res, 41:*784-789, 1962.

49. F. Brudevold, R. Aasenden, H. G. McCann, III, and H. G. McCann, "Use of an Enamel Biopsy Method for Determination of *in Vivo* Uptake of Fluoride from Topical Treatments," *Caries Res, 3:*119-133, 1969.

50. B. R. Bhussry, "Chemical and Physical Studies of Enamel from Human Teeth. III. Specific Gravity, Nitrogen Content and Histologic Characteristics of Opaque White Enamel," *J Dent Res, 37:*1054-1059, 1969.

51. M. F. Little, T. R. Dirksen, and G. Schlueter, "The Ca, P, Na, and Ash Content at Different Depths in Caries," *J Dent Res, 44:*362-365, 1965.

52. G. N. Jenkins, "The Mechanism of Action of Fluoride in Reducing Caries Incidence," *Int Dent J, 17:*552-563, 1967.

53. O. Backer-Dirks, "Posteruptive Changes in Dental Enamel," *J Dent Res, 45:*503-511, 1966.

8

FOOD-CARIES INTER-RELATIONSHIPS

James T. Barenie
Basil G. Bibby

C ENTURIES AGO the wise men of various cultures, in different parts of the world, decided independently that dental decay was the result of food coming in contact with the teeth. If proof of this was needed, it was provided by experiments that showed if contact between caries-producing food and the teeth was avoided by feeding animals through stomach tubes, no caries developed.[1] That bacterial action on food is also needed for the occurrence of caries has been shown by the inability of caries-producing diets to initiate caries in bacteria-free animals.[2]

Beyond the knowledge that food is necessary for the development of caries, present understanding of food-caries interrelationships is vague. This absence of reliable information is due both to a lack of comprehensive scientific effort in the area and also to the complexity of food-caries relationships. It has been demonstrated that even though food is necessary for the initiation of caries, all foods do not promote caries to the same degree. In fact, in various test systems it has been found that some foods or their components give rise to caries, some are caries-inactive, and still others are caries-preventive.[3] Therefore, within a meal or even within a single food there can exist several factors that may promote or retard the development of dental caries.

Further complicating the understanding of the food factors related to dental decay are the diverse mechanisms through which foods can influence caries susceptibility. Nutrients may act systemically during the developmental period to alter the morphology or composition of teeth, thereby rendering them more or less susceptible to decay. At a systemico-local level foods may alter the composition or rate of flow of saliva with consequent modification of the caries process. Locally, retained food can exert direct or indirect effects on the tooth surface. Direct actions on the tooth surface include enamel demineralization by inherent acids, fluoride deposition, or formation of a protective barrier such as a fatty coating. The indirect actions relate to effects on the dental plaque. Foods, by altering the bacterial content, metabolism, and local buffering action of the plaque, can change the immediate environment of the tooth surface.

Available information indicates that nutritional deficiencies or imbalances during tooth development, other than lack of fluoride, play minor roles in determining the intrinsic resistance of teeth to caries attack in either man or animals. There are indications that imbalances can modify the morphology and structure of animal teeth, but clear correlations between such changes and caries have not been offered. Some inadequacies during tooth development such as protein deficiency in rodents suggest that complex metabolic disturbances result in teeth with greater susceptibility to caries. However, some of the reported effects of nutritional factors on animal caries may be attributed to modifications in the frequency of eating or physical properties of the experimental diets rather than to the development of caries-resistant or caries-susceptible teeth. Thus, the preponderance of evidence indicates that nutrition during the developmental period is not an overriding factor determining caries susceptibility.

This chapter will (1) review some of the known food-caries relationships, (2) make specific suggestions for clinicians providing patients with dietary counseling, and (3) propose areas where future research could be beneficial in providing knowledge to ameliorate the caries problem.

SPECIFIC NUTRIENT GROUPS AND DENTAL CARIES
Carbohydrates

Most research has implicated the carbohydrates as that portion of the diet contributing most to the initiation and progression of dental caries. Almost all epidemiological studies show high caries rates in association with high sugar consumption and low caries rates when little sugar is eaten. Further, it has not been possible to produce experimental dental decay without a fairly high content of carbohydrate in the diet. That contact between the carbohydrate and the teeth is necessary has been shown by the absence of caries in animals fed a cariogenic diet through stomach tubes.

However, all carbohydrates do not seem to have the same potential for tooth destruction. Experiments testing the cariogenic effects of starches indicate the starches do not cause as much decay as equivalent amounts of simple sugars.[4] There seems to be conclusive evidence in both animal and human studies that readily fermentable simple sugars such as sucrose, glucose, or fructose are necessary in order for high caries rates to occur. Some authors have gone further by specifically implicating sucrose as the "arch criminal" of dental caries.[5] Clinical surveys show that dental caries is most active in populations that eat large amounts of sucrose-containing foods. However, this does not mean that sucrose is the sole cause of dental caries. It could also mean that sucrose is the cheapest and most available sweetening agent in modern communities. In fact, animal studies have shown other simple sugars quite capable of promoting dental caries.[6, 7]

The role sugars play in the caries process seems to be more complicated than the simple provision of a substrate which is readily metabolized by microorganisms yielding acids that subsequently demineralize the tooth. Studies of some human population groups indicate that teeth developing during periods of sugar restriction may have an innate caries resistance,[8, 9] but these studies have been interpreted differently by some investigators.[10] Animal studies[11, 12] have provided additional evidence that the ingestion of sugars during tooth development may influence the caries susceptibility of teeth. Sognnaes,[11] studying the effects of high dietary carbohydrate levels in rodents, found that increased carbohydrate ingestion during tooth development resulted in an increased susceptibility to caries as seen in Figure 8-1. It is possible, therefore, that carbohydrates may act during the development of teeth to alter caries susceptibility of human teeth.

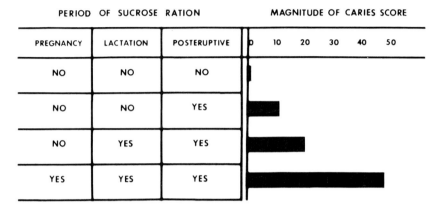

PERIOD OF SUCROSE RATION			MAGNITUDE OF CARIES SCORE					
PREGNANCY	LACTATION	POSTERUPTIVE	0	10	20	30	40	50
NO	NO	NO						
NO	NO	YES						
NO	YES	YES						
YES	YES	YES						

Figure 8-1. Influence of sucrose ration on caries susceptibility of hamsters. Adapted from R. F. Sognnaes, *J Amer Dent Assn*, 1948.

Recently, much attention has been directed to the role that mono- and disaccharides, particularly sucrose, play in providing substrates from which the oral bacteria elaborate polysaccharides.[13] The importance in caries causation of extracellular and intracellular polysaccharides produced by different microorganisms has not yet been determined. It is suggested that these polysaccharides might be utilized as an energy source, resulting in additional or prolonged acid production after dietary sugars are cleared from the mouth. Extracellular polysaccharide formation might further influence the caries process by aiding in the implantation and adhesion of bacterial plaques and/or by inhibiting diffusion of acids and buffering agents.

While epidemiological surveys have shown that dental caries is most active in groups consuming large amounts of carbohydrates, the caries activity does not seem to be related to the total sugar intake per se. Instead, the factors which seem to be of paramount importance are the *frequency* of sugar ingestion and the *adhesiveness* of the sugar-containing food. That the frequency of eating sweet foods has as much or more importance than the total sugar consumption was convincingly demonstrated by the Vipeholm study.[14] Correlations in other groups of children between high caries incidence and the increased frequency

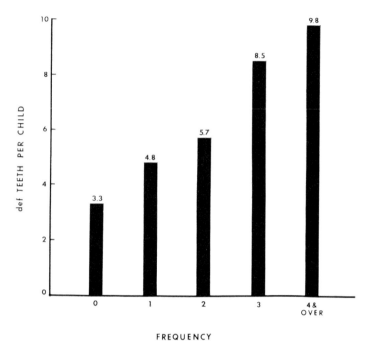

Figure 8-2. Effect of between-meal eating on caries activity in children. From R. L. Weiss and A. H. Trithart, *Amer J Pub Hlth,* 1960.

of between-meal eating also emphasize the importance of this factor. Weiss and Trithart[15] reported a direct and almost linear relationship between caries increments and frequency of ingestion of sugar-containing snacks as seen in Figure 8-2.

Evidence gleaned from clinical experience, the Vipeholm study and observations that liquid diets are less cariogenic[16] indicates that the adhesiveness of food to teeth or the prolonged retention of food in the oral cavity is related to the caries process. The amount of food retained depends upon the food's adhesiveness to the teeth, its cohesiveness, and its speed of dissolution in the mouth. Retention will further vary depending on tooth surface morphology, salivary flow, and activity of oral musculature.

Proteins and Amino Acids

Attempts to relate dietary intake of proteins to dental caries experience in humans are inconclusive, but it is generally believed that proteins may be caries-retarding. Studies are available which show marked caries reductions after caries-susceptible individuals are placed on high-protein diets. In one such study, Becks et al.[17] altered the diets to contain large amounts of meat, eggs, milk, and milk products. After one year on these modified diets, over 60 percent of patients who had previously suffered from rampant caries showed no new decay. However, in this study as in others of its type, the additional protein was supplied at the expense of the carbohydrate portion of the diet. Similar problems of interpretation have arisen when human population groups deficient in dietary protein have been studied. Hurtarte and Scrimshaw[18] reported on the low caries incidence in children deficient in dietary protein; however, the diet was also deficient in refined carbohydrate. These investigations are examples in which multiple dietary modifications cloud the interpretation of the caries-related effects of a single factor.

While the effect of protein on human caries experience is confusing, it is generally agreed that certain proteins and amino acids can reduce caries in animals. However, in many animal experiments testing the effects of diminished or supplemented protein levels, the carbohydrate portion of the diet was also manipulated. There is some evidence available to suggest a possible developmental influence of proteins on caries susceptibility. Experiments[19, 20] have shown that depriving pregnant rats of protein will result in offspring with an increased caries susceptibility. However, other evidence suggests proteins exert their caries-reducing effects through a local postdevelopmental mechanism.

Most investigators have utilized casein, the principal milk protein, in studying the posteruptive effects of protein on animal caries. Osborn et al.[21] compared the effect of the proteins casein and gluten on rat caries and found that rats on a diet of gluten had twice the caries scores of animals eating casein as the major protein source. They postulated that the greater amounts of lysine and glutamic acid present in casein may have been responsible for the lower caries scores. Earlier studies[22, 23] had also demonstrated the caries-reducing effects of casein. The effects of protein may be related to laboratory experiments which have shown that protein can bind to enamel with a resultant reduction in enamel solubility.[24, 25]

Interest has been focused on specific amino acid components of proteins to determine if they might be responsible for effects on caries susceptibility. Shaw[26] has tested the effect of casein and an equivalent amino acid mixture on rat caries. He found that the amino acid mixture gave significantly greater caries reduction for smooth surfaces. It was proposed that the sticky physical nature of casein might bind cariogenic substances to the tooth surface, thereby negating some of the beneficial effects provided by casein's components. Other investigations[27, 28] with the amino acid lysine have given conflicting evidence on its effect in animal caries, but it is generally thought that lysine is caries-reducing. No conclusive evidence is available concerning the effect of other amino acids on caries.

Fats

It has been postulated that the low caries incidence recorded in Eskimo settlements before exposure to civilized dietary regimens was due to the high fat content of the natural diet. Unfortunately, it is just as easy to attribute the low caries activity to a lack of refined carbohydrates. Rosebury and Karshan[29] studied the dietary habits of Eskimos in three Alaskan settlements. Differences in the degree of "Westernization" of the diet as well as differences in caries incidence existed between the three settlements. However, no simple relationship between the amount of fat or any other major component of the diet and the degree of dental decay existing in each settlement could be established.

Boyd[30] reported on caries incidence in two groups of diabetic children. One group received twice as much fat in their diet as did the second group. The caloric value of the fat was replaced by additional carbohydrate in the second group, but no significant difference in caries scores occurred between the two groups.

Although human studies relating fats and caries are inconclusive, there is sufficient evidence existing to conclude that fats reduce caries in animal test systems. Several investigators,[31, 32] studying caries reductions in animals attained through the use of vitamin D preparations, came to the conclusion that both vitamin D and the oils present were responsible for significant caries reduction. The greatest reductions in caries were attained when the vitamin D was given as the animal type of sterol in the form of cod-liver oil. Later studies utilizing diets with high fat concentrations have consistently shown significant reductions in dental caries.[33-35] In some studies such as that by Schweigert,[33] the fat content of the diet was increased at the expense of normal sucrose levels. Altering the diet in this way makes it difficult to interpret the results, because either lowered sucrose levels or higher fat levels could be responsible for the caries reductions. However, previous studies by Schweigert et al.[36] had shown that high caries scores could be produced by diets with low sucrose levels. In the fat addition studies, large amounts of sucrose remained in the diet, yet caries reductions were greater than those in investigations where sucrose levels were decreased. It can be concluded, therefore, that the addition of fat was responsible for the caries reductions.

In another study, Gustafson et al.[37] fed hamsters diets containing 25 percent of a fat (hydrogenated arachis oil, lard, or arachis oil) and compared the caries scores to a control group of hamsters receiving no fat in the diet. All of the groups received a diet containing 45 percent sucrose. The hamsters ingesting the hydrogenated arachis oil exhibited a caries reduction of 83 percent. The hamsters on lard or arachis oil diets exhibited caries reductions of 72 and 64 percent, respectively.

While at least one study gives some evidence of a preeruptive caries-inhibitory effect due to fat,[38] most studies seem to indicate a posteruptive local effect is responsible for the protection. Gustafson et al.[37] found a significantly greater amount of sucrose could be dissolved in fifteen seconds from food particles of the nonfat diet than could be dissolved from food particles of the fat diet. This suggests that fat may form a coating over food particles, inhibiting dissolution of food. Walsh and Green[39] have suggested fats may prevent the demineralization of enamel. They postulated that the formation of a hydrophobic layer of fat on the enamel surface may prevent or retard the dissolution of enamel by certain acids. It has also been suggested that fats may prevent caries by altering the oral flora[40] or by decreasing the oral retention of food residues.[41]

Vitamins

Early investigators hoped to find a causal relationship between various vitamin deficiencies and dental caries; however, it now seems that the role played by vitamin deficiencies in the caries process is minor. It is known that vitamins A, C, and D are necessary during tooth development in order for proper formation and mineralization to occur. While definitive relationships between the caries susceptibility of teeth developing during the occurrence of deficient or ideal levels of these vitamins have not been established for man, it is easy to believe that a more perfectly formed tooth would be less susceptible to decay.

Whether vitamins affect the caries process by influencing the oral microorganisms is not known, but theoretically, vitamin deficiencies could limit microbial metabolism, thus reducing acid production and possibly caries rates. However, little information is available indicating that vitamin deficiencies result in reduced caries incidence in humans, and in any case, it would be unrealistic to recommend vitamin deprivation because of the debilitating effects to the human host.[42] Attempts to reduce caries in man through vitamin supplementation have generally failed. Of the vitamins tested, pyridoxine (vitamin B_6) seems to hold the most promise for preventing caries. Several investigators have reported significant caries reductions in animals and humans using pyridoxine supplements.[43-45] It has been postulated that pyridoxine exerts this effect by stimulating that portion of the oral flora which produces less lactic acid. With the increased number of these organisms, there is a resultant decline in the number of lactic acid-producing organisms.[46]

Phosphates

Numerous studies have shown that the addition of phosphates to the diet of animals results in significant reductions in dental decay.[47, 48] Several types of inorganic and organic phosphates have been found to exert this cariostatic effect. Of the phosphates tested in animal studies, sodium trimetaphosphate, sodium orthophosphate, and dibasic calcium orthophosphate have given the greatest caries reductions. It has generally been found that the more insoluble the phosphate compound, such as the calcium phosphates, the less likely it is to produce significant inhibition of dental caries.

Unfortunately, the dramatic effects of inorganic phosphates in preventing caries in animals are not paralleled in man. In two investigations in which phosphates were added to flour that was incorporated into baked goods eaten by subjects, no caries-protective effect could be established.[49, 50] Phosphate supplementation of breakfast cereals eaten by children has been reported to result in a 20 to 40 percent reduction of decay,[51] but a more recent study by Peterson found no beneficial effect to be gained from eating phosphate-supplemented cereals.[52] Another trial involving phosphates utilized chewing gum as the vehicle.[53] The phosphate-enriched gum seemed to offer no greater benefit than a sugarless gum since children chewing these gums demonstrated similar reductions in caries compared to children chewing sugar-containing gum. The apparent inability of phosphates to reduce caries in man may be related to (1) the lower phosphate to food ratios used in the human tests, (2) differences in the frequency of phosphate intake, or (3) differences between the oral environments of test animals and man.

While the inorganic phosphates tested in man have shown mixed effectiveness, a product having the registered trademark Anticay®* has demonstrated consistent caries reductions in the order of 20 percent.[54] Anticay is composed of approximately 85 percent organic calcium sucrose phosphate esters and 15 percent

---

* CSR Research Laboratores, Roseville, NSW, Australia.

inorganic calcium orthophosphate. It is added to foods so that it represents 1 percent by weight of the carbohydrate present in the food. Anticay has been approved as an additive to foods in Australia, and it has demonstrated few problems in changing the taste or texture of the foods to which it is added. Similar products are now being tested in the United States.

Fluoride

The ingestion of optimal fluoride concentrations is the easiest and most effective known method of preventing decay. The value and safety of communal fluoride programs is certain—as evidenced by the 80 million people drinking fluoridated water in the United States. In spite of this evidence, an even greater number of people are not receiving the benefits of fluoride for various social, political, and economic reasons. In order to protect a larger part of the population from caries, the dental practitioner must continue efforts to obtain communal fluoridation in fluoride deficient areas because of the obvious advantages provided by this public health measure. During the last twenty-five years, the role of the dentist in promoting communal water fluoridation seems to have been that of an educator or an aloof expert. During this period, fluoridation programs suffered many setbacks that possibly could have been averted if alternative motivational techniques had been utilized. Knutson,[55] in evaluating progress of fluoridation programs, has suggested that future success may well depend more on the role of the dentist as a politician than as an educator.

While communal fluoridation offers numerous advantages, it seems likely that large segments of the population will not receive these benefits for many years. The dentist treating patients residing in fluoride deficient areas must be prepared to prescribe systemic fluoride on an individual basis for caries prevention. It has been suggested that fluoride can be added to milk, salt, flour, vitamins, etc., to establish optimal fluoride ingestion, but it appears the easiest and most certain method of delivery would be in the form of a fluoride tablet, solution, or lozenge. These supplements taken alone or combined with food or drink offer versatility of administration that should sufficiently meet most individual requirements.

The 1958 report of the Council on Dental Therapeutics of the American Dental Association[56] recommended that when drinking water is devoid of fluoride, children three years of age and older should receive 1.0 mg of fluoride ion per day in supplement form. Children two to three years of age should receive 0.5 mg of fluoride ion per day, and children below this age should have all food and drink prepared using water supplemented to contain 1.0 ppm fluoride. Other recommendations made by the Council concerning supplemental fluoride prescriptions included:

1. Fluoride prescriptions should bear the warning: "CAUTION: Store out of reach of children."
2. Prescriptions should not be made for more than 264 mg of sodium fluoride.
3. Fluoride supplements should only be prescribed when the fluoride ion concentration of the drinking water is less than 0.7 ppm. The amount of fluoride in the supplement should be adjusted to account for any naturally occurring water-borne fluoride.
4. Only parents expected to follow directions carefully should be allowed to carry out an individual supplementation program.

Trace Elements

The conclusive evidence that small amounts of fluoride can markedly influence caries experience has stimulated investigation of the effects of other trace elements on the caries process. Large regional differences in trace element concentration of soil, water, and food exist, and these differences, working alone or perhaps in conjunction with another variable such as fluoride, may be responsible for altered caries susceptibility.

In a review article by Lossee and Ludwig,[57] attention was focused on how the trace elements molybdenum, strontium, and selenium may affect human caries experience. The simultaneous existence of reduced caries incidence and high levels of water-borne molybdenum or strontium has led several investigators to believe that these trace elements may exert a beneficial influence in reducing dental caries.[58–61] Investigations on the effects of selenium by Hadjimarkos et al.[62, 63] have related high levels of this element to increased caries experience. Although there are indications that these trace elements as well as others such as boron, lithium, and vanadium may modify the incidence of caries, only fluoride has been clearly shown to reduce caries.

RELATED FOOD INTERREACTIONS IN THE ORAL CAVITY

Food-Saliva Relationships

Understanding the role played by saliva in the caries process has proved an elusive quest. It is known that food stimuli can alter the flow and composition of saliva, but the exact changes have not been accurately measured. It is difficult to measure these changes because many factors can alter saliva, including (1) the rate of salivary flow, (2) the duration and type of stimulus responsible for the salivary flow, (3) the glands from which the saliva is secreted, (4) the time of day, and (5) contamination of saliva from sources such as food, plaque, and crevicular fluid. Because of variables such as these, most studies on saliva have failed to adequately standardize the sampling technics. Certain conclusions have been made, however, concerning the effects foods have on saliva.

Food can affect saliva through a local reflex mechanism and perhaps by systemic pathways. Highly flavored foods or those requiring vigorous chewing act through the local reflex mechanism to change the rate of flow and composition of saliva. Systemic manifestations of food influences are represented by nutrients such as proteins, which can alter the blood urea concentration, thus affecting the salivary urea level. Although the exact systemic mechanisms of action are unknown, some nutrients can alter saliva, possibly in such a way that caries susceptibility would be influenced.

It has been found that the buffering capacity of the saliva is enhanced by increasing salivary flow. It has also been suggested that foods change the buffering capacity of saliva. Ericsson reported that proteins and vegetables raised the buffering capacity of saliva, while carbohydrates reduced it.[64] Unfortunately, the rate of flow was not measured in this study, and it is possible flow alterations were responsible for the findings.

While the relationship between xerostomia and rampant caries is well known, more subtle variations in salivary flow have not been shown to have pronounced effects on caries experience. Slack and Martin[65] have shown that increasing salivary flow can result in tooth cleanliness equivalent to that provided through toothbrushing. Although this increased salivary flow was not obtained from normal foodstuffs, it provided evidence of beneficial effects obtained by increasing salivary flow. Diminished salivary flow has been related to dehydration and the consumption of exclusively liquid diets.[66] The decreased salivary flow associated with liquid diets might favor caries development, but this would probably be offset by the decreased cariogenicity of liquid diets.

The salivary content of ions such as calcium, phosphate, and fluoride could affect the caries process. However, in a review by Dawes,[67] it was pointed out that because of homeostatic regulation there is little change in the blood or saliva concentration of these ions, despite additional dietary ingestion.

Although there is reason to believe that the amount of saliva and its chemistry are related to caries, there is no clear evidence to show that changes in food or nutrition can modify saliva so that it could offset acid action in the mouth or make the teeth more or less resistant to decay. While the reflex responses of the salivary glands influence the quantity and quality of saliva, no practical way of using this response for the prevention of caries has been propounded, other than attempting to stimulate a flow of saliva with high buffering power at the end of a meal.

Food and Oral Microorganisms

Food is capable of influencing the oral flora through systemic and local pathways. Examples of systemic pathways include certain nutritional deficiency states such as iron or vitamin B deficiencies in which oral manifestations as well as alterations in the oral flora occur.[68] Although food acting systemically can affect the oral microorganisms, it is much more likely that the presence of food in the oral cavity is responsible for influencing the bacterial population. Thus, the composition and consistency of foods and the frequency with which they are eaten may affect the oral microorganisms.

Changes in the diet do not appear to bring about absolute alterations in the makeup of the bacterial spectrum of the mouth; neither the complete elimination of some species nor the extensive overgrowth of others has been documented. Jay[69] reported that patients with high initial lactobacillus counts placed on a restricted carbohydrate diet showed remarkable reductions in the number of lactobacilli present. However, observations in man and monkeys[70] have shown that while the lactobacillus count changes in response to food intake, the streptococcal population is less affected.

Although the streptococcal population of the plaque is generally unaffected by dietary variation, it is of interest that the portion of the streptococcal population that forms extracellular polysaccharide is modified by diet. Bowen[70] has shown that the number of polysaccharide-forming streptococci in monkeys declines when dietary carbohydrate is restricted. Krasse[71] has further shown that the presence of certain sugars in the diet, notably sucrose and lactose, favors the implementation of such cariogenic streptococci in hamsters. The stimulation of extracellular polysaccharide formation by sucrose results in a heavier plaque containing a smaller total bacterial population, and one in which the nutritionally deprived organisms in its depth have a different metabolism from those on the surface. While both the number of polysaccharide-forming bacteria and the amount of polysaccharide formed are responsive to sucrose intake, it must be borne in mind that the property of stimulating formation of extracellular polysaccharide is not limited to sucrose.

That alterations of microbial metabolism or growth by dietary means might modify the caries attack is indicated by reported effects of pyridoxine. Strean et al.[43, 46] have demonstrated that alterations in the oral flora as well as caries reductions occur if diets are supplemented with pyridoxine. Although the oral microorganisms can be influenced by dietary alterations as shown above, there is not sufficient evidence to establish the significance of major nutrients such as proteins, fats, or minerals on bacterial growth or metabolism.

Tooth-Cleansing Ability of Foods

The use of fibrous foods to cleanse teeth while eating has often been recommended by dentists as an effective plaque and caries control measure. There is little scientific evidence that any significant cleansing action or caries prevention is exerted by fibrous foods.

Howitt et al.[72] studied an inmate of San Quentin Prison who volunteered to subject himself to various dietary and toothbrushing regimens. To their surprise the investigators found that while eating either a "sticky carbohydrate" or a "detergent" diet, an increase in retained debris was observed beyond that occurring with the normal prison diet. The greatest increase of debris occurred while consuming the detergent diet, which was composed mainly of raw fruits and vegetables. Further efforts to increase the detergent effect of the diet did not result in an improvement in oral hygiene when compared to the "sticky carbohydrate" diet.

A study by Knighton,[73] often quoted as demonstrating the detergent qualities of food, measured the ability of chewing and brushing to remove yeast cells, previously eaten in the form of a cake, from the oral cavity. Salivary samples were taken to measure the retained yeast cells. It was found that by chewing paraffin, gum, apples, oranges, bananas, or candy it was possible to remove more organisms than was possible utilizing toothbrushing. However, the experimental design was such that total oral clearance was measured rather than the removal of toothborne organisms.

Slack and Martin[65] reported the results of a two-year study comparing a group of apple-chewing children to a nonchewing control group. The children chewing apples had significantly better gingival health and encouraging reductions in caries increments. However, the previous caries experience of the control and test groups was significantly different, thus placing some doubt on the conclusiveness of the study.

Clark et al.[74] compared the cleansing ability of toothbrushing to apple chewing. In their experiments, the average cleaning efficiency attained by chewing apples was 90 percent. Toothbrushing resulted in only a 60 percent cleaning efficiency. However, in this study also, the experimental design measured total oral clearance rather than removal of adherent dental plaque. While trying to measure the cleaning potential of fibrous foods, Clark et al. found that one of the most important factors in toothcleaning was the stimulation of salivary flow. They therefore attempted the development of a nonchewable tablet containing salivary stimulants. The stimulated salivary flow was found to be as effective as toothbrushing in removing the test food residue.

Arnim[75] compared the ability of fibrous foods, personal oral hygiene (brushing, dentifrices, flossing, and oral irrigation), and mouthwashes to cleanse the tooth surfaces. Utilizing disclosing solutions, photographs, and planimeter measurements, he measured the removal of bacterial plaque from the labial surfaces of anterior teeth. The fibrous foods were chewed for three hours, and special efforts were made to chew vigorously as well as to rub the food particles against the teeth. The test foods eaten in the three-hour period were sugar cane, apples, celery, lettuce, and carrots. The results showed that "no teeth were cleaned perceptibly on approximal surfaces by chewing, nor were they thoroughly cleansed on any surface, save possibly the occlusal."[75] The measurements made on the labial surfaces showed that only from 3 to 19 percent of the surface had been cleaned.

In a more recent study,[76] eighteen male dental students were studied for the effects of chewing carrots on the plaque, gingiva, and gingival exudate. Nine of the students chewed three carrots three times a day for eighteen days as the sole method of oral hygiene. The nine remaining students chewed no carrots and used no oral hygiene methods. The results, as shown in Figure 8-3, demonstrated no significant difference in the plaque index between the control and experimental groups at any time in the investigation.

The use of foods that require chewing such as apples, carrots, or celery may be beneficial at the tooth surface by stimulating

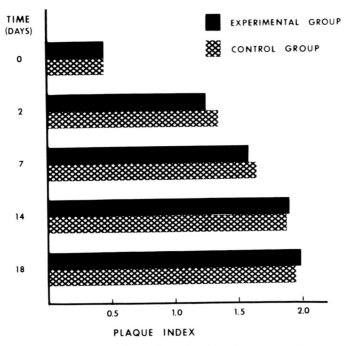

Figure 8-3. Mean plaque index values for dental students obtained at the start and after two, seven, fourteen, and eighteen days without active oral hygiene. Adapted from J. Lindhe and P. Wicen, *J Periodont Res,* 1969.

an increased flow of protective saliva. This action of supposedly detergent foods could be of more value than their doubtful effect in removing plaque. However, the time and effort of both the patient and trained dental personnel could no doubt be spent in more valuable preventive measures. If efforts to use fibrous foods are encouraged in a preventive program, their value may come from replacement of more cariogenic foods. The use of fibrous foods, however, should not be recommended as a replacement for more proven cleansing technics.

PRACTICAL APPLICATION OF FOOD-CARIES RELATIONSHIPS FOR CARIES PREVENTION

Although dentists have some background in the science of nutrition, it is questionable whether they have sufficient knowledge or whether it is their proper place to provide overall nutritional guidance. Instead, it is felt that specific dietary counseling as it relates to oral health is indicated, but patients with systemic problems exhibiting oral manifestations are best treated by referral to a physician. Most dental patients are in need of caries-preventive dietary advice; the nature of the advice depends upon the individual's oral and systemic condition. The majority of dental patients should receive the basic dietary advice that would aid in a caries-preventive program. A more select group of patients could receive intensive dietary analysis as well as more comprehensive dietary recommendations.

The basic dietary counseling all patients should receive as part of a preventive program would include a brief explanation of the caries process and the essential role that food, especially sucrose, plays in the process. The detrimental effects of frequent ingestion of adhesive refined carbohydrates should be stressed. Recommendations to limit the frequency of carbohydrate ingestion would be of more benefit than attempts to only limit the amount of sugar ingested. A brief verbal history may be helpful to determine the presence of pernicious eating habits which should be eliminated or for which more acceptable substitutes could be recommended. Substitutes could include foods containing less fermentable carbohydrates as well as less cariogenic liquid substitutes. Frequently suggested substitutes include fresh fruits and vegetables, nuts, cheeses, milk, and sucrose-free confections. While this type of dietary advice is not based upon a comprehensive dietary analysis, the recommendation of acceptable substitutes and a reduction in the frequency of sucrose intake are practical suggestions that can be followed by most patients. Supplemental fluorides should be recommended for patients residing in fluoride-deficient areas.

More comprehensive dietary counseling would be indicated when patients are suffering from rampant caries, when patients are highly motivated toward prevention, or when prevention is essential as in patients with hemophilia. Jay[77] and Nizel[78] have been prominent promoters of dietary analyses and regimens intended to prevent decay as well as provide nutritional adequacy.

The reader is referred to these sources for a listing of specific technics and diets recommended for large-scale alterations in dietary regimens. Such programs are based upon the sound scientific knowledge that restriction in the ingestion of readily fermentable carbohydrates will reduce dental caries. The beneficial effects of dietary counseling on caries occurrence were shown by Howe et al.[79] They found that in 189 patients considered to be cooperative in following dietary recommendations an average decrease in caries incidence of 56 percent occurred. These dramatic results were confirmed by Becks et al.[17] in a study involving 790 patients suffering with rampant decay (ten new carious surfaces per year). By reducing the intake of refined carbohydrates, over 80 percent of the patients showed less than two new carious surfaces per year.

Although the benefits to be gained from dietary counseling are well established, the utilization of this preventive therapy is minimal. Doyle[80] contends that the lack of financial reward as well as the likelihood of the advice being unheeded are the principal reasons for the limited utilization of nutritional counseling by dental practitioners. Further, although the dental benefits of restricted diets are established, the emotional effects on a child are not. A joint committee of the American Academy of Pediatrics and the American Society of Dentistry for Children[81] reported: "It is worth remembering that special dietary programs have other implications in childhood. If a child is compelled to eat a diet that is different from that of the other children even in his own home, and if the diet is different from the school meal, other children will make life miserable for the child in question. The result may be damaging to the sense of security. This factor should be carefully considered in relation to whatever advantages may be obtained by special diets."

Bearing in mind the difficulty in obtaining cooperation in large-scale dietary alterations, the amount of time involved in bringing about such changes as well as proper follow-up guidance, and the possible deleterious effects on the child's emotional complexion, it seems wise to limit the application of this type of therapy.

AREAS FOR FUTURE FOOD-CARIES RESEARCH

It is a logical conclusion that the most promising road to wide-spread prevention of caries would be to concentrate efforts on its most widespread cause—people's eating habits. It is probably true that given all the advantages that can be obtained from dietary counseling, fluoride, occlusal sealants, advanced dental care, and meticulous oral hygiene, a select fraction of the population will be able to demonstrate appreciable success in the prevention of dental caries. However, disease prevention for a favored minority of the population is no longer an acceptable social goal. Instead, methods must be sought that will benefit the population at large while requiring little or no effort on the part of the individual.

In the effort to discourage between-meal eating of destructive foods, neither education nor legislation can be expected to accomplish much until more is known about the social, psychological, and physiological reasons for snacking or sucrose addiction. What is needed are motivational technics that might be used on a mass-media basis and that are capable of altering an individual's desire for satisfaction of a deep-seated drive such as appetite.

An alternative approach of substituting less cariogenic candies and snacks for those of higher cariogenicity or of incorporating cariostatic agents into known cariogenic foodstuffs seems to hold more promise for reducing dental caries. While it is known that sucrose is the principal cause of caries, it is not known for certain how to replace it or combine it to produce candies or foods that will have competitive taste and cost appeal, without which any program of food substitution will be largely ineffective. Further, continuing research must discover what foodstuffs, as distinct from sucrose used in a pure state, contribute to the accumulation or removal of plaque; which foods produce more acid in plaque or destroy more enamel; and which foods contain protective factors. Studies testing the effects of food additives on human caries experience are needed to establish whether additives such as orthophosphates, trimetaphosphates, organic phosphates, trace elements, or pyridoxin, which have shown promise in laboratory and animal studies, have any value for large-scale caries prevention in man.

REFERENCES

1. O. W. Kite, J. H. Shaw, and R. F. Sognnaes, "The Prevention of Experimental Tooth Decay by Tube-feeding," *J Nutr,* 42:89-105, 1950.
2. F. J. Orland, J. R. Blayney, R. W. Harrison, R. F. Ervin, J. A. Reyniers, P. C. Trexler, H. A. Gordon, and M. Wagner, "Experimental Caries in Germfree Rats Inoculated with Enterococci," *JADA,* 50:259-272, 1955.
3. R. M. Stephan, "Effects of Different Types of Human Foods on Dental Health in Experimental Animals," *J Dent Res,* 45:1551-1561, 1966.
4. W. G. Shafer, "The Caries-Producing Capacity of Starch, Glucose, and Sucrose Diets in the Syrian Hamster," *Science,* 110:143-144, 1949.
5. E. Newbrun, "Sucrose, the Arch Criminal of Dental Caries," *J Dent Child,* 36:239-248, 1969.
6. T. H. Grenby and J. B. Hutchinson, "The Effects of Diets Containing Sucrose, Glucose or Fructose on Experimental Dental Caries in Two Strains of Rats," *Arch Oral Biol,* 14:373-380, 1969.
7. R. M. Green and R. L. Hartles, "The Effect of Diets Containing Different Mono- and Disaccharides on the Incidence of Dental Caries in the Albino Rat," *Arch Oral Biol,* 14:235-241, 1969.
8. R. Harris, "Biology of the Children of Hopewood House, Bowral, Australia. 4. Observations of Dental-Caries Experience Extending Over 5 Years (1957-1961)," *J Dent Res,* 42:1387-1399, 1963.
9. R. F. Sognnaes, "Analysis of Wartime Reduction of Dental Caries in European Children," *Am J Dis Child,* 75:792-821, 1948.
10. T. M. Marthaler, "Epidemiological and Clinical Dental Findings in Relation to Intake of Carbohydrates," *Caries Res,* 1:222-238, 1967.
11. R. F. Sognnaes, "Caries-Conducive Effect of a Purified Diet When Fed to Rodents During Tooth Development," *JADA,* 37:676-692, 1948.
12. R. R. Steinman and M. I. Haley, "The Biological Effect of Various Carbohydrates Ingested During the Calcification of the Teeth," *J Dent Res,* 24:211-214, 1957.
13. R. J. Fitzgerald and H. V. Jordan, "Polysaccharide Producing Bacteria and Caries," In R. S. Harris (Ed.), *Art and Science of Dental Caries Research* (New York, Acad Pr, 1968), pp. 79-86.
14. B. E. Gustafsson, C. E. Quensel, L. S. Lanke, C. Lundquist, H. Grahnen, B. E. Bonow, and B. Krasse, "The Vipeholm Dental Caries Study. The Effect of Different Levels of Carbohydrate Intake on

Caries Activity in 436 Individuals Observed for Five Years," *Acta Odontol Scand, 11:*232-364, 1964.

15. R. L. Weiss and A. H. Trithart, "Between-Meal Eating Habits and Dental Caries Experience in Preschool Children," *Am J Public Health, 50:*1097-1104, 1960.

16. G. Gustafson, E. Stelling, E. Abramson, and E. Brunius, "Experimental Dental Caries in Golden Hamsters. V. The Cariogenic Effect of Different Carbohydrates in Dry and Moist Diets," *Odontol Tid, 63:* 506-523, 1955.

17. H. Becks, A. L. Jensen, and C. B. Millarr, "Rampant Dental Caries: A Five Year Clinical Survey," *J Dent Res, 23:*210-211, 1944.

18. A. Hurtarte and N. S. Scrimshaw, "Dental Findings in a Nutritional Study of School Children in Five Guatemalan Highland Villages," *J Dent Res, 34:*390-396, 1955.

19. P. J. Holloway, J. H. Shaw, and E. A. Sweeney, "Effects of Various Sucrose : Casein Ratios in Purified Diets on the Teeth and Supporting Structures of Rats," *Arch Oral Biol, 3:*185-200, 1961.

20. J. H. Shaw, "Influence of Marginal and Complete Protein Deficiency for Varying Periods During Reproduction on Growth, Third-Molar Eruption and Dental Caries in Rats," *J Dent Res, 48:*310-316, 1969.

21. M. O. Osborn, J. F. Carey, and A. K. Fisher, "Effect of Dietary Protein and Fat on Dental Caries in the Rat," *J Dent Res, 45:*1564, 1966.

22. B. S. Schweigert, E. Potts, J. H. Shaw, M. Zepplin, and P. H. Phillips, "Dental Caries in the Cotton Rat. VIII. Further Studies on the Dietary Effects of Carbohydrate, Protein and Fat on the Incidence and Extent of Carious Lesions," *J Nutr, 32:*405-412, 1946.

23. L. A. Bavetta and F. J. McClure, "Protein Factors and Experimental Rat Caries," *J Nutr, 63:*107-117, 1957.

24. E. I. Pearce and B. G. Bibby, "Protein Adsorption on Bovine Enamel," *Arch Oral Biol, 11:*329-336, 1966.

25. M. E. Weiss and B. G. Bibby, "Some Protein Effects on Enamel Solubility," *Arch Oral Biol, 11:*59-63, 1966.

26. J. H. Shaw, "Influence of Casein Replacement by Amino Acid Mixture on Experimental Dental Caries in Rats and on the Periodontal Syndrome in Rice Rats," *J Dent Res, 45:*1810-1814, 1966.

27. F. J. McClure, "Wheat Cereal Diets, Rat Caries, Lysine and Minerals," *J Nutr, 65:*619-631, 1958.

28. M. L. Dodds, "Protein and Lysine as Factors in the Cariogenicity of a Cereal Diet," *J Nutr, 82:*217-223, 1964.

29. T. Rosebury and M. Karshan, "Dental Caries Among Eskimos of the Kuskokwim Area of Alaska. III. A Dietary Study of Three Eskimo Settlements," *Am J Dis Child, 57:*1343-1362, 1939.

30. J. D. Boyd, "Dental Caries as Influenced by Fat Versus Carbohydrate in the Diet," *Am J Dis Child,* 67:278-281, 1944.

31. T. Rosebury and M. Karshan, "Susceptibility to Dental Caries in the Rat. VIII. Further Studies of the Influence of Vitamin D and of Fat and Fatty Oils," *J Dent Res,* 18:189-202, 1939.

32. E. C. McBeath and W. A. Verlin, "Further Studies on the Role of Vitamin D in the Nutritional Control of Dental Caries in Children," *JADA,* 29:1393-1397, 1942.

33. B. S. Schweigert, J. H. Shaw, M. Zepplin and C. A. Elvehjem, "Dental Caries in the Cotton Rat. VI. The Effect of the Amount of Protein, Fat and Carbohydrate in the Diet on the Incidence and Extent of Carious Lesions," *J Nutr,* 31:439-447, 1946.

34. H. Granados, J. Glavind, and H. Dam, "Observations on Experimental Dental Caries. The Effect of Purified Rations with, and without Dietary Fat," *Acta Pathol Microbiol Scand,* 25:453-459, 1948.

35. J. H. Shaw, "Effects of Dietary Composition on Tooth Decay in the Albino Rat," *J Nutr,* 41:13-24, 1950.

36. B. S. Schweigert, J. H. Shaw, P. H. Phillips, and C. A. Elvehjem, "Dental Caries in the Cotton Rat. III. Effect of Different Dietary Carbohydrates on the Incidence and Extent of Dental Caries," *J Nutr,* 29:405-411, 1945.

37. G. Gustafson, E. Stelling, E. Abramson, and E. Brunius, "Experiments with Various Fats in a Cariogenic Diet. IV. Experimental Dental Caries in Golden Hamsters," *Acta Odontol Scand,* 13:75-84, 1955.

38. G. J. Cox, "Dental Caries Today," *Penn Dent J,* 15:307-310, 1948.

39. J. P. Walsh and R. W. Green, "The Influence of Some Surface-Active Substances on Decalcification of the Enamel Surface," *J Dent Res,* 29:270-277, 1950.

40. W. L. Williams, H. P. Broquist, and E. E. Snell, "Oleic Acid and Related Compounds as Growth Factors for Lactic Acid Bacteria," *J Biol Chem,* 170:619-630, 1947.

41. B. G. Bibby, H. J. V. Goldberg, and E. Chen, "Evaluation of Caries-Producing Potentialities of Various Foodstuffs," *JADA,* 42:491-509, 1951.

42. S. Dreizen, "Vitamins and Dental Caries," in R. F. Gould (Ed.), *Dietary Chemicals vs. Dental Caries* (Washington, D.C., Am Chem Soc Pub, 1970), pp. 33-45.

43. L. P. Strean, F. T. Bell, E. W. Gilfillan, G. A. Emerson, and E. E. Howe, "The Importance of Pyridoxine in the Suppression of Dental Caries in School Children and Hamsters," *NYS Dent J,* 24:133-137, 1958.

44. R. W. Hillman, P. G. Cabaud, and R. A. Schenone, "The Effects of

Pyridoxine Supplements on the Dental Caries Experience of Pregnant Women," *Am J Clin Nutr*, 10:512-515, 1962.

45. W. H. Bowen, "Effects of Foods on Oral Bacterial Populations in Man and Animals," *J Dent Res*, 49:1276-1281, 1970.

46. L. P. Strean, "The Importance of Pyridoxine in Effecting a Change in Microflora of the Mouth and Intestines," *NYS Dent J*, 23:85-87, 1957.

47. A. E. Nizel and R. S. Harris, "The Effects of Phosphates on Experimental Dental Caries: A Literature Review," *J Dent Res*, 43:1123-1136, 1964.

48. P. H. Keyes, "Research in Dental Caries," *JADA*, 76:1357-1373, 1968.

49. I. I. Ship, and O. Mickelsen, "The Effects of Calcium Acid Phosphate on Dental Caries in Children: A Controlled Clinical Trial," *J Dent Res*, 43:1144-1149, 1964.

50. H. M. Averill and B. G. Bibby, "A Clinical Test of Additions of Phosphate to the Diet of Children," *J Dent Res*, 43:1150-1155, 1964.

51. G. K. Stookey, R. A. Carroll, and J. C. Muhler, "The Clinical Effectiveness of Phosphate-Enriched Breakfast Cereals on the Incidence of Dental Caries in Children: Results After Two Years," *JADA*, 74:752-758, 1967.

52. J. K. Peterson, "North Dakota Field Test of Cariostatic Effect of 1% Sodium Dihydrogen Phosphate and Disodium Hydrogen Phosphate Added to Presweetened Breakfast Cereals," *J Dent Res*, 48:1308, 1969.

53. S. B. Finn and H. C. Jamison, "The Effect of a Dicalcium Phosphate Chewing Gum on Caries Incidence in Children: 30-Month Results," *JADA*, 74:987-995, 1967.

54. B. M. Smythe, "ANTICAY—A New Food Additive to Help Reduce Dental Caries," *Fd Technol Aust*, 23:56-61, 1971.

55. J. W. Knutson, "Water Fluoridation After 25 Years," *JADA*, 80:765-769, 1970.

56. Council on Dental Therapeutics, American Dental Association, "Prescribing Supplements of Dietary Fluorides," *JADA*, 56:589-591, 1958.

57. F. L. Losee and T. G. Ludwig, "Trace Elements and Caries," *J Dent Res*, 49:1229-1236, 1970.

58. T. G. Ludwig, W. B. Healy, and F. L. Losee, "An Association Between Dental Caries and Certain Soil Conditions in New Zealand," *Nature*, 186:695-696, 1960.

59. R. J. Anderson, "The Relationship Between Dental Conditions and the Trace Element Molybdenum," *Caries Res*, 3:75-87, 1969.

60. H. Lodrup, "The Low Rate of Dental Decay in Bonn on Rhein, and the Conclusions that Can Be Drawn from It," *Nor Tannlaegeforen Tid*, 63:35-50, 1953.

61. F. L. Losee and B. L. Adkins, "A Study of the Mineral Environment of Caries-Resistant Navy Recruits," *Caries Res, 3:*23-31, 1969.

62. D. M. Hadjimarkos, C. A. Storvick, and L. F. Remmert, "Selenium and Dental Caries. An Investigation Among School Children of Oregon," *J Pediatr, 40:*451-455, 1952.

63. D. M. Hadjimarkos, "Selenium: A Caries-Enhancing Trace Element," *Caries Res, 3:*14-22, 1969.

64. Y. Ericsson, "Clinical Investigations of the Salivary Buffering Action," *Acta Odontol Scand, 17:*131-165, 1959.

65. G. L. Slack and W. J. Martin, "Apples and Dental Health," *Brit Dent J, 105:*366-371, 1958.

66. H. D. Hall, J. J. Merig, Jr., and C. A. Schneyer, "Metrecal® Induced Changes in Human Saliva," *Proc Soc Exp Biol Med, 124:*532-536, 1967.

67. C. Dawes, "Effects of Diet on Salivary Secretion and Composition," *J Dent Res, 49:*1263-1273, 1970.

68. B. Krasse, "The Effect of Nutrition on Saliva and Oral Flora," *Symp Swed Nutr Found, 3:*21-29, 1965.

69. P. Jay, "The Reduction of Oral Lactobacillus Counts by the Periodic Restriction of Carbohydrate," *Am J Ortho Oral Surg, 33:*162-184, 1947.

70. W. H. Bowen and D. E. Cornick, "Effects of Carbohydrate Restriction in Monkeys *(M. irus)* With Active Caries," *Helv Odontol Acta, 11:* 27-31, 1967.

71. B. Krasse, "The Effect of the Diet on the Implantation of Caries-Inducing Streptococci in Hamsters," *Arch Oral Biol, 10:*215-221, 1965.

72. B. F. Howitt, W. C. Fleming, and F. V. Simonton, "A Study of the Effects Upon the Hygiene and Microbiology of the Mouth of Various Diets, Without and With the Use of the Toothbrush," *Dent Cosmos, 70:*575-588, 1928.

73. H. T. Knighton, "Effects of Various Foods and Cleansing Agents on the Elimination of Artificially Inoculated Yeast from the Mouth," *JADA, 29:*2012-2018, 1942.

74. R. H. Clark, D. I. Hay, C. J. Schram, and B. J. Wagg, "Removal of Carbohydrate Debris from the Teeth by Salivary Stimulation," *Brit Dent J, 111:*244-248, 1961.

75. S. S. Arnim, "The Use of Disclosing Agents for Measuring Tooth Cleanliness," *J Periodontol, 34:*227-245, 1963.

76. J. Lindhe and P. Wicen, "The Effects on the Gingivae of Chewing Fibrous Foods," *J Periodont Res, 4:*193-201, 1969.

77. P. Jay, A. M. Beeuwkes, and H. M. Benson, *Dietary Program for the Control of Dental Caries.* Ann Arbor, Overback, 1955.

78. A. E. Nizel, *The Science of Nutrition and Its Application in Clinical Dentistry,* 2nd ed. Philadelphia, Saunders, 1966.

79. P. R. Howe, B. S. White, and M. D. Elliott, "The Influence of Nutritional Supervision on Dental Caries," *JADA*, 29:38-43, 1942.

80. W. A. Doyle, "Utilization of Dietary Counseling in a Private Office," *Dent Clin North Am*, *July*:517-524, 1965.

81. Report of the Joint Committee of the American Academy of Pediatrics and the American Society of Dentistry for Children, "Dental Caries and a Consideration of the Role of Diet in Prevention," *Pediatrics*, 23:400-407, 1959.

9

THE EFFECTIVENESS OF ORAL HYGIENE METHODS IN THE CONTROL OF DENTAL CARIES

Louis W. Ripa

THE CARIES-DIRECTED GOAL of oral hygiene procedures is the removal of all easily fermentable carbohydrates, plaque, and other debris from the tooth surfaces. This is a logical approach based upon the chemicoparasitic theory of dental decay. By eliminating bacteria and their nutrients from the tooth surface, a caries-conducive dietobacterial milieu cannot establish itself and generate the acid conditions necessary for demineralization of the tooth surface.

Methods of oral hygiene advocated as providing some degree of oral cleanliness include manual and automatic toothbrushing, flossing, mouth rinsing, and oral irrigation. Certain fibrous foods have also been recommended as aids in caries control because of their supposed cleaning ability.

MANUAL TOOTHBRUSHING

Regular toothbrushing removes oral debris and is beneficial in limiting gingivitis and periodontal disease.[1, 2] A similar relationship between toothbrushing and caries, however, is difficult to document. Several studies, reviewed by Bibby,[3] have failed to establish a significant correlation between toothbrushing habits and the incidence of dental caries.

Koch and Lindhe[4] assessed the effect of daily supervised tooth-brushing using a nontherapeutic dentifrice in Swedish school children ages nine to eleven years. After three years of super-vised brushing, the children were assessed for gingivitis,[5] for dental plaque,[6] and for dental caries. Two years after discon-tinuing supervision, the oral condition of the children was again reassessed.

Immediately following the three-year supervised brushing pe-riod, the mean gingival index of the control group* was found to be three times that of the supervised brushing group; the plaque index for the control group was twice that of the super-vised brushing group (see Table 9-I). These results indicate the beneficial effects of toothbrushing on oral cleanliness and gin-gival health. However, two years following discontinuation of supervised toothbrushing, there were no differences between the two groups in either the gingival condition or plaque scores. Furthermore, at neither examination did supervised brushing demonstrate an effect on caries. The supervised group brushing with a nontherapeutic dentifrice experienced caries increments similar to the control group at both examinations. These results seem to indicate that routine toothbrushing with a nonthera-peutic dentifrice has a beneficial effect on oral cleanliness and the state of the gingiva; however, the observed improvement in oral hygiene is of questionable value in preventing dental caries.

Another recent investigation in an older age group was unable to correlate frequency of brushing with caries incidence. Dale[7] examined 736 Australian soldiers, ages seventeen to nineteen, for dental caries and questioned them about the number of times per day that they brushed. The subjects were placed in one of four categories based upon their answers regarding brushing fre-quency. As seen in Table 9-II, there was no significant difference in dental caries (DMFT or DMFS) between any of the groups.

---

* The control group did not participate in any type of supervised oral hygiene procedures.

TABLE 9-I

THE EFFECTS OF SUPERVISED TOOTHBRUSHING WITH A NONTHERAPEUTIC DENTIFRICE ON GINGIVITIS, PLAQUE ACCUMULATION AND DENTAL CARIES IN CHILDREN

1st Examination

Group	*Gingival Index*		*Plaque Index*		*DMFS Increment (1965-1966)*	
	Mean	*S.E.*	*Mean*	*S.E.*	*Mean*	*S.E.*
Supervised brushing	0.33	0.03	0.84	0.06	8.32	0.63
Control	0.96	0.11	1.54	0.10	8.98	0.71

2nd Examination

Group	*Gingival Index*		*Plaque Index*		*DMFS Increment (1966-1968)*	
	Mean	*S.E.*	*Mean*	*S.E.*	*Mean*	*S.E.*
Supervised brushing	0.50	0.06	1.50	0.08	14.36	0.93
Control	0.49	0.06	1.46	0.10	13.96	0.85

1st examination—after three years of supervision in the "treatment" group.
2nd examination—two years following termination of supervision.
From G. Koch and J. Lindhe, "The State of the Gingiva and the Caries-Increment in School Children During and After Withdrawal of Various Prophylactic Measures," in W. D. McHugh (Ed.), *Dental Plaque* (Edinburgh, Livingstone, 1970), pp. 271-281.[4]

Oral Hygiene in Oral Health

TABLE 9-II

TOOTHBRUSHING FREQUENCY AND ITS RELATIONSHIP TO
DENTAL CARIES PREVALENCE

| | | Toothbrushing Frequency/Day | | | |
		0	1	2	3
No. of Patients		67	327	188	31
DMFT	Mean	18.69	19.47	19.11	17.19
	S.D.	6.03	5.94	6.28	5.36
DMFS	Mean	53.15	62.14	59.88	48.00
	S.D.	29.72	36.06	35.64	14.18

From W. J. Dale, "Toothbrushing Frequency and Its Relationship to Dental Caries and Periodontal Disease," *Aust Dent J, 14*:120-123, 1969.[7]

The group that never brushed had a caries experience similar to the group that brushed three times or more a day.

The lack of an expected correlation between toothbrushing and caries incidence in Dale's study may be associated with the inadequate brushing technics of the average individual. Most patients brush the easily accessible labial, facial, and occlusal surfaces of the teeth but neglect the proximal and lingual areas. This does not, however, explain the results obtained by Koch and Lindhe in their supervised brushing study. Their findings indicate that even under a controlled situation of improved oral cleanliness, dental caries is not affected. It may be that brushing, even under the most rigorous circumstances, cannot remove plaque and debris, especially from the sheltered proximal areas and the pit and fissure occlusal sites,[8] sufficiently to affect the development of dental caries.

Hendon et al.[9] compared the cleaning efficiency of the Bass method of brushing (without flossing), the vertical method, and the patient's own (*ad libitum*) method on artificial plaque placed interproximally in the mouths of six dental students. Single gold molar crowns were designed with a proximal slot fitted to receive a slab of human enamel. One crown was cemented in each participant, and the enamel slabs were inserted after first being coated with Pulpdent Paste® (methyl cellulose and calcium hydroxide) colored red with basic fuchsin dye. The colored Pulpdent served as an artificial plaque. After a timed brushing period, the slab was removed, and the area of artificial plaque that had been brushed off was calculated. It was found that the patients' *ad libitum* technics removed more material than either the Bass or vertical methods in which special instruction had been given (Table 9-III). However, in no instance did the toothbrush bristles penetrate completely to the contact area.

Although artificial plaque was used in this study, the results are worth reviewing since it is one of the few reports in which cleaning of the interproximal area was specifically examined and a quantitative method of assessment was used, rather than relying on subjective clinical impressions. Highly motivated patients (dental students) who had received detailed instruction in accepted toothbrushing technics were unable to remove all of the artificially placed material. In order for the dentist to scientifically prescribe oral hygiene programs involving toothbrushing, it must be ascertained whether the average patient, with well-executed brushing habits, can control plaque and other debris on his teeth to a level that will reduce caries.

TABLE 9-III

MEAN PERCENT ARTIFICIAL PLAQUE REMOVED (BY AREA) FROM PROXIMAL ENAMEL SLABS BY DIFFERENT TOOTHBRUSHING TECHNICS

| Patients | Technic | | |
	Vertical	Bass	Ad libitum
1	75.69	82.39	74.44
2	80.52	71.89	83.99
3	85.62	83.81	87.09
4	75.03	74.32	80.58
5	55.46	60.81	62.12
6	63.55	71.41	71.79

From G. E. Hendon, S. E. Keller, and L. R. Manson-Hing, "Clearance Studies of Proximal Tooth Surfaces, Part I," *Ala J Med Sci*, 6:213-227, 1969.[9] (Courtesy of Doctors Hendon, Keller, and Manson-Hing, and the *Alabama Journal of Medical Science*)

FLOSSING

The use of dental floss or tape has been advocated as an effective method of cleaning interproximal tooth surfaces.[10, 11] Bass, in fact, incorporates flossing as an essential part of his oral hygiene technic.

Most recommendations for the use of floss are empirical, based upon subjective clinical impressions of the ability of floss to remove plaque and debris from interproximal areas. Keller and Manson-Hing,[11] however, using the enamel slab technic of Hendon et al.,[9] but with a four-day natural plaque build-up, demonstrated the most effective interproximal tooth-cleaning method was the use of a manual toothbrush with a dentifrice, followed by the use of dental floss. In a follow-up study using the same experimental design, these investigators further concluded that, contrary to the usual recommendation, there was no significant difference in the cleaning efficiency of waxed or unwaxed floss.

AUTOMATIC TOOTHBRUSHING

Within the past decade many different brands of electric toothbrushes have appeared on the market. Generally, these automatic brushes have either an oscillating action in which the brush rotates back and forth in a 60 degree arc, or they have a horizontal vibrating motion.

The effectiveness of automatic toothbrushes has been reviewed by Ash[12] and Parfitt.[13] Both stress that the influence of automatic toothbrushes on gingival health can be more easily assessed than the effect on dental caries. This is because dental caries is a relatively slow disease, and evaluation of therapeutic agents and devices to prevent caries would take several years, while gingivitis is the result of local irritation, the removal of which produces rapid results.

The author knows of no reported study that has evaluated the effectiveness of automatic toothbrushes on dental caries. There have been a number of studies in which these devices have been reviewed for their effect on gingival health and the removal of plaque and oral debris. Such studies compare electric toothbrushing with manual brushing. The two commercial products that have been most frequently evaluated are the General Electric® and Broxodent® automatic toothbrushes. Reviews of these studies[12, 13] had similar conclusions regarding the effectiveness of electric toothbrushing devices:

(1) Electric toothbrushes are not more effective than manual brushes for the average patient.

(2) A toothbrush, whether automatic or manual, must be employed skillfully. The effectiveness of the device is a direct function of the ability of the patient who uses it and the motivation of the patient to clean particular surfaces. Thus, one type of brush may be more effective for one individual than for another.

(3) Proper use of electric toothbrushes caused no more trauma to gingival tissues than proper use of a manual toothbrush.

(4) When electric brushing was compared with manual brushing, there was no difference in interproximal cleaning ability. However, when manual brushing coupled with flossing was compared with electric toothbrushing, the former combined method proved more effective for cleaning interproximal areas.[11]

FORCED WATER JET

There are two types of forced water jets available for use in the mouth. One pumps water electrically in a pulsating fashion; the other type is attached to the faucet and gives a continuous stream of water. With the pulsating or intermittent type, the force of the jet can be varied from 5 to 50 pounds per square inch (psi).[13] The pressure of the faucet type is controlled by the water pressure in the line and the amount of opening of the faucet valve.

The water jet will remove soft debris from about and between the teeth. Parfitt[13] concluded from *in vitro* tests using glass plates that forces of 20 to 40 psi were required to remove soft debris similar to materia alba. This force is within the working range of the commercial products available. Keller and

Manson-Hing[11] found that a combination of intermittent water jetting and toothbrushing was more effective in removing four-day plaque from a test interproximal site than was toothbrushing alone. Others[14] have found that water jets will not remove adherent plaque or pellicle, nor are they effective in removing calculus.

There have been no trials in which the use of a water jet as a caries control adjunct has been evaluated. On an empirical basis the use of a water jet can be recommended only as a subordinate aid in a total caries control program and should not replace the traditional tooth-cleaning methods of toothbrushing and flossing. In terms of caries control programs, the water jet may have its greatest use as a vehicle for transporting anti-cariogenic agents such as fluoride solutions[15] into intimate contact with the teeth. Such an approach deserves future clinical evaluation.

MOUTHWASHES

Mouthwashes have been known since Biblical times and were originally used for reasons of religion, hygiene, or halitosis. With the discovery of bacteria and the subsequent era of antisepsis in medicine, mouthwashes were recommended for their possible antibacterial effects. Most commercial mouthwashes, however, have only a transient effect on bacteria. McCormick[16] has stated that:

> Antiseptic and antibiotic mouthwashes are probably more harmful than helpful by altering the balance of the oral flora in an indiscriminating way. Unfortunately, the general public can easily be misled into believing that an antibacterial mouthwash is a panacea. . . . Studies of the effects of antibacterial mouthwashes on the oral flora have generally overlooked the fact that the salivary bacteria and plaque bacteria may be different in numbers and type. Krasse[17] has shown that salivary bacterial samples are different from bacterial samples taken from pits, plaque, and periodontal pockets. . . . Thus, a study that shows that salivary bacteria are reduced in number by a mouthwash cannot predict whether or not there will be an accompanying change in dental caries or periodontal disease.

Both fluoride mouthwashes[18-24] and "remineralizing" calcium phosphate mouthwashes[25] have been tested for their anticariogenic potential (Table 9-IV). These agents attempt to chemical-

TABLE 9-IV

RESULTS OF CLINICAL TRIALS IN WHICH TOPICAL FLUORIDE WAS ADMINISTERED BY MOUTH RINSING

Study	Agent	Applications/Duration Supervision*	No. Patients	Age	Results
Bibby, Zander, McKelleget, Labunsky (1946)	.01% NaF acidulated mouthwash pH 4	3 × week/1 yr. us	54 control 31 treated	Sophomore dental students	Not significant
Roberts, Bibby, Wellock (1948)	.01% NaF acidulated mouthwash pH 4	2 × week/1 yr. s	169 control 187 treated	6th grade	30% caries increase
Torell and Siberg (1962)	Neutral 0.2% NaF solution	1 × month/1 yr. s	1019 control 912 treated	Approx. 7-9	13% to 27% less dental care received by treated group
Torell and Ericsson (1965)	Neutral 0.05% NaF solution	1 × day/2 yrs. us	196 control 160 treated	Approx. 11	50% caries reduction
Torell and Ericsson (1965)	Neutral 0.2% NaF solution	2 × month/2 yrs. s	196 control 172 treated	Approx. 11	21% caries reduction

* us = unsupervised; s = supervised.

ly alter the enamel of the teeth rather than to affect the oral microflora.

Recently, self-application programs involving fluoride mouthwashes have produced promising results in terms of caries reduction. In a clinical trial by Torell and Siberg,[22] Swedish school children, ages seven to nine, rinsed once a month with a neutral 0.2 percent NaF solution under the supervision of a dental nurse. The investigators claimed 13 to 27 percent less dental care was needed in the group of children that rinsed compared to untreated children enrolled in the same school classes the previous year. Only proximal surfaces of anterior teeth were assessed.

In 1965, Torell and Ericsson[23] reported the results of a study designed to evaluate several methods of fluoride therapy including self-application mouth-rinsing technics. A neutral 0.05 percent NaF solution was used daily following toothbrushing for a two-year period. The rinsing was performed at home without supervision. Another group of children rinsed once every two weeks with a 0.2 percent neutral NaF solution. This group rinsed at school under the supervision of a dental nurse. After two years, the group that rinsed daily without supervision using 0.05 percent NaF had approximately 50 percent less new caries than the control group, while the group that rinsed fortnightly with 0.2 percent NaF under supervision had a 21 percent caries reduction. The difference between the two groups is significant and indicates the importance of *frequency* of fluoride contact as a prime determinant of success.

The formulae and directions for use for these two NaF formulations are presented in Figures 9-1 and 9-2. It is preferred that plastic containers be used for storage. Commercial buffered acid fluoride phosphate mouthwashes are also available,* and Figure 9-3 is a prescription for one commercial product. The manufacturer states that it can be used to provide both topical and systemic fluoride effects. In other words, while the mouthwashes mentioned above were meant to be swished and expec-

---

* Phos-Flur Oral Rinse/Supplement, Hoyt Laboratories, Needham, Massachusetts 02194.

Sodium fluoride mouthwash (0.2%)

Use once every two weeks

℞	Sodium fluoride	0.2 gm
	distilled water	100 cc

Directions: Rinse mouth with 1 tsp. of mouthwash for 60 seconds once every two weeks after brushing teeth carefully after supper.

Caution: Store out of reach of children. Do not use for preschool children. Carefully supervise young school age children.

Figure 9-1. Example of a prescription for a sodium fluoride mouthwash recommended for use every two weeks. The mouth should be rinsed and the solution expectorated.

Sodium fluoride mouthwash (.05%)

Use daily

℞	Sodium fluoride	0.2 gm
	distilled water	400 cc

Directions: Rinse mouth with 1 tsp. of mouthwash for 60 seconds daily after brushing teeth carefully after supper.

Caution: Store out of reach of Children. Do not use for preschool children. Carefully supervise young school age children.

Figure 9-2. Example of a prescription for a sodium fluoride mouthwash recommended for daily use. The mouth should be rinsed and the solution expectorated.

Commercial fluoridated mouthwash

Use daily

℞	Phos-Flur,® acidulated fluoride phosphate mouthwash
Dispense:	250 ml
Directions:	Rinse mouth with 1 tsp. of mouthwash for 60 seconds daily after brushing teeth carefully after supper. Rinse and swallow.
Caution:	Keep out of reach of children.

Figure 9-3. Example of a prescription for a proprietary mouthwash. The manufacturers recommend the solution be used daily and that it be rinsed and swallowed in a non-fluoridated community.

torated, the manufacturers recommend that Phos-Flur® be swished and swallowed. This is contraindicated when the fluoride content of the drinking water is 0.7 ppm fluoride or more, and it will have no systemic benefit to the teeth of children beyond the age of twelve (except for third molars). The manufacturer also suggests that the dosage be halved when the drinking water contains 0.4 to 0.7 ppm fluoride.

While fluoride-containing therapeutic mouthwashes appear to represent a positive method of caries control, this method should only be prescribed and relied upon when the patient is well motivated and cooperation is assured.

A therapeutic dextranase mouthwash has also been proposed. Dextrans are high-molecular weight glucose polymers, produced by certain human oral microorganisms. Human strains of dextran-producing streptococci have been shown to cause caries in gnotobiotic animals.[26] Fitzgerald and coworkers[27] have found that the addition of the enzyme dextranase, which is capable of dispersing dextran-containing plaque, to the diets of hamsters inoculated with known cariogenic dextran-producing streptococci causes a significant reduction of plaque and caries. Dextranase has been tested in humans for its ability to alter plaque composition and amount.[28-30] These studies have not proved very successful in humans and would be difficult to adapt to a private practice situation. Furthermore, although dextranase was found to inhibit caries in test animals, there has been no published report on the effect of dextranase on caries in human subjects.

DETERGENT FOODS

It has been recommended that detergent foods such as apples, celery, and carrots be eaten at the end of meals. These are termed "Nature's toothbrushes" when brushing is impossible or impractical.

Arnim[31] evaluated the effect of detergent foods (apples, celery, lettuce, and carrots) on tooth cleanliness, based upon the food's ability to remove plaque material stainable by erythrocin disclosing tablets. He found that the proximal and gingival areas of the teeth were not cleansed by this method. Since plaque accumulations in these sites have been associated with caries and gingivitis, he concluded that chewing fibrous foods was of no value in limiting dental disease.

Slack and Martin[32] evaluated the effect of daily apple chewing on an initial group of 195 school children, ages six to fifteen. Directions stated that apples were to be served at the end of each meal and after eating anything between meals. The apples were especially selected for their firmness. Unfortunately, the test group decreased to ninety children in two years; the initial caries incidence in the control group and the apple group were so different at the initial examination that future comparison was made invalid. Slack and Martin concluded, however, that the gingival condition of the apple-chewing group of children was significantly better than in the control group. Definitive conclusions regarding caries incidence could not be made. Two years after discontinuation of the apple chewing, sixty-seven children in the former apple-chewing group were reexamined. No differences in either caries or gingival condition could be found between them and the remaining control group of children.[33]

It would appear that the empirical recommendation that fibrous foods improve dental health by promoting oral cleanliness and preventing dental caries is largely unfounded.

THERAPEUTIC DENTIFRICES

Historically, the primary function of a dentifrice has been to clean and polish the accessible surfaces of the teeth. Manufacturers, however, have added to certain dentifrice formulations ingredients which they claim will effect a reduction in dental caries. Those dentifrices that contain an active agent purported to be effective as a caries preventive are termed "therapeutic" dentifrices.

Because of their anticipated effect upon bacterial growth or bacterial carbohydrate metabolism, dentifrices containing antibiotics,[34, 35] ammonium phosphate and urea,[36, 37] chlorophyll or anionic detergents[38-40] have, at one time or another, been advocated as therapeutic pastes. These types of "therapeutic" dentifrices, however, have been largely replaced by dentifrices with a fluoride additive in the belief that the fluoride contact will provide protection to the enamel surface by making it more resistant to acid attack. *In vitro* tests have demonstrated that fluoride-containing therapeutic pastes will lower the acid solubility of enamel and protect it from extensive demineralization and artificial caries or "white spot" production.[41, 42]

Sodium fluoride was the first fluoride to be incorporated into a dentifrice. However, three independent clinical trials[43-45] conducted between 1945 and 1955 failed to show any cariostatic effect for a sodium fluoride-containing dentifrice. The negative findings were believed due to the incompatibility of the dentifrice abrasive, calcium carbonate or calcium orthophosphate, with sodium fluoride.[46] The fluoride reacted with the calcium-polishing compounds within the dentifrice tube and was unavailable for reaction with the calcium of the tooth.

In 1954, a dentifrice formulation that employed stannous fluoride as the active ingredient and calcium pyrophosphate as the abrasive was reported.[47, 48] Muhler et al. found that heating dicalcium phosphate, a common dentifrice abrasive, could make it relatively compatible with stannous fluoride. The heat-treated calcium phosphate salt, called calcium pyrophosphate ($Ca_2P_2O_7$), permitted the fluoride ions to remain relatively active in the dentifrice and, thus, to be available for reaction with the tooth enamel. The results of three initial studies conducted by Muhler et al.[45, 47-50] (Table 9-V) demonstrated the effectiveness of the dentifrice as a caries preventive agent. However, a decreased effectiveness with increased duration of the studies was noted. The altered effect was attributed to a partial inactivation of the therapeutic agent upon prolonged storage.[50] A new formulation containing stannous pyrophosphate ($Sn_2P_2O_7$) in addition to stannous fluoride and calcium pyrophosphate was tested. The added compound was supposed to furnish a reservoir of stannous ions to replace those in the stannous fluoride that may have been inactivated by other constituents of the formulation.[51] The commercial dentifrice formulation, Crest®,* received a Group B classification in 1960 from the American Dental Association's Council on Dental Therapeutics,[52] and a Group A classification in 1964.[53] A Group A product is considered an accepted dental remedy and may carry the Council's Seal of Acceptance. Table 9-V lists the clinical trials conducted in North America designed to test specifically the efficacy of this dentifrice formulation.[51, 54-66]

Studies of stannous fluoride dentifrices have also been conducted in England (see review by Duckworth[67]) and Sweden.[68] With one exception,[58] all of the North American studies listed in Table 9-V have reported statistically significant results with use of the Crest formulation. Based upon the ten North American studies of one to three years' duration where brushing was *unsupervised* (listed in Table 9-V), the average (DMFS) caries reduction using this formulation was 30 percent.[51, 54, 56, 60, 62-68] The average reduction obtained from those studies of one to two years' duration in which brushing was *supervised* was 32 percent.[57, 67, 68, 71, 72]

Other stannous fluoride and sodium fluoride-containing dentifrices, which have the noncalcium abrasive, sodium metaphos-

---

* Procter and Gamble Co., Cincinnati, Ohio.

TABLE 9-V

DENTIFRICE STUDIES USING STANNOUS FLUORIDE WITH A COMPATIBLE CALCIUM PHOSPHATE ABRASIVE SYSTEM (NORTH AMERICAN STUDIES ONLY)

Study	Dentifrice	Initial Age	Supervision	Duration	% Reduction	
					DMFT	DMFS
Muhler et al.[45]	SnF_2-$Ca_2P_2O_7$	5-15	No	6 mos.	53.4	71.5
Muhler et al.[47]	SnF_2-$Ca_2P_2O_7$	5-15	No	1 yr.	50.6	49.3
Muhler et al.[48]	SnF_2-$Ca_2P_2O_7$	5-15	No	6 mos. 1 yr.	45.4 33.9	44.7 36.0
Muhler et al.[49]	SnF_2-$Ca_2P_2O_7$	17-36	No	6 mos. 1 yr.	55.0 53.7	50.4 41.6
Muhler et al.[50]	SnF_2-$Ca_2P_2O_7$	17-36	No	24 mos.	30.0	34.0
Muhler[54]	SnF_2-$Ca_2P_2O_7$, $Sn_2P_2O_7$	6-18	No	6 mos. 1 yr. 18 mos. 2 yrs. 3 yrs.	42.2 28.2 31.4 24.5 23.7	25.8 18.5 24.3 19.2 22.4
Gish and Muhler[55]	SnF_2-$Ca_2P_2O_7$,$Sn_2P_2O_7$†	6-14	No	12 mos.	15.8 (28.6)*	38.3 (31.1)*
Gish and Muhler[56]	SnF_2-$Ca_2P_2O_7$,$Sn_2P_2O_7$†	6-14	No	24 mos.	23.1 (25.7)*	35.4 (29.5)*
Muhler[57]	SnF_2-$Ca_2P_2O_7$, $Sn_2P_2O_7$	5-17	No	6 mos. 12 mos.		37.1 33.0
Kyes et al.[58]	SnF_2-$Ca_2P_2O_7$, $Sn_2P_2O_7$	17-24	No	1 yr. 2 yrs.	+31 14	.5 14

Zacherl and McPhail[59, 60]	SnF₂-Ca₂P₂O₇, Sn₂P₂O₇	Approx. 6-8	No	10 mos. 18 mos. 30 mos.	36.3 36.4 35.5	39.2 42.1 40.4
		Approx. 11-13	No	10 mos. 18 mos. 30 mos.	22.7 34.8 37.3	34.1 38.7 43.5
Horowitz et al.[61]	SnF₂-Ca₂P₂O₇, Sn₂P₂O₇	6-10	No	1 yr. 2 yrs. 3 yrs.	+8.8 9.1 16.7	+5.1 2.1 16.9
			Supervised 1×/day in school plus unsupervised home brushing	1 yr. 2 yrs. 3 yrs.	10.8 13.1 16.3	9.9 11.8 20.9
Jordon and Peterson[51]	SnF₂-Ca₂P₂O₇, Sn₂P₂O₇	8-11	Supervised 1×/day in school plus unsupervised home brushing	1 yr.	35.5	33.9
Jordon and Peterson[62]	SnF₂-Ca₂P₂O₇, Sn₂P₂O₇	8-11	Supervised 1×/day in school plus unsupervised home brushing	2 yrs.	15.8	20.5
			No	2 yrs.	15.9	12.4
Peffley and Muhler[63]	SnF₂-Ca₂P₂O₇, Sn₂P₂O₇	10-19	Semisupervised 3×/day in military school	5 mos. 10 mos.	103 93	58.4 57.0
Bixler and Muhler[64]	SnF₂-Ca₂P₂O₇, Sn₂P₂O₇	11-18	Semisupervised 3×/day in military school	8 mos.	55 (46)*	52 (38)*

(Continued on next page)

TABLE 9-V—*Continued*

Study	Dentifrice	Initial Age	Supervision	Duration	% Reduction DMFT	DMFS
Bixler and Muhler[65]	SnF_2-$Ca_2P_2O_7$, $Sn_2P_2O_7$	11-23	Semisupervised 3×/day in military and boarding schools	8 mos. 19 mos.		60 54
Thomas and Jamison[66]	SnF_2-$NaPO_4$, $CaHPO_4$	7-16	Semisupervised 2-3×/day in orphanages	24 mos.	38.8	30.6
	SnF_2-$Ca_2P_2O_7$, $Sn_2P_2O_7$	7-16	Semisupervised 2-3×/day in orphanages	24 mos.	22.8	30.4

* = 2 examiners.
† = Fluoridated community.
SnF_2 = Stannous fluoride.
$Ca_2P_2O_7$ = Calcium pyrophosphate.
$Sn_2P_2O_7$ = Stannous pyrophosphate.
$CaHPO_4$ = Dicalcium phosphate.

TABLE 9-VI

DENTRIFICE STUDIES USING SODIUM MONOFLUOROPHOSPHATE
AS THE ACTIVE THERAPEUTIC AGENT

Study	Dentifrice	Initial Age	Supervision	Duration	% Reduction	
					DMFT	DMFS
Mergele[76]	MFP-IMP-SNLS	9-13	No	3 yrs.	8.8	17.4
	SnF_2-$Ca_2P_2O_7$				6.4	13.2
	SNLS-CaHPO₄ *				+1.0	3.5
Naylor & Emslie[77]	MFP-CaHPO₄-SNLS	11-12	No	3 yrs.	8.4	14.5
	SnF_2-IMP				13.9	18.1
Fanning et al.[78]	MFP-IMP-SNLS	11-13	No	2 yrs.		20.2
	SnF_2-IMP					21.9
Møller et al.[79]	MFP-IMP-SNLS	10-12	1×/day	30 mos.		18.9
Thomas & Jamison[80, 81]	MFP-IMP-SNLS	8-16	2×/day	2 yrs.	37.1	34.1
Mergele[82]	MFP-IMP-SNLS	7-21	3×/day	22 mos.	19	21
	SnF_2-IMP				12	9

* F area (Houston, 1 ppmF).
MFP-IMP-SNLS = sodium monofluorophosphate, insoluble sodium metaphosphate, sodium N-lauroyl sarcosinate.
MFP-CaHPO₄-SNLS = sodium monofluorophosphate, dicalcium phosphate, sodium N-lauroyl sarcosinate.
SnF_2-$Ca_2P_2O_7$ = stannous fluoride, calcium pyrophosphate.
SnF_2-IMP = stannous fluoride, insoluble sodium metaphosphate.
SNLS-CaHPO₄ = sodium N-lauroyl sarcosinate, dicalcium phosphate.

phate, have been clinically tested, e.g. Cue®, Super Stripe®, and Fact®.* The elimination of calcium in the abrasive system was designed to make the therapeutic agent and abrasive compatible. This type of formulation proved effective[69–71] and received Group B classification from the American Dental Association.[72–74] Group B classification means the dentifrice is provisionally accepted, lacking sufficient evidence to justify classification in Group A, but for which there is reasonable evidence of usefulness and safety.† In spite of their accepted caries-preventive potential, some of these dentifrices have failed to be competitive on the commercial market.

The Council on Dental Therapeutics has also given Group A recognition to a toothpaste containing monofluorophosphate as the active therapeutic agent.[75] This paste, Colgate MFP®,‡ uses sodium metaphosphate as the noncalcium abrasive. Table 9-VI lists the results of clinical trials in which the caries preventive potential of this paste is evaluated against nontherapeutic control dentifrices, and in some cases, against a stannous fluoride-calcium pyrophosphate dentifrice as an active control.[76–82] These trials, reporting caries reductions ranging from 17 percent to 34 percent, indicate the therapeutic value of this dentifrice.

SUMMARY

Methods of achieving oral cleanliness have been discussed in this chapter. While classic toothbrushing methods can clean the teeth sufficiently to produce a limiting effect on gingivitis, the same claim cannot be made for dental caries. Toothbrushing with a nontherapeutic dentifrice, as routinely practiced by the average individual, does not limit caries incidence. While floss and water jets are aids in achieving better tooth cleanliness, they have not been evaluated for their effect on dental caries.

The principal value of toothbrushing in a caries control program appears to be as a method for providing frequent fluoride

---

* Colgate Palmolive Co., Lever Brothers Co., and Bristol Myers Co., respectively.
† Classification nomenclature has since been changed: Group A products are now listed as "Accepted," and Group B products as "Provisionally Accepted."
‡ Colgate Palmolive Co.

applications to the teeth through the use of an effective therapeutic dentifrice. The Council on Dental Therapeutics of the American Dental Association has recognized the caries preventive potential of two commercial dentifrices, Crest and Colgate MFP, by granting them a Group A classification.* These dentifrices can reduce caries by approximately 30 percent when used under ordinary home conditions. While it is attractive to assume that trials in which brushing was supervised would produce greater caries reductions by insuring frequent contact of the therapeutic agent with tooth enamel, this has not been substantiated by the results of the clinical trials herein reviewed.

Mouthwashes which are supposed to affect bacteria produce only transient effects on the oral microflora. Fluoride-containing therapeutic mouthwashes, used daily, have been found to reduce caries by as much as 50 percent. Remineralizing calcium phosphate mouthwashes also show some promise. While dextranase has produced caries reductions in laboratory animals inoculated with known cariogenic bacteria, no studies have been published to date in which the effect of dextranase on human caries has been evaluated. The effect of dextranase mouthwashes on human plaque has been disappointing.

Since routine tooth-cleaning procedures do improve the health of the oral soft tissues, they should be recommended on that basis. However, because no tooth-cleaning methods presently available have been found to reduce dental caries in an average population, the dentist must seek methods of caries control using therapeutic agents and technics that have proven beneficial in repeated clinical trials.

REFERENCES

1. D. R. Hoover and W. Lefkowitz, "Reduction of Gingivitis by Toothbrushing," *J Periodontol*, 36:193-197, 1965.
2. R. R. Lobene, "Evaluation of Altered Gingival Health from Permissive Powered Toothbrushing," *JADA*, 69:585-588, 1964.
3. B. G. Bibby, "Do We Tell the Truth About Preventing Caries?," *J Dent Child*, 33:269-279, 1966.

---

* A third dentifrice, Macleans Flouride® (Beecham Products), has recently been classified "Accepted" by the Council on Dental Therapeutics.

4. G. Koch and J. Lindhe, "The State of the Gingiva and the Caries-Increment in School Children During and After Withdrawal of Various Prophylactic Measures," In W. D. McHugh (Ed.), *Dental Plaque* (Edinburgh, Livingstone, 1970), pp. 271-281.

5. H. Löe and J. Silness, "Periodontal Disease in Pregnancy, I. Prevalence and Severity," *Acta Odontol Scand*, 21:533-551, 1963.

6. J. Silness and H. Löe, "Periodontal Disease in Pregnancy," *Acta Odontol Scand*, 22:121-135, 1964.

7. W. J. Dale, "Toothbrushing Frequency and its Relationship to Dental Caries and Periodontal Disease," *Austr Dent J*, 14:120-123, 1969.

8. B. Gillings and M. Buonocore, "Thickness of Enamel at the Base of Pits and Fissures in Human Molars and Bicuspids," *J Dent Res*, 40:119-133, 1961.

9. G. E. Hendon, S. E. Keller, and L. R. Manson-Hing, "Clearance Studies of Proximal Tooth Surfaces, Part I," *Ala J Med Sci*, 6:213-227, 1969.

10. C. C. Bass, "The Optimum Characteristics of Dental Floss for Personal Oral Hygiene," *Dent Items of Int*, 70:921-934, 1948.

11. S. E. Keller and L. R. Manson-Hing, "Clearance Studies of Proximal Tooth Surfaces, Part III and IV: *In Vivo* Removal of Interproximal Plaque," *Ala J Med Sci*, 6:399-405, 1969.

12. M. M. Ash, Jr., "A Review of the Problems and Results of Studies on Manual and Power Toothbrushes," *J Periodontol*, 35:202-213, 1964.

13. G. J. Parfitt, "Therapeutic Devices," *Ann NY Acad Sci*, 135:360-373, 1968.

14. R. D. Emslie, "The Value of Oral Hygiene," *Brit Dent J*, 117:373-383, 1964.

15. M. Massler, "Teen-age Cariology," *Dent Clin North Am*, 13:405-423, 1969.

16. J. McCormick, "A Critical Review of the Literature on Mouthwashes," *Ann NY Acad Sci*, 135:374-385, 1968.

17. B. Krasse, "The Effect of Caries-Inducing Streptococci in Hamsters Fed Diets With Sucrose or Glucose," *Arch Oral Biol*, 10:223-226, 1965.

18. B. G. Bibby, H. A. Zander, M. McKelleget and B. Labunsky, "Preliminary Reports on the Effect on Dental Caries of the Use of Sodium Fluoride in a Prophylactic Cleaning Mixture and a Mouthwash," *J Dent Res*, 25:207-211, 1946.

19. J. F. Roberts, B. G. Bibby, and W. D. Wellock, "The Effect of an Acidulated Fluoride Mouthwash on Dental Caries," *J Dent Res*, 27:297-500, 1948.

20. W. S. Weisz, "The Reduction of Dental Caries Through the Use of a Sodium Fluoride Mouthwash," *JADA*, 60:438-456, 1960.

21. I. L. Shannon, "Laboratory Studies in the Development of a Stannous Fluoride Mouthwash," *J S Calif Dent Assoc*, 32:167-172, 1964.

22. P. Torell and A. Siberg, "Mouthwash With Sodium Fluoride and Potassium Fluoride," *Odontol Rev* (Malmo), *13*:62-72, 1962.

23. P. Torell and Y. Ericsson, "Two-Year Clinical Tests With Different Methods of Local Caries-Preventive Fluorine Applications in Swedish School Children," *Acta Odontol Scand, 23*:287-322, 1965.

24. R. Lundstam, "Teachers Administering Mouthwash With Fluorides in Jamtland, Sweden," *Sverige Tandlakarforb Tid, 56*:681-682, 1964.

25. J. McCormick and T. Koulourides, "A Study of Neutral Calcium, Phosphate, and Fluoride Remineralizing Mouthwashes," *IADR Abstracts*, No. 402, 1965.

26. R. J. Gibbons, K. S. Perman, P. Knoettner, and B. Kapsimalis, "Dental Caries and Alveolar Bone Loss in Gnotobiotic Rats Infected With Capsule Forming Streptococci of Human Origin," *Arch Oral Biol, 11*:549-560, 1966.

27. R. J. Fitzgerald, P. H. Keyes, T. H. Stoudt, and D. M. Spinell, "The Effects of a Dextranase Preparation on Plaque and Caries in Hamsters, a Preliminary Report," *JADA, 76*:301-304, 1968.

28. R. C. Caldwell, H. J. Sandham, W. V. Mann, Jr., S. B. Finn, and A. J. Formicola, "The Effect of Dextranase Mouthwash on Dental Plaque in Young Adults and Children," *JADA, 82*:124-131, 1971.

29. R. R. Lobene, "A Clinical Study of the Effect of Dextranase on Human Dental Plaque," *JADA, 82*:132-135, 1971.

30. P. H. Keyes, M. A. Hicks, B. M. Goldman, R. M. McCabe, and R. J. Fitzgerald, "Dispersion of Dextran Bacterial Plaques on Human Teeth With Dextranase," *JADA, 82*:136-141, 1971.

31. S. S. Arnim, "The Use of Disclosing Agents for Measuring Tooth Cleanliness," *J Periodontol, 34*:227-245, 1963.

32. G. L. Slack and W. J. Martin, "Apples and Dental Health," *Brit Dent J, 105*:366-370, 1958.

33. G. L. Slack and W. J. Martin, "Apples and Dental Health: Follow-up Examination," *Brit Dent J, 110*:350-352, 1961.

34. T. J. Hill and A. H. Kneisner, "Penicillin Dentifrice and Dental Caries Experience in Children," *J Dent Res, 28*:263-266, 1949.

35. H. A. Zander, "Effect of a Penicillin Dentifrice on Caries Incidence in School Children," *JADA, 40*:569-574, 1950.

36. D. W. Kerr and R. G. Kesel, "Two-Year Caries Control Study Utilizing Oral Hygiene and an Ammoniated Dentifrice," *JADA, 42*:180-188, 1951.

37. G. N. Davies and R. M. King, "The Effectiveness of an Ammonium Ion Toothpowder in the Control of Dental Caries," *J Dent Res, 30*:645-655, 1951.

38. L. S. Fosdick, "Clinical Experiment on the Use of Sodium N-Lauroyl Sarcosinate in the Control of Dental Caries," *Science, 123*:988-989, 1956.

39. O. Backer-Dirks, G. W. Kwant, and J. L. Starmans, "Effect of a Sodium Lauroyl Sarcosinate Dentifrice: A Clinical Investigation," *Dent Abstracts*, 5:371, 1960.

40. J. Hayden and R. L. Glass, "Relative Efficacy of Sodium N-Lauroyl Sarcosinate in Reducing Dental Caries," *J Dent Res*, 38:671-672, 1959.

41. M. G. Buonocore and A. J. Gwinnett, "Chemical, Polarized Light, and Microradiographic Study of the Effects of Various Toothpastes on 'White Spot' Formation *In Vitro*," *J Oral Ther*, 3:321-329, 1967.

42. L. W. Ripa and M. G. Buonocore, "The Effectiveness of Dentifrice Protection on *In Vitro* "White Spot" Formation: Microradiographic, Polarized Light and Chemical Investigation," *IADR Abstracts*, No. 175, 1967.

43. B. G. Bibby, "Test of the Effect of Fluoride Containing Dentifrices on Dental Caries," *J Dent Res*, 24:297-303, 1945.

44. K. C. Winkler, O. Backer-Dirks, and J. van Amerongen, "A Reproducible Method for Caries Evaluation. Test in a Therapeutic Experiment With a Fluoridated Dentifrice," *Brit Dent J*, 95:119-124, 1953.

45. J. C. Muhler, A. W. Radike, W. H. Nebergall and H. G. Day, "A Comparison Between the Anti-cariogenic Effects of Dentifrices Containing Stannous Fluoride and Sodium Fluoride," *JADA*, 51:556-559, 1955.

46. Y. Ericsson, "Fluorides in Dentifrices; Investigations Using Radioactive Fluorine," *Acta Odontol Scand*, 19:41-77, 1961.

47. J. C. Muhler, A. W. Radike, W. H. Nebergall, and H. G. Day, "The Effect of a Stannous Fluoride-Containing Dentifrice on Caries Reduction in Children," *J Dent Res*, 33:606-612, 1954.

48. J. C. Muhler, A. W. Radike, W. H. Nebergall, and H. G. Day, "Effect of a Stannous Fluoride-Containing Dentifrice on Caries Reduction in Children. II. Caries Experience After One Year," *JADA*, 50:163-166, 1955.

49. J. C. Muhler, A. W. Radike, W. H. Nebergall, and H. G. Day, "The Effect of a Stannous Fluoride-Containing Dentifrice on Dental Caries in Adults," *J Dent Res*, 35:49-53, 1956.

50. J. C. Muhler and A. W. Radike, "Effect of a Dentifrice Containing Stannous Fluoride on Dental Caries in Adults. II. Results at the End of Two Years of Unsupervised Use," *JADA*, 55:196-198, 1957.

51. W. A. Gordan and J. K. Peterson, "Caries-inhibiting Value of a Dentifrice Containing Stannous Fluoride: First Year Report of a Supervised Toothbrushing Study," *JADA*, 54:589-594, 1957.

52. Council on Dental Therapeutics, "Evaluation of Crest Toothpaste," *JADA*, 61:272-274, 1960.

53. Council on Dental Therapeutics, "Reclassification of Crest Toothpaste," *JADA*, 69:195-196, 1964.
54. J. C. Muhler, "Effect of a Stannous Fluoride Dentifrice on Caries Reduction in Children During a Three-Year Study Period," *JADA*, 64: 216-224, 1962.
55. C. W. Gish and J. C. Muhler, "Effectiveness of a SnF₂-Ca₂P₂O₇ Dentifrice on Dental Caries of Children Whose Teeth Calcified in a Natural Fluoride Area. I. Results at the End of 12 Months," *JADA*, 71:60-65, 1965.
56. C. W. Gish and J. C. Muhler, "Effectiveness of a SnF₂-Ca₂P₂O₇ Dentifrice on Dental Caries in Children Whose Teeth Calcified in a Natural Fluoride Area. II. Results at the End of 24 Months," *JADA*, 73:853-855, 1966.
57. J. C. Muhler, "A Clinical Comparison of Fluoride and Antienzyme Dentifrices," *J Dent Child*, 37:501-502, passim 511-514, 1970.
58. F. M. Keyes, N. J. Overton, and T. W. McKean, "Clinical Trials of Caries Inhibitory Dentifrices," *JADA*, 63:189-193, 1961.
59. W. A. Zacherl and C. W. B. McPhail, "Evaluation of a Stannous Fluoride-Calcium Pyrophosphate Dentifrice," *J Can Dent Assoc*, 31:174-180, 1965.
60. W. A. Zacherl and C. W. B. McPhail, "Final Report on the Efficacy of a Stannous Fluoride-Calcium Pyrophosphate Dentifrice," *J Can Dent Assoc*, 36:262-264, 1970.
61. H. S. Horowitz, F. E. Law, M. B. Thompson, and S. R. Chamberlin, "Evaluation of a Stannous Fluoride Dentifrice for Use in Dental Public Health Programs," *JADA*, 72:408-422, 1966.
62. W. A. Jordan and J. K. Peterson, "Caries-Inhibiting Value of a Dentifrice Containing Stannous Fluoride: Final Report of a Two-Year Study," *JADA*, 58:42-44, 1959.
63. G. E. Peffley and J. C. Muhler, "The Effect of a Commercial Stannous Fluoride Dentifrice Under Controlled Brushing Habits on Dental Caries Incidence in Children; Preliminary Report," *J Dent Res*, 39: 871-874, 1960.
64. D. Bixler and J. C. Muhler, "Experimental Clinical Human Caries Test Design and Interpretation," *JADA*, 65:482-488, 1962.
65. D. Bixler and J. C. Muhler, "Effectiveness of a Stannous Fluoride-Containing Dentifrice in Reducing Dental Caries in Children in a Boarding School Environment," *JADA*, 72:653-658, 1966.
66. A. E. Thomas and H. C. Jamison, "Effect of SnF₂ Dentifrices on Caries on Children: Two-Year Clinical Study of Supervised Brushing in Children's Homes," *JADA*, 73:844-852, 1966.
67. R. Duckworth, "Fluoride Dentifrices. A Review of Clinical Trials in the United Kingdom," *Brit Dent J*, 124:505-509, 1968.
68. P. Torell and Y. Ericsson, "Two-Year Clinical Tests With Different

Methods of Local Caries-Preventive Fluorine Application in Swedish School Children," *Acta Odontol Scand, 23*:287-322, 1965.

69. A. H. Segal, R. H. Stiff, W. A. George, and A. Picozzi, "Cariostatic Effect of a Stannous Fluoride-Containing Dentifrice on Children: Two-Year Report of a Supervised Toothbrushing Study," *J Oral Ther, 4*:175-180, 1967.

70. F. Brudevold, N. W. Chilton, and W. D. Wellock, "A Preliminary Comparison of a Dentifrice Containing Fluoride and Soluble Phosphate and Employing a Calcium-Free Abrasive With Other Types of Fluoride Dentifrices. First Year Report of a Clinical Study," *J Oral Ther, 1*:1-6, 1964.

71. F. Brudevold and N. W. Chilton, "Comparative Study of a Fluoride Dentifrice Containing Soluble Phosphate and a Calcium-Free Abrasive: Second-Year Report," *JADA, 72*:889-894, 1966.

72. Council on Dental Therapeutics, "Evaluation of Cue Toothpaste," *JADA, 69*:197-198, 1964.

73. Council on Dental Therapeutics, "Evaluation of Fact Toothpaste," *JADA, 71*:930-931, 1965.

74. Council on Dental Therapeutics, "Evaluation of Super Stripe Toothpaste," *JADA, 72*:1515, 1966.

75. Council on Dental Therapeutics, "Council Classifies Colgate With MFP (Sodium Monofluorophosphate) in Group A," *JADA, 79*:937-938, 1969.

76. M. Mergele, "Report II.—An Unsupervised Brushing Study on Subjects Residing in a Community With Fluoride in the Water," *Bull Acad Med NJ, 14*:251-255, 1968.

77. M. N. Naylor and R. D. Emslie, "Clinical Testing of Stannous Fluoride and Sodium Monofluorophosphate Dentifrices in London School Children," *Brit Dent J, 123*:17-23, 1967.

78. E. A. Fanning, T. Gotjamanos, and N. J. Vowles, "The Use of Fluoride Dentifrices in the Control of Dental Caries: Methodology and Results of a Clinical Trial," *Austr Dent J, 13*:201-206, 1968.

79. I. J. Møller, J. J. Holst, and E. Sørensen, "Caries-Reducing Effect of a Sodium Monofluorophosphate Dentifrice," *Brit Dent J, 124*:209-213, 1968.

80. A. Thomas and H. Jamison, "Effect of a Combination of Two Cariostatic Agents on Caries in Children: Two-Year Clinical Study of Supervised Brushing in Children's Homes," *Bull Acad Med NJ, 14*:241-246, 1968.

81. A. Thomas and H. Jamison, "Effect of a Combination of Two Cariostatic Agents in Children: Two-Year Clinical Study of Supervised Brushing in Children's Homes," *JADA, 81*:118-124, 1970.

82. M. Mergele, "Report I. A Supervised Brushing Study in State Institution Schools," *Bull Acad Med NJ, 14*:247-250, 1968.

10

TOPICAL METHODS OF CARIES CONTROL USING FLUORIDES AND ADHESIVES

Louis W. Ripa and Michael G. Buonocore

INTRODUCTION

C OMMUNAL WATER FLUORIDATION is an inexpensive and relatively simple method of providing therapeutic doses of fluoride to the teeth. It has the advantage of requiring minimal motivation for the patient to accept treatment, and it will reduce caries by approximately 50 to 60 percent. All other caries preventive measures require a greater degree of patient cooperation. Professionally administered topical fluoride and adhesive applications require that patients present themselves to a dental office at regular intervals and that they accept the suggested therapy. Fluoride administered in pills, lozenges, mouthwashes, and the like requires that the patient conscientiously adhere to the preventive regimen that has been prescribed.

Communal water fluoridation is a community health effort because of the large numbers of people involved. Its effects cannot be controlled by an individual dentist or patient. The information presented in this chapter stresses the technics that are applicable to an individual program of caries prevention. Such a program can be implemented both in the dental office and in the patient's home. These technics may supplement communal water fluoridation where it exists. Where the benefits of communal water fluoridation are not available, these technics, if followed

309

assiduously, can themselves produce significant reductions in caries experience.

TOPICAL FLUORIDE APPLICATIONS IN THE DENTAL OFFICE

This section is concerned with caries prevention using topical fluoride agents applied by the dentist or hygienist in the dental office; some of the many fluoride studies are reviewed, and factors are discussed which are pertinent to the selection and use of topical fluorides.

Which fluoride compound and what method of application is best for use in the dental office? Unfortunately, at this time the results of numerous clinical studies do not indicate one particular fluoride agent as being superior to another. Furthermore, since many variables influence the results of clinical trials of fluoride agents, it is difficult to compare the results of two or more different clinical studies.

The Fluoride Agent

Three topical fluoride compounds are available to the dental practitioner, sodium fluoride (NaF), stannous fluoride (SnF_2) and acidulated fluoride phosphate (AFP).

Sodium Fluoride

Topical application of sodium fluoride was first investigated in the 1940s by Bibby and simultaneously by Knutson and co-workers of the U.S. Public Health Service. Sodium fluoride was initially used by Bibby in concentrations of 0.1 percent applied three times a year at intervals of four months.[1] Knutson and Armstrong, working for the Public Health Service, increased the concentration to 2 percent and also increased the number of yearly applications.[2-4] The Public Health Service recommended that at the first appointment the patient should receive a cursory cleaning with pumice, after which the teeth are isolated and a 2 percent solution of sodium fluoride applied. A second, third, and fourth application, each *not* preceded by prophylaxis, was recommended at intervals of approximately one week. The series was recommended at ages three, seven, ten, and thirteen. These ages were selected so that groups of teeth would be treated as they erupted, thus affording maximum protection through early contact with fluoride.

There have been a number of studies using sodium fluoride, mostly in nonfluoride areas. Some of these studies are presented in Table 10-I.[1, 5-8] In one of the first studies using sodium fluoride, Bibby[1] obtained a 45.9 percent reduction after one year and 27.6 percent reduction after two years. In a study conducted by the U.S. Public Health Service[5] in which a 2 percent sodium fluoride solution was used, two, four, or six applications were given per year to three different groups of children. Because a maximum effect was obtained using four annual applications, this was the treatment regimen adopted.

Numerous studies by different investigators throughout the world have confirmed the caries-preventive effects of sodium fluoride applications.[8-12] Reductions of 30 to 40 percent have been fairly consistently reported. By averaging results from twenty-eight studies using topical neutral sodium fluoride, Buonocore and Bibby indicated a net reduction in caries of 33 percent could be obtained with this agent.[13]

Although the efficacy of topical applications of sodium fluoride in areas without communal water fluoridation has been established, the effectiveness of a similar preventive program to

TABLE 10-I

STUDIES EMPLOYING TOPICAL NaF IN PERMANENT TEETH: NONFLUORIDE AREAS

Study	Initial Age	% F Conc.	No. Applications	Years After Initial Application	% Reduction DMFT	% Reduction DMFS
Bibby[1]	10-13	0.1	3	1		45.9
			6	2		27.6
Galagan & Knutson[5]	7-15	2	2	1	21.7	13.5
			4	1	40.7	33.7
			6	1	41.0	28.3
Bergman[6]	11-12	2	4	3		43.0
Law et al.[7]	7-13	2	4	1	35.2	35.8
Torell & Ericsson[8]	10	2	4	2		19.8

TABLE 10-II

STUDIES EMPLOYING TOPICAL NaF IN PERMANENT TEETH:
FLUORIDE AREAS

Study	Initial Age	% F Conc.	No. Applications	Years After Initial Application	% Reduction DMFT	% Reduction DMFS
Downs & Pelton[14]	6-18	2	4	1	0.4	0
Galagan & Vermillion[15]	7-16	2	4	1	8.9	

the teeth of children born and reared in an optimal fluoride area is not conclusively established.

The results of two studies[14, 15] utilizing sodium fluoride in a fluoride area on permanent teeth are reported in Table 10-II. Downs and Pelton[14] conducted their investigations in Sterling, Colorado, and Cheyenne, Wyoming; and Galagan and Vermillion[15] in Tucson, Arizona. Both investigations were negative; however, both research teams suggested further study in this area.

Stannous Fluoride

In the 1950s, Muhler and coworkers at the University of Indiana recognized the caries-inhibiting potential of stannous fluoride. Subsequently, stannous fluoride was introduced as a new topical agent for caries control and was also included as the therapeutic ingredient in a commercial dentifrice (Crest). The results of clinical trials by this group of investigators indicated that annual or biannual applications of an 8 percent stannous fluoride solution could produce caries reductions greater than the 30 to 40 percent figure associated with 2 percent sodium fluoride applications (Table 10-III).[16] In trials in which 2 percent NaF and 8 percent SnF_2 were evaluated concurrently, stannous fluoride demonstrated superior reductions.[17-21]

Other investigators have also found stannous fluoride to be an effective anticaries agent; however, the reductions that these investigators obtained using stannous fluoride have generally been less than those originally reported (Table 10-III).[7, 22-26] Buono-

TABLE 10-III

STUDIES EMPLOYING TOPICAL SnF₂ IN PERMANENT TEETH:
NONFLUORIDE AREAS

Study	Initial Age	% SnF₂ Conc.	No. Applications	Years After Initial Application	% Reduction DMFT	% Reduction DMFS
Mercer & Muhler[16]	6-14	8	1	1	50	51
Gish et al.[17]	7	8	1	8 mos.	21*	26*
Gish et al.[18]	7	8	1	1	59*	56*
Gish et al.[20]	7	8	1	1	31*	31*
	7	8	2	2	17*	24*
	7	8	3	3	35*	39*
	7	8	4	4	32†	30†
Gish et al.[21]	7	8	2	2	28*	26*
	7	8	3	3	30*	23*
	7	8	4	4	20†	25†
	7	8	5	5	30†	35†
Peterson & Williamson[22]	9-13	8	2	2	26.2	24.2
Harris[23]	7-12	8	6	3	23.3	—
Law et al.[7]	7-13	8	1	3	23.6	—
Cartwright et al.[24]	6-19	8	4	2	—	37
Horowitz & Lucye[25]	8-10	8	2	2	8	8
Wellock et al.[26]	8-12	8	1	1	9	0
		1.23% (NaF + HF),	1	1	55	71
Salter et al.[27]	6-7	8	1	1	64.7	55.8
			2	1	29.4	29.5

* = Compared to 4 applications of 2% NaF.
† = Compared to 2 series of 4 applications of 2% NaF spaced at 3-yr. intervals.

core and Bibby[13] reviewed the results of fourteen studies using topical stannous fluoride. They found an average caries reduction of 36 percent. This is comparable to the average figure of 33 percent that they computed for sodium fluoride.

Variations in results between independent clinical studies are not unusual. Differences are partially attributable to different study design including such factors as age of patients, criteria and methods of assessing caries, methods and frequency of application of the therapeutic agents, and length of the study. The consistently higher findings of the Indiana group, however, may be associated with their claim that stannous fluoride topical applications can produce an arrestment of early carious lesions.[28-30]

Arrestment of a lesion will lead to a reversal in clinical diagnosis between the initial examination and the subsequent one. That is, a lesion originally diagnosed as carious, if it arrests, will be diagnosed as sound at a later examination. Reversals tend to favor the stannous fluoride-treated group by elevating the percent reduction. Whether stannous fluoride treatments will arrest early lesions is not entirely clear. *In vitro* studies, for instance, have shown that the tin moiety in stannous fluoride solutions can alter the radiographic interpretation of early lesions by increasing the radiodensity of the demineralized enamel.[31, 32] If the same change occurs in the clinical situation, a carious lesion might be masked radiographically rather than actually be arrested.

As with sodium fluoride, there have been few studies in which the effectiveness of a topical application of stannous fluoride has been assessed in an area with communal water fluoridation. Muhler[33, 34] reported a 49 to 54 percent reduction when 8 percent stannous fluoride was applied to the teeth of six- to seventeen-year-old children in Indianapolis, a fluoridated community (Table 10-IV). Horowitz and Heifetz,[35, 36] however, obtained a *clinically* nonsignificant reduction of 21 percent when stannous fluoride was applied to children in Chattanooga, Tennessee. The

TABLE 10-IV

STUDIES EMPLOYING TOPICAL SnF₂ IN PERMANENT TEETH:
FLUORIDE AREAS

Study	Initial Age	% SnF₂ Conc.	No. Applications	Years After Initial Application	% Reduction DMFT	DMFS
Muhler[33]	6-17	8	1	.5	35	36
			2	1	35	31
Muhler[34]	6-17	8	3	1.5	36	36
			4	2	46	35
			5	2.5	54	49
Horowitz & Heifetz[35, 36]	Approx. 7-9	8	1	1	16.9	10.0
			2	2	20.4	12.7
			3	3	20.9	21.1

protocol of these two studies differed in several respects: (1) the age range of the children, (2) the number of topical applications given each year, and (3) the use of radiographs in caries diagnosis. Consequently, direct comparison of these two studies is difficult. Interpretation is further complicated by the fact that when the Indianapolis study began, the water supply had been fluoridated for only six years. Thus, presumably only the six-year-old children in the study groups had a lifetime exposure to fluoridated water.

Acidulated Fluoride Phosphate

The use of an acidulated fluoride solution is based on the known information that slightly decalcified enamel will acquire more fluoride than sound enamel. Brudevold et al. developed a solution of sodium fluoride that was acidulated with orthophosphoric acid and buffered to a pH of approximately 3 in order to slightly demineralize the enamel surface, thereby enhancing fluoride uptake.[37] Several clinical studies utilizing acidulated fluoride phosphate systems have been reported since Brudevold's original *in vitro* investigation in 1963 (Table 10-V). The original clinical report by Wellock and Brudevold[38] was conducted on 296 public school children in Massachusetts. Single annual acidulated fluoride phosphate applications resulted in reductions of 55 to 71 percent after one year. Second year reductions were of a similar magnitude. Pameijer et al.[39] compared the cariostatic effects of neutral 2 percent sodium fluoride and acidulated fluoride phosphate using a half-mouth technic of application. They reported a 51 percent caries reduction for the acidulated fluoride phosphate-treated teeth compared to the teeth treated with the neutral sodium fluoride. Wellock et al.[26] and Cartwright et al.[24] obtained reductions of approximately 50 percent with the acidulated, buffered sodium fluoride solution, while Muhler et al.,[40] using acidulated stannous fluoride solutions at pH 3 and 6, obtained reductions of similar magnitude.

Recent studies, however, have reported less spectacular results. In a three-year continuing study, Horowitz[41-43] applied an aqueous solution of acidulated fluoride phosphate once a year and

TABLE 10-V

STUDIES OF TOPICALLY APPLIED ACIDULATED
PHOSPHATE-FLUORIDE SYSTEMS IN PERMANENT TEETH:
NONFLUORIDE AREAS

Study	Initial Age	Agent	No. Applications	Years After Initial Appointment	% Reduction DMFT	% Reduction DMFS
Wellock & Brudevold[38]	8-11	1.23% (NaF + HF)	1	1	55	71
		0.1 M H_3PO_4, pH approx. 3	2	2	67	70
Pameijer et al.[39]	4-10	2% NaF, 0.15 M H_3PO_4, pH 3.6	4	3-15 mos.		51*
Wellock et al.[26]	8-12	1.23% (NaF + HF)	1	1	44	46
		0.1 M H_3PO_4, pH 3.0-3.5	2	2	44	52
Cartwright et al.[24]	6-9	1.23% (NaF + HF) 0.1 M H_3PO_4, pH 2.8	4	2	49	
Muhler et al.[40]	6-13	8% SnF_2 + 8% NaH_2PO_4, pH 3.0	2	1	65.5	67.0
		3.6% NaF + 1.8% K_2HPO_4, pH 6.0	2	1	51.2	51.5
Averill et al.[44]	7-11	2% NaF, 0.1 NaH_2PO_4 + H_3PO_4, pH 4.4	4	2	11.6	+2.3
Cons et al.[45]	6-11	1.23% (NaF + HF) 0.1 M H_3PO_4, pH 3	3	3	16	+1
Ingraham & Williams[49]	6-10	1.23% (NaF + HF)	2	2	18.2	10.9
		0.1 M H_3PO_4, pH 3	2	2	23.9†	13.1†
Horowitz[41]	10-12	1.23% (NaF + HF)	1	1	17.0	22.4
		0.1 M H_3PO_4, pH 3	2	1	28.3	27.1
Horowitz[42]	10-12	1.23% (NaF + HF)	2	2	25.7	33.0
		0.1 M H_3PO_4 pH 3	4	2	32.9	35.9
Horowitz[43]	10-12	1.23% (NaF + HF)	3	3	26.8	30.0
		0.1 M H_3PO_4, pH 3	6	3	40.3	42.6
De Paola et al.[46]	6-8	1% NaF, 0.1 M H_3PO_4, pH 3.8	3	1	23	21
		0.25% NaF, 0.03 M H_3PO_4, pH 3.8‡	6	2	6	11
			9	3	1	3

* Compared to half-mouth treatments with 2% NaF.
† Agent changed during 2nd and 3rd years of study.
‡ Acidulated phosphate fluoride solution applied in rubber trays with paper liners.

twice a year to groups of Hawaiian school children. The group receiving the single annual application had approximately 30 percent less caries compared to the control group of children who received only a standard prophylaxis. The group that received fluoride applications every six months had approximately 40 percent less caries. Averill et al.[44] and Cons et al.[45] in two- and three-year studies, respectively, were unable to detect a significant caries inhibition with acidulated fluoride phosphate solutions. DePaola[46] sprayed the teeth of six- to eight-year-old children with a milder acidulated fluoride solution three times a year for three years. At the conclusion of the study, an insignificant 3 percent reduction in carious tooth surfaces was recorded; however, the permanent teeth erupting during the study showed an 18 percent reduction.

Much of the fluoride that enters the enamel when acidulated solutions are used will quickly leach out.[47] High concentrations of fluoride extend into the first 25 to 50 μ of enamel; however, much of the fluoride is quickly lost within the first twenty-four hours following application. That which is not retained is believed to be unreacted fluoride plus soluble reaction products, principally calcium fluoride. Since the optimal enamel-fluoride concentration that will impart maximum caries protection is not known, the significance of the fluoride loss is not understood. Unsuccessful attempts have been made to hinder the leaching process by coating the tooth with cavity varnish, silicone grease, or petroleum jelly following topical fluoride applications.

Concentration of the Fluoride

Sodium Fluoride

Sodium fluoride is usually used in a 2 percent concentration. It can be prepared by mixing 2 gm of sodium fluoride in 100 ml of distilled water. The solution can be kept in a closed plastic container for long periods without deterioration.

Stannous Fluoride

Stannous fluoride is usually used in an 8 percent concentration. It must be prepared fresh for each patient and used immediately. For the preparation of stannous fluoride solution, a pharmacist can dispense 0.8 gm stannous fluoride into No. 0 gelatin capsules which are kept sealed until used. When the topical fluoride is to be applied, the contents of one capsule are added to 10 ml of distilled water and shaken. A 25 ml polyethylene bottle is suitable for the preparation of the solution. Any solution not used during the treatment must be discarded because it becomes inactivated.

Acidulated Fluoride Phosphate

The acidulated fluoride phosphate solutions may be purchased commercially. One commercial product (Luride®*) has 1.23 percent of fluoride as sodium fluoride, buffered to a pH of approximately 3 with 0.1 M phosphoric acid.

Physical Consistency of the Fluoride

Fluoride preparations are available in aqueous solutions, as viscous gels, and are incorporated within prophylaxis pastes. To date, aqueous solutions have been most commonly employed, and the efficacy of using fluoride in an aqueous vehicle has been established in numerous clinical trials. All of the investigations cited in Tables 10-I through 10-V used the aqueous form of the particular fluoride agent tested.

Recently, acidulated fluoride phosphate has become commercially available in gel form. The gel has essentially the same formulation as the aqueous solution, with the addition of hydroxyethyl cellulose for viscosity. Fluoride gels have the advantage of a quick, easy application technic via a tray that is adjusted to conform to the dental arches. Since both upper and lower arches may be treated simultaneously, the time of application is reduced by half.

Clinical trials have been reported in which the patient applies the fluoride gel to his own teeth using custom-fitted trays or mouth guards. Because of the simplicity of the self-application technic and the minimum commitment in terms of time and supervisory personnel, the applications can be repeated on a

---

* Hoyt Laboratories, Needham, Massachusetts.

TABLE 10-VI

STUDIES OF TOPICALLY APPLIED ACIDULATED PHOSPHATE-FLUORIDE GEL SYSTEMS

Study	Initial Age	Method of Application	No. Applications	Years After Initial Application	% Reduction	
					DMFT	DMFS
Bryan & Williams[43]	8-12	foam rubber trays	1	1	45.0	28.4
Ingraham & Williams[40]	6-10	wax or foam rubber trays	2	2	52.3	41.2
Swejda et al.[50]	Approx. 7	foam rubber trays	1	1	+0.3	+0.5
Cons et al.[45]	6-11	wax trays	3	3	24.6	17.8
Horowitz[41]	10-12	cotton-lined wax trays	1	1	11.9	13.7
Horowitz[42]	10-12	cotton-lined wax trays	2	2	12.2	21.6
Horowitz[43]	10-12	cotton-lined wax trays	3	3	15.5	24.4

daily basis if desired. Results of self-application trials will be described later in this chapter.

Investigations in which fluoride gels have been used in trays under conditions similar to that employed in the private dental office have not been promising (Table 10-VI). Bryan and Williams[48] applied an acidulated phosphate fluoride gel in foam rubber trays to 121 Tennessee school children, ages eight to twelve. After one year, one application resulted in a 28.4 percent reduction, based on DMF surfaces. Ingraham and Williams[49] reported a 41 percent reduction using a similar technic. Szwejda et al.,[50] on the other hand, reported a 17.8 percent reduction (DMFS) when an acidulated phosphate fluoride gel was applied annually in foam rubber or wax trays for one and three years, respectively. Horowitz[41-43] reported annually the results of a three-year study on ten to twelve-year-old Hawaiian children treated with single annual applications of acidulated phosphate fluoride in cotton-lined wax trays. After three years, a 24.4 percent reduction in DMF surfaces was reported. While one is able to conclude from these studies that a tray-applied, acidulated phosphate fluoride can be an effective cariostatic agent, the level of efficacy has not yet been demonstrated to be comparable to the aqueous form of this same agent.

A fluoride-containing prophylaxis paste is attractive because of the ease and time-saving potential of the technic. The classical topical application procedure requires a thorough prophyaxis, followed by a topical application of a fluoride solution to each tooth. If a fluoride-containing prophylaxis paste is efficacious, the time-consuming topical application step could be eliminated. It is also possible that the combined use of fluoride-containing prophylaxis pastes and topical solutions could act synergistically to effect a caries reduction greater than that obtained if either were used alone.

The first clinical trial of a fluoride-containing prophylaxis paste was reported by Bibby et al.[51] They mixed hydrogen peroxide, pumice, and a 4 percent solution of sodium fluoride and applied the resultant paste to the teeth of two groups of Massachusetts school children twice and three times a year. Although

TABLE 10-VII

STUDIES USING FLUORIDE-CONTAINING PROPHYLAXIS PASTES ALONE

Study	Initial Age	Agent	No. Applications	Years After Initial Application	% Reduction DMFT	DMFS
Bibby et al.[51]	6-15	4% NaF, pumice, H_2O_2	2	1		25
	6-14	4% NaF, pumice, H_2O_2	3	1		42
Peterson et al.[54]	10-13	17.5% SnF_2, silex	4	2	35.1(38.8)	41.9(34.2)
Scola and Ostrom[55]	17-24	17.5% SnF_2, lava pumice	1	1	12	12
Scola and Ostrom[56]	17-24	17.5% SnF_2, lava pumice	2	2	26	12
Bixler and Muhler[57]	5-18	8.9% SnF_2, lava pumice	2	1	30.6	34.6
Bixler and Muhler[58]	5-18	8.9% SnF_2, lava pumice	4 / 6	2 / 3	30.0 / 32.5	34.2 / 35.0
Gish and Muhler[59]	6-14	8.9% SnF_2, lava pumice*	2	1	29.3(45.1)	39.6(41.7)
Horowitz and Lucye[25]	8-10	8.9% SnF_2, lava pumice	2	2	+7.9	+5.9
Peterson et al.[60]	11-13	2.1% F ($KF \cdot H_2O$), H_3PO_4, lava pumice*	2	2	19.0(7.8)	15.1(12.3)
	10-13	2.1% F ($KF \cdot H_2O$), H_3PO_4, lava pumice	2	2	13.5(12.2)	15.7(15.3)

( ) = results of 2nd independent examiner.
* = fluoride community.

reductions of 25 to 42 percent were reported in the respective groups, in a later trial supervised by Bibby, similar reductions were not obtained.[52]

In 1961, the U.S. Air Force developed a prophylaxis paste containing stannous fluoride, silicone, and silex abrasive which effectively reduced acid solubility of tooth enamel *in vitro*.[53] Clinical tests by Peterson et al.[54] produced reductions of 35 to 41 percent when applied at six-month intervals for two years.

Within the past ten years, a series of trials was conducted using lava pumice as the abrasive and either 8.9 percent stannous fluoride, 17.5 percent stannous fluoride, or acidulated potassium or sodium fluoride as the therapeutic agent (Table 10-VII). Scola and Ostrom[55, 56] reported one and two-year results of annual applications of a 17.5 percent stannous fluoride, lava pumice mixture. Significant reductions were not obtained when tested on seventeen to twenty-four-year-old naval personnel. Bixler and Muhler[57, 58] applied an 8.9 percent stannous fluoride lava pumice mixture every six months to children residing in a nonfluoride community, while Gish and Muhler[59] made similar applications in a fluoridated area. Although substantial reductions were announced in all three reports (see Table 10-VII), Horowitz and Lucye[25] failed to obtain any reduction using this same agent. The protocol of the first group of investigators required application of the therapeutic paste at six-month intervals, while Horowitz and Lucye applied the fluoride-containing prophylaxis paste at twelve-month intervals.

Peterson et al.[60] tested an acidulated potassium fluoride-lava pumice paste on children in both fluoridated and nonfluoridated communities. Two independent investigators failed to document significant reductions in either group. The authors suggested the pumice abrasive might have adversely affected the acidulated fluoride solution.

The lack of replicate positive findings from clinical trials in which the efficacy of a fluoride-containing prophylaxis paste is tested is discouraging. Vrbic et al.[61] have suggested, on the basis of laboratory investigation, that the abrasivity of prophylaxis systems might actually remove the fluoride-rich outer enamel lay-

TABLE 10-VIII

STUDIES USING FLUORIDE CONTAINING PROPHYLAXIS PASTES PLUS TOPICAL FLUORIDE

Study	Initial Age	Agent	Years After Initial Application	% Reduction DMFT	% Reduction DMFS
Bixler and Muhler[57, 58]	5-18	8.9% SnF₂—lava pumice prophy, + 8% SnF₂ topical	1 2	46.1(40.1) 35.3(46)	47.6(41.9) 38.5(43.1)
Gish and Muhler[59]	6-14	8.9% SnF₂—lava pumice prophy, + 8% SnF₂ topical*	1	68.4(57.9)	75.4(57.6)
Horowitz and Lucye[25]	8-10	8.9% SnF₂—lava pumice prophy, + 8% SnF₂ topical	2	+3	1
Peterson et al.[54]	10-13	17.5% SnF₂—silex prophy + 8% SnF₂ topical	2	29.3	32.2
Scola and Ostrom[55, 56]	17-24	17.5% SnF₂—lava pumice prophy + 10% SnF₂ topical	1 2	47 52	43 41

( ) = Results of 2nd independent examiner.
* = fluoride community.

er, thus decreasing rather than increasing the fluoride content of treated teeth. Zuniga and Caldwell[62] have shown that various abrasive systems, with or without fluoride, when applied *in vitro* to tooth enamel for thirty seconds at 200 gm vertical force, will abrade an average of 2.37 μ from a sound enamel surface and 6.89 μ from a "white spot" area.

Commercially available fluoride-containing prophylaxis pastes have been marketed and are available to the practitioner. One such paste contains acidulated phosphate fluoride and silicone dioxide; another contains stannous fluoride-zirconium silicate. Laboratory data have indicated favorable fluoride uptake and decreased enamel solubility are associated with the use of these agents.[63, 64] Confirmatory clinical evidence supporting the use of one of these agents has been reported in studies testing self-application brushing technics, which are described later in this chapter.

Table 10-VIII summarizes the results of trials in which a fluoride-containing prophylaxis paste was applied together with a topical fluoride application. By averaging the percent reductions listed in Table 10-VIII, a reduction of 42 percent (DMFS) for this combined therapeutic approach is obtained. This figure is higher than the 30 to 40 percent reduction generally associated with topical fluoride applications that include cleaning with a nontherapeutic paste. With one exception, however, the design of these studies did not include a treatment group which received a standard prophylaxis and topical fluoride application. Therefore, direct comparison between the classical method of cleaning with topical fluoride application and fluoride-prophylaxis with topical fluoride cannot be made. In the one investigation which included such a comparison, neither treatment group derived any benefits from the fluoride therapy.[25]

Application of Topical Fluoride
Sodium Fluoride

As originally recommended by the U.S. Public Health Service, the treatment technic utilizing sodium fluoride includes an initial prophylaxis with pumice. The upper and lower quadrants on one side of the mouth are isolated with cotton rolls and dried. A 2 percent solution of sodium fluoride is applied with a cotton-tipped applicator. After all surfaces are visibly wet, they are allowed to dry for three to four minutes. A second, third, and fourth application, each not preceded by a prophylaxis, are given at intervals of approximately one week. The series of treatments are recommended at ages three, seven, ten, and thirteen in order to treat newly erupting groups of teeth.

This treatment regimen does not coordinate with the recall schedules of most dental offices and is one reason why more dentists do not use sodium fluoride for topical applications in their office.

Stannous Fluoride

The recommended procedure for the topical application of stannous fluoride includes an initial *thorough* prophylaxis. Each tooth surface is cleaned with pumice for five to ten seconds, and unwaxed dental floss is used to clean interproximal areas. A quadrant or half-mouth is isolated with cotton rolls, and a *freshly prepared* 8 percent solution of stannous fluoride is applied with cotton applicators. The solution is applied continuously, keeping the teeth moist for four minutes. The recommended frequency of stannous fluoride treatments depends upon the individual patient's susceptibility. Generally, two applications are given a year. In children with a very low caries incidence, one application a year may be sufficient, while in highly susceptible patients, two or more applications per year are required. After treatment the patient may expectorate but is instructed not to eat, drink, or rinse for at least thirty minutes.

Acidulated Fluoride Phosphate

The preferred treatment procedure for acidulated fluoride phosphate topical solutions is the same as that for stannous fluoride, but the acidulated solution is stable when kept in a plastic container and need not be prepared fresh for each patient.

SUMMARY

A logical extension of water fluoridation is the use of fluoride applied topically to the teeth by professionals or semiprofessionals. Numerous studies have demonstrated the efficacy of sodium fluoride, stannous fluoride, and acidulated fluoride phosphate when applied topically to the teeth of individuals residing in locales where the benefits of community water-borne fluoride are not available. In these areas, sodium fluoride and stannous fluoride, applied as advocated, can reduce caries by 30 to 40 percent (Tables 10-I and 10-III). Acidulated fluoride phosphate has not had as long a period of investigation as the other two agents; however, it also appears to be effective at the 30 to 40 percent level or above (Table 10-V). The efficacy of topical fluoride applications in individuals residing in a community with water fluoridation has yet to be demonstrated unequivocally (Tables 10-II and 10-IV). This does not mean that such treatments should be discontinued. It indicates that until further documentation becomes available, fluoride applications administered to individuals exposed to community water fluoride should be decided on the basis of individual need, rather than provided routinely.

Since there is a lack of evidence to indicate that one of the fluoride agents has a clear-cut superiority in effectiveness, the choice of agent must ultimately depend on knowledge of the advantages and disadvantages associated with their use, the preference of the individual operator and the adaptability of the procedure to dental office routine (Table 10-IX). Sodium fluoride, for instance, has the advantage of possessing a relatively long shelf life and has an acceptable taste to the patient. It has the disadvantage, however, of being recommended for use by the Public Health Service in a treatment regimen of four applications given within one month's time at ages three, seven, ten, and thirteen. This type of treatment arrangement does not fit in well with most office scheduling procedures. The dentist, however, may elect to use biannual applications as recommended for stannous fluoride and acidulated fluoride phosphate.

The recommended treatment frequency for stannous fluoride, which can be given in single yearly, or semiannual application, conforms to standard private office routine. Stannous fluoride has several disadvantages. The aqueous solution is unstable, un-

TABLE 10-IX

COMPARISON OF TOPICAL FLUORIDE AGENTS

	NaF	*SnF₂*	*AFP*
Efficacy	33% reduction	36% reduction	> 36% reduction
Application	4×/yr. at ages 3, 7, 10, 13; but may be applied like other agents	2×/yr. or as indicated	2×/yr. or as indicated
Stable	Yes	No	Yes
Adaptable to office recall	No/yes	Yes	Yes
Cost	Inexpensive	Inexpensive	Rel. expensive
Taste	Acceptable	Unpleasant	Flavored
Tooth discoloration	No	Yes	No
Gingival reaction	No	Occasionally	None reported

dergoing hydrolysis and oxidation to stannous hydroxide and stannic ion. Because this reaction reduces the agent's effectiveness, a fresh solution must be prepared for each treatment. The 8 percent stannous fluoride solution is astringent, and its disagreeable taste makes it unacceptable to many children. The addition of flavoring agents to mask the unpleasant taste is not recommended. Pigmentation of teeth following topical application of this agent has been reported. Pigmentation generally appears in association with carious lesions and hypocalcified areas and around margins of restorations. While the pigmented areas have been cited as evidence of caries arrestment, they can be esthetically unsightly.

Acidulated fluoride phosphate solutions also have the advantage of being recommended for semiannual or annual applications. This treatment frequency can be integrated with most standard office recall procedures. The solution is stable when kept in plastic containers and need not be prepared fresh for each patient. Some of the commercial preparations contain additives to improve the taste of the material.

Fluoride gels have lately become available and are generally used in a tray system. Prophylaxis pastes containing fluoride are also available. As indicated in Table 10-VI, of the five studies where a fluoride gel was applied either once or twice a year, as would be done in a dental practice, three did not show clinically significant reductions in dental caries. Clinical trials of different fluoride-containing prophylaxis pastes gave variable results (Table 10-VII) and the trials to determine the clinical efficacy of commercially available fluoride-containing prophylaxis pastes when applied topically by a dentist or hygienist are equivocal.

The use of either a fluoride gel-tray system or a fluoride-containing prophylaxis paste alone is attractive in that the time required for the classical prophylaxis-topical fluoride treatment, usually thirty minutes, could be decreased by nearly half. Current investigation, however, does not justify a change in the two-step therapeutic regimen at this time. A gel-tray method of application does not appear to be effective, based upon available evidence, when applied once or twice a year. A fluoride-containing prophylaxis paste should not be substituted for the topical fluoride application, although such a paste may be used in place of the nonfluoride-containing prophylaxis agent. Following a thorough cleaning and polishing, teeth should be isolated with cotton rolls, air dried, and a four-minute application of topical fluoride administered meticulously with cotton-tipped applicators. Either a single quadrant or a half-mouth (upper and adjacent lower quadrant) may be isolated, depending upon the operator's ability to keep the teeth free of saliva. All surfaces must be wetted with the fluoride solution. Unwaxed floss may be used to draw the solution interproximally. An aqueous solution of sodium fluoride, stannous fluoride, or acidulated fluoride phosphate should be used for the topical treatment, the selection being based upon the considerations outlined in Table 10-IX.

SELF-ADMINISTRATION OF TOPICAL FLUORIDE

Clinical trials have been conducted in which the fluoride-containing therapeutic agent is applied to the teeth by the patient himself. The traditional self-application technic is via toothbrushing with a therapeutic dentifrice. The methods discussed in this section differ from the classical toothbrushing approach in that (1) the therapeutic agent is usually more concentrated than that found in a dentifrice; (2) the agent may be a standard topical fluoride solution, a fluoride-containing prophylaxis paste, a mouthwash, or a gel; and (3) the method of application may involve technics other than toothbrushing.

There are three methods by which the patient may apply a concentrated fluoride solution directly to his own teeth. He may scrub his teeth with a toothbrush that has been dipped in a fluoride solution or to which a fluoride-containing prophylaxis paste has been applied. He may rinse with a fluoride solution, or he may wear custom-fitted mouth trays which hold a topical fluoride solution in intimate contact with the teeth. Compared to the traditional methods of individual applications by a dentist or hygienist, the self-administration technics have the advantage of reducing the time and cost of treating a large group of patients. Successful self-administration procedures are especially suited to the public health programs where large groups of children are treated. These methods may also be of value in treating caries-prone patients where home applications by the patient might supplement other forms of caries preventive care.

Self-Administration of Topical Fluoride by Brushing

Studies in which groups of children have applied topical fluoride solutions, gels, or fluoride-containing prophylaxis pastes on their teeth by brushing have been conducted in Sweden,[65, 66] Canada[67, 68] and the United States[69-71] (Table 10-X). With few exceptions, the results of these trials have been discouraging. In the Swedish studies, individual groups of children brushed with 1 percent or 0.5 percent sodium fluoride solutions, with zirconium fluoride and with ferric fluoride.[65, 66] Four, nine, or ten applications were made over a two-year period. Brushing with 1 percent sodium fluoride solution nine times during two years produced a 25 to 30 percent caries reduction in the maxillary teeth only.[65] The lack of a significant reduction in the lower arch was attributed to a possible dilution of the fluoride solution by the saliva. Results also indicated that the more frequent

TABLE 10-X

SELF-ADMINISTRATION OF TOPICAL FLUORIDE BY BRUSHING

Study	Initial Age	Agent	Total Applications/ Duration	Supervision	Results
Berggren and Welander[65] ...	9-13	1% NaF solution	9/2 yrs.	Yes	25-30% reduction in maxillary teeth; no significant reduction in mandibular teeth
Berggren and Welander[66] ...	10	0.5% NaF solution	10/2 yrs. 4/2 yrs.	Yes	29% caries reduction 17% caries reduction
		zirconium fluoride	10/2 yrs. 4/2 yrs.		17% caries reduction no reduction
		ferric fluoride	10/2 yrs. 4/2 yrs.		33% caries reduction 8% caries reduction
Bullen, McCombie, Hole[67] ...	6	Acidulated phosphate fluoride solution, 1.23% NaF, pH 3.0	4-5/1 yr.	Yes	38.5% reduction in permanent molars and incisors; 4.3% reduction in primary teeth
Bullen, McCombie, Hole[68] ...			7-9/2 yrs.		15.0% reduction in permanent molars and incisors; no statistically significant difference in deciduous teeth
Heifetz, Horowitz, Driscoll[69, 70] ...	Approx. 12-13	Nontherapeutic prophylaxis paste followed by 0.6% acidulated fluoride-phosphate solution, pH 3	5/1 yr.	Yes	2.7% caries reduction
		0.6% acidulated fluoride phosphate solution, pH 3			1.9% caries reduction
		nontherapeutic prophylaxis paste followed by 1.23% acidulated fluoride phosphate gel, pH 3			10-14% caries reduction

Author	Age	Method	Frequency/Duration	Fluoridated community	Results
	12-13	laxis paste followed by 0.6% acidulated fluoride-phosphate solution, pH 3			3% caries reduction
		0.6% acidulated fluoride phosphate solution, pH 3			8% caries reduction
		nontherapeutic prophy-laxis paste followed by 1.23% acidulated fluoride phosphate gel, pH 3			
Goaz, McElwaine, Biswell, White[72]	6-14	6% sodium monofluoro-phosphate solution	Daily/ 14 mos.*	No	39.4% reduction in the relative increment of decay, 42.1% reduction in the number of new decayed and filled surface (primary and permanent teeth)
Goaz, McElwaine, Biswell, White[73]	6-14	6% sodium monofluoro-phosphate solution	Daily/ 21 mos.*	No	46.7% reduction in the relative increment of decay, 46.6% reduction in the number of new decayed and filled surfaces (primary and permanent teeth)
Lang, Thomas, Taylor, Rothhaar[79]	6-10	9.0% stannous fluoride-zirconium silicate prophylaxis paste	3/18 mos.†	Yes	37.8-42.1% caries reduction based upon DMFS increments; 27.1-40.6% reduction bond upon DMFT increments (3 examiners)
Gish, Mercer[80]	6-15	9.0% stannous fluoride-zirconium silicate prophylaxis paste	4/24 mos.	Yes	16% reduction based on DMF surface increment in fluoride community; 42% reduction based on DMF surface increment in nonfluoride community
Muhler, Kelley, Stookey, Lindo, Harris[77]	6-14	9.0% stannous fluoride-zirconium silicate prophylaxis paste	1/1 yr.	Yes	40.6% reduction in new DMF teeth; 63.9% reduction in new DMF surfaces

* = community fluoridated for 10 years. † = fluoridated community.

application regimen (ten times during two years versus five times) was associated with greater reductions.[66]

The Canadian studies employed an acidulated phosphate fluoride solution (1.23 percent NaF, pH 3.0), brushed on the teeth of six-year-old children four or five times during the school year.[67, 68] Toothbrushes labelled with the name of each child were issued to each participating first grade classroom teacher. Every six weeks, public health nurses visited the classrooms and supervised the toothbrushing drills. Children dipped their toothbrushes into the fluoride solution and brushed according to accepted procedure. A 38.5 percent caries reduction in permanent molars and incisors was obtained after the first year.[67] A less promising 15.0 percent reduction was reported after the second year.[68] No statistically significant differences in caries activity between control and treated primary teeth were observed.

First and second-year results from a United States Public Health Service study in New Orleans were also discouraging.[69–71] Children brushed five times a year using either a 0.6 percent acidulated phosphate fluoride solution or a 1.23 percent acidulated phosphate fluoride gel. Three different technics were used (see Table 10-X). The maximum benefit, 10 to 14 percent caries reduction, was obtained after two years in the group that brushed with a prophylaxis paste followed by the acidulated phosphate-fluoride gel. Because of the lack of meaningful benefits and the attrition of the study groups, the project, originally designed to continue for three years, was terminated after the second year.

Goaz et al. evaluated the effectiveness of daily brushings with a 6 percent solution of sodium monofluorophosphate on children in a fluoridated community.[72, 73] The brushings were done at home and, therefore, were not under the direct supervision of the investigators. After fourteen months, a 39.4 percent reduction in the relative increment of decay (R.I.D.) was reported with a 42.1 percent reduction in the number of new decayed and filled surfaces (ΔDFS).[72] After twenty-one months, the R.I.D. and ΔDFS were approximately 50 percent.[73] Although these reductions are high, the unusual method of reporting caries reductions makes evaluation difficult. The high number of reversals in both control and treated groups reported in this study and the pooling of primary and permanent teeth in the results must also be considered. Also, because of the age range of the subjects and the date when fluoridation of the community water supplies began, not all permanent teeth received the same fluoride exposure during their developmental period. There have been no further clinical investigations using sodium monofluorophosphate solutions in a self-application technic.

A zirconium silicate ($ZrSiO_4$) prophylaxis paste containing 9 percent stannous fluoride has been introduced as a possible effective caries-preventive agent in mass self-administration programs.[74-76] Approximately 5 gm of the therapeutic paste is applied to a nylon toothbrush, and the child scrubs each quadrant in sequence for approximately five minutes. Rinsing is allowed after each quadrant is completed.[77] Muhler summarized the results obtained in several unpublished trials with this agent. Although reductions were impressive, the opportunity to evaluate the results fully was not available because of the review nature of the article.[78] The three reports[77, 79, 80] summarized in Table 10-X, however, indicate the possible efficacy of the stannous fluoride-zirconium silicate prophylaxis paste when utilized in a self-administration program. Lang et al.[79] supervised the self-application of SnF_2-$ZrSiO_4$ in six to ten-year-old children residing in a fluoridated community. Three applications were made at six-month intervals, and evaluation was performed by three different examiners. After eighteen months, reductions of 37.8 to 42.1 percent, based upon DMFS increments, were recorded. In another trial by Gish,[80] this agent was also self-applied every six months by children ingesting water-borne fluoride; the reduction was only 16 percent. In nonfluoridated communities, Muhler et al.[77] reported a 63.9 percent reduction based upon DMF surface increments twelve months after a single self-application; Gish and Mercer[80] reported a 42 percent reduction after four applications spaced at six-month intervals. The promising caries reductions obtained, especially in nonfluoridated areas, should stimulate additional trials of this agent to conclusively establish its efficacy when used in a self-application brushing program.

Self-Administration of Fluoride Solutions by Mouth Rinsing

The use of mouth rinses as a vehicle to apply fluoride in a self-administered therapeutic program was first reported by Bibby et al. in 1946.[51] Although this initial study and a second study[81] reported two years later failed to produce significant results, the fluoride-rinsing method was revived in the 1960's in a series of clinical trials, many of which were conducted in the Scandinavian countries and the United States.[8, 82-89] In a previous chapter, several of these trials have been described (see Chapter 9) and therapeutic concentrations and regimens recommended. Particularly significant was the report by Torell and Ericsson[8] in which two different therapeutic regimens were tested. One group of children rinsed daily using a neutral 0.05 percent sodium fluoride solution without supervision. A second group rinsed every two weeks under supervision with a neutral 0.2 percent sodium fluoride solution. After two years, the group that rinsed with a lower fluoride concentration on a daily basis exhibited a 50 percent caries reduction, compared to a 21 percent reduction in the group that rinsed with the high concentration every two weeks. These data suggest the importance of frequency of application in determining the success of a fluoride therapeutic program.

Self-Administration of Topical Fluoride by Mouthpieces

Englander et al.[90] reported high caries reductions when children applied custom-fitted mouthpieces containing an acidulated sodium fluoride gel (pH 4.5) or a neutral sodium fluoride gel (pH 7.0) to their maxillary and mandibular teeth over a twenty-one-month period (Table 10-XI). The study, conducted in a fluoride-deficient community (Cheektowaga, New York; 0.3 ppm F), involved six-minute self-administrations of the therapeutic agent each day of the school year. Individual sets of polyvinyl mouthpieces were constructed and distributed to the children. The children put five to ten drops of sodium fluoride gel (1 to 2 mg fluoride) into each mouthpiece. Both mouthpieces were inserted by the children and worn for six minutes. Saliva and excess gel which oozed from the mouthpiece periphery were expectorated into paper towels. After treatment, the children rinsed their mouths, washed their applicators, and stored them in cardboard boxes. The applications were performed in school under the supervision of dental hygienists. After twenty-one months, the average child had given himself 245 treatments. At the conclusion of the study the group that used the acidulated fluoride had 64 percent less carious teeth, and the group that used the neutral sodium fluoride had 67 percent less carious teeth than the nontreated control group (Table 10-XI). Twenty-three months after discontinuation of treatment, the children were reexamined to determine if a residual fluoride effect had been maintained.[91] Of the original 500 children in the control and treatment groups, 379 were available for reexamination and were evaluated. There were approximately 70 percent less carious teeth in each of the treated groups compared to the control (Table 10-XI).

The results of self-administration of topical fluoride by mouthpiece were also evaluated in a fluoridated community.[92] Children, ages 11 to 15 in Charlotte, North Carolina (1.0 ppm F), applied acidulated sodium fluoride gel by mouthpiece under the supervision of dental assistants. Applications were made three days a week for three school years. The mean number of applications was 255, similar to the 245 applications recorded in the Cheektowaga study. At the end of the study, the DMFS increment in the nontreated control group of children was 2.20. In the treatment group of 337 children, the increment was 1.57; this represented a caries reduction of 28.6 percent (Table 10-XI). These results, of course, are not as dramatic as those obtained in the nonfluoride community and may reflect the initial low caries scores of the groups, the high level of dental care in the community, and the initial fluoride content of the teeth. Interpretation of the data is further complicated by the use of two examiners, one of whom did not observe statistically different caries scores between the control and treated children that he examined.

Primary teeth exfoliated during the course of these studies

TABLE 10-XI

SELF-ADMINISTRATION OF TOPICAL FLUORIDE BY MOUTHPIECES

Study	Initial Age	Agent	Applications/Duration	% Reduction DMFS	% Reduction DMFT
Englander et al.[90]	11-14	Acidulated NaF gel, 1.1% NaF, 0.1 M PO₄ pH 4.5	daily/21 mos.	75	64
		Neutral NaF gel, 1.1% NaF, pH 7.0	daily/21 mos.	80	67
Englander et al.[91]	11-14	Acidulated NaF gel, 1.1% NaF, 0.1 M PO₄ pH 4.5	No additional treatment; 44-month effect*	70	70
		Neutral NaF gel, 1.1% NaF, pH 7.0	No additional treatment; 44-month effect*	69	70
Englander et al.[92]	11-15	Acidulated NaF gel, 1.1% NaF, 0.1 M PO₄ pH 4.5	3× week/27-31 mos. (fluoride community)	28.6	

* 44 months includes 21 months treatment, 23 months no treatment.

TABLE 10-XII

FLUORIDE UPTAKE BY SURFACE LAYERS OF ENAMEL IN SELF-ADMINISTRATION
FLUORIDE-MOUTHPIECE STUDIES

Circumstance	Group	No. of Teeth	Average No. Treatments	F (ppm) by Layer			
				(5-10 μ)*	(15-20 μ)	(30-40 μ)	(60-80 μ)
Cheektowaga, 0.3 ppm F, during 21-month treatment regimen: primary teeth[90, 93, 94]	Control	39	0	632	269	142	65
	Acidulated NaF gel, 1.1% NaF, 0.1 M PO₄, pH 4.5	7	15	1293	679	323	141
		8	123	2607	1934	1334	1076
		8	231	4261	2873	2151	1774
	Neutral NaF gel, 1.1% NaF, pH 7.0	3	17	694	329	194	100
		8	125	1312	645	259	120
		4	221	1702	624	280	173
Cheektowaga, 0.3 ppm F, 6 to 9 mos. following discontinuation of treatment; primary teeth[91]	Acidulated NaF gel, 1.1% NaF, 0.1 M PO₄, pH 4.5	6	243	2782	2179	1373	1140
Charlotte, 1.0 ppm F, during 3 yr. treatment regimen: permanent teeth[92, 95, 96]	Control	12	0	1653	929	500	264
	Acidulated NaF gel, 1.1% NaF, 0.1 M PO₄, pH 4.5	11	123	2759	1345	775	473
		9	219	2542	1489	804	504

* Approx. depth from surface (microns).

and permanent teeth extracted for orthodontic reasons were collected and evaluated for uptake of fluoride.[90-96] In both the fluoridated and nonfluoridated communities, there was a significant increase in fluoride concentrations in all outer layers of enamel analyzed (Table 10-XII), compared to nontreated control teeth. A seven-fold increase in fluoride concentration was observed in primary teeth which had been treated with the acidulated solution in the nonfluoride area. Discontinuation of treatment appeared to produce a decrease in fluoride concentration, especially in the outer layer of enamel, but, as seen in Table 10-XI, the anticariogenic potential of the treatments was not affected. Fluoride uptake in the teeth treated with the neutral sodium fluoride gel was less than that of the teeth treated with the acidulated gel. Again, this discrepancy did not appear to affect the anticariogenic potential of the neutral gel, as demonstrated by the percent reductions recorded in Table 10-XI.

Use of Self-Administration Technics in the Private Dental Office

For those patients in a private dental office who can be motivated to practice frequent, self-administered fluoride therapy, the use of mouth rinses or mouthpieces is recommended. These technics have the advantage of providing frequent contact between the fluoride agent and the teeth, thus increasing the total fluoride content in the outer layers of enamel and providing maximum protection against caries.

It must be remembered that since the patient administers the fluoride himself, without professional or semiprofessional supervision, a high degree of cooperation is required. The technic can be used for any well-motivated patient but is especially indicated for patients who exhibit a high caries incidence and for whom additional caries protection is needed.

The methods and prescription for recommending fluoride mouth rinses are described in Chapter 9. If a mouthpiece technic is used, the equipment required and procedure are as follows.

Supplies and Equipment

1. Omnivac II® vacuum adapter*
2. Omnidental® mouthguard material and cast lubricant*

3. Thera-Flur® (24 ml) acidulated fluoride phosphate gel†
   (prescription required)

Procedure

1. Take alginate impressions of the maxillary and mandibular
   arches.
2. Pour casts in stone or plaster.
3. Spray hardened casts with lubricant.
4. Impress polyvinyl sheet on maxillary and mandibular casts
   (use Omnivac vacuum adapter and Omnidental mouthguard material) (Figure 10-1a).
5. Trim maxillary and mandibular mouthpieces to a horse-
   shoe shape.
6. Give patient mouthpieces and either a prescription for
   acidulated fluoride phosphate gel (Figure 10-2) or a 24 ml
   bottle from office inventory.

The patient is told to put five to ten drops in each mouthpiece
for five to six minutes while engaged in a seated activity such as
watching television (Figures 10-1b and 10-1c). Application
should be each weekday for one year. Used daily, the bottle of
fluoride gel will last approximately five weeks, after which a new
supply is required. New mouthpieces may have to be constructed
during the year, depending upon the age of the patient and
stage of dentition development. The patient should be cautioned to expectorate any excess into a glass or cup rather than
swallowing it. Urinalysis of patients who participated in both
mouthguard application studies described above indicated that
any excess fluoride was not swallowed by the participants.

After the caries attack is controlled, it may be advisable, on an
empirical basis, to continue applications in order to maintain
the high fluoride levels in the treated teeth. Discontinuation of
therapy will depend upon the caries incidence of the patient at
future appointments and should be decided by the dentist on an
individual basis.

---

* Omnidental Corp., Harrisburg, Pennsylvania.
† Hoyt Laboratories, Needham, Massachusetts.

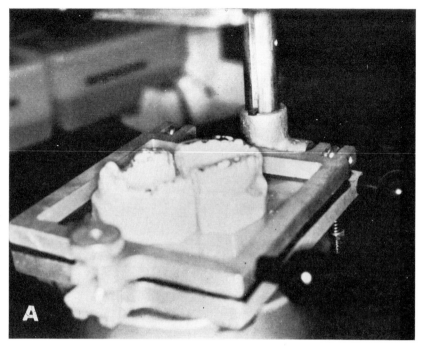

Figure 10-1a. Polyvinyl sheet being impressed on maxillary and mandibular casts.

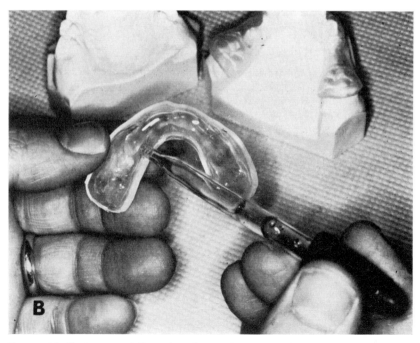

Figure 10-1b. Drops of fluoride solution being evenly distributed in horse-shoe-shaped mouthpieces.

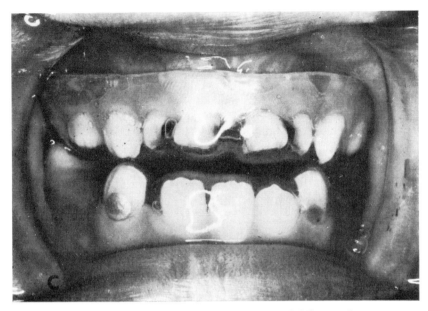

Figure 10-1c. Mouthpieces positioned in child's mouth.

ADHESIVES FOR PIT AND FISSURE CARIES CONTROL

The rationale for pit and fissure caries control resides in the fact that these areas are especially susceptible to caries and present a major dental problem.[97-104] Typical of the situation are the findings of Knutson, Klein, and Palmer[102] that 43 percent of all carious or filled surfaces found in 4,416 elementary

---

R   Thera-Flur® acidulated fluoride phosphate gel

Dispense: 24 ml

Sig.   5 to 10 drops of each mouthguard maintained in mouth for 6 minutes for 5 days per week. Rinse mouth after use.

Figure 10-2. Prescription for acidulated fluoride phosphate gel for use in self-administration program utilizing mouthpieces.

school children were on the occlusal surfaces of the permanent teeth. Day and Sedwick[103] found that 45 percent of the caries in the permanent teeth of thirteen-year-old children involved the occlusal surfaces. These findings are of particular significance since the occlusal surfaces represent only 12.5 percent of the total surfaces at risk at these ages. The deciduous dentition in children one to three years of age, as reported by Hennon et al.,[98] presents a similar picture in that two thirds of the caries reported for the primary molar teeth were occlusal lesions.

Even with water fluoridation, occlusal caries remains a significant problem in that the benefits to these surfaces are not as great as those provided to the interproximal surfaces.[105-108] In fact, although water fluoridation may result in an absolute reduction in both occlusal and proximal lesions, as shown by Horowitz and Peterson,[108] the relative percentage incidence of occlusal caries may actually rise because of the more selective protection afforded the proximal surfaces by fluoride. Findings indicate, for instance, that in a nonfluoride area the caries incidence on the proximal surfaces is about the same as that found on the occlusal surfaces. However, in a fluoride community, because of the selective protection afforded the proximal surfaces, the *relative* incidence of occlusal caries may actually rise, while that of proximal caries declines, resulting in a wide differential between the two.

Recognition of the problem has resulted in various attempts to prevent pit and fissure caries. Hyatt's[109] prophylactic odontotomy, which required drilling and filling of all pits and fissures with amalgam, and Bodecker's[110-112] "eradication of enamel fissures," which was largely based on the removal but not the filling of the fissures, were subject to considerable criticism. A major objection to the former method resulted from the fact that since all fissures did not decay, it was considered presumptuous to drill and/or fill all fissures. These technics, moreover, were not true preventive measures in that both required mechanical intervention similar to that used in restorative procedures. Other technics not involving drilling were those of Miller[113, 114] who used red copper cement and silver nitrate, and Ast[115] who employed zinc chloride with potassium ferrocyanide; none of these technics proved successful.

More recently, adhesives have been employed to seal pits and fissures for caries control. Adhesives require no drilling but rather slight chemical and physical modification of the enamel surface to render it more receptive to bonding. This modification or conditioning of the surface appears to be best achieved by short exposure of the enamel to acid. Among the first reports of adhesive sealing was that of Cueto and Buonocore[116, 117] who utilized methyl-2 cyanoacrylate monomer with a siliceous filler to seal pits and fissures of permanent molars and bicuspids. A caries reduction of 86.3 percent was obtained after one year. The second-year results reported by Ripa, Buonocore, and Cueto[118, 119] showed an 82.5 percent caries reduction.

A report by Ripa and Cole,[120] who sealed teeth of handicapped children, confirmed the effectiveness of the methyl-2 cyanoacrylate-siliceous filler formulation. This work differed from those previously reported[116–119] in that a single yearly application of the adhesive was made rather than six-month interval applications. While considerable loss of adhesive coverage was observed in these studies, protection against caries was nevertheless quite high.

Two other studies involving the use of cyanoacrylates in combination with methylmethacrylate polymer powder[121] and various metal powders[122] were reported by Takeuchi et al. Although of less than one year duration, these studies showed good evidence of a treatment effect. Only one study, that of Parkhouse and Winter,[123] failed to report positive results with the cyanoacrylates. These authors not only changed the ratio of monomer to filler in the adhesive but also used a different conditioning solution to prepare the enamel for bonding than that employed by Cueto and Buonocore.[116, 117] In spite of the early loss of adhesive from the treated teeth observed by Parkhouse and Winter, the decay rate was no greater than on control teeth. This important observation, which is in agreement with those of other studies, attests to the fact that conditioning of the pit and fissure areas

TABLE 10-XIIIA

CLINICAL SEALANT STUDIES: ADDUCTS OF
BISPHENOL A AND GLYCIDYL METHACRYLATE:
ULTRAVIOLET LIGHT POLYMERIZED SYSTEM

Investigator	Duration (Mos.)	% Retained Sealant*	Reduction†
Buonocore[150]	12	99	100
Buonocore[151]	24	87	99
McCune et al.[152]	12	88	81-85‡
Horowitz et al.[153]	24	73	67
Horowitz et al.[154]	48	50	41
Going[155]	36	56	47
Rock[147]	12	54	65
Rock[148]	24	80	99
Luoma et al.[157]	6	99	92
Meurman et al.[158]	18	95	88
Risager & Poulsen[159]	12	69	§
Gourley[160]	12	87	65
Gourley[161]	24	78	58

* Completely covered teeth only.
† Permanent teeth only.
‡ Two investigators.
§ Caries data not presented in the usual fashion.

with acid does not appear to increase their susceptibility to caries.

Because of their difficult and sometimes unpredictable handling characteristics and the fact that the cyanoacrylates tend to decompose by hydrolysis in the presence of moisture, new adhesives were sought.

Several clinical trials were instituted using agents whose base formulation represented the reaction product of bisphenol A and

TABLE 10-XIIIB

CLINICAL SEALANT STUDIES: ADDUCTS OF
BISPHENOL A AND GLYCIDYL METHACRYLATE:
AUTO-POLYMERIZING SYSTEMS

Investigator	Time (Mos.)	% Retained Sealant*	% Caries Reduction†
Roydhouse[125]	36	—	29
Rock[147]	12	52	81
Rock[148]	24	52	65
Wilson et al.[149]	6	74	78

* Completely covered teeth only.
† Permanent teeth only.

glycidyl methacrylate (BIS-GMA).[124] The materials tested were either self-polymerizing upon mixing with a catalyst-accelerator system or they required ultra-violet light for acceleration. Tables 10-XIIIA and 10-XIIIB list the results of controlled clinical trials using self-polymerizing and ultra-violet light polymerized BIS-GMA systems respectively. In the study by Roydhouse,[125] acid pretreatment of the enamel (see discussion below) was not used. In all of the other studies the occlusal surfaces were first pretreated with acid to make them more receptive to bonding. The caries reductions, as presented in the tables, are quite dramatic, ranging as high as 100 percent one year following treatment in two separate and independent studies.

Because of the diverse conditions under which clinical trials are performed, it is hazardous to make generalizations about the sealant studies. Nevertheless, the results of the clinical trials using both the earlier cyanoacrylate system and the BIS-GMA system have been almost uniformly favorable. In 1972, the American Dental Association's Council on Dental Materials and Devices expanded their testing program to include pit and fissure sealants.[126] Shortly thereafter, provisional acceptance was granted to two commercial sealants with BIS-GMA base formulations, Nuva-Seal®* (an ultraviolet light polymerized system) and Epoxylite 9075®† (a self-polymerizing system).[127, 128] While the use of these products is considered a preventive measure, the products themselves are not considered preventive materials since they contain no active agent such as fluoride. In 1974, the Council on Dental Materials and Devices reaffirmed its position on pit and fissure sealants and continued both Nuva-Seal and Epoxylite 9075 in the provisionally accepted category.[129] In addition to these two products, provisional acceptance has also been granted to a third commercial sealant, Delton.®‡ Thus, in approximately one decade, occlusal sealing went from the clinical investigation phase to one of commercial availability and product review and acceptance.

---

* The L. D. Caulk Co., Division of Dentsply International Inc., Milford, Delaware.
† Lee Pharmaceuticals, S. El Monte, California.
‡ Johnson & Johnson, New Brunswick, N.J.

Natural enamel surfaces are not conducive to bonding in that they can be considered as fully reacted, low-energy substrates. The optimal bonding of adhesives to teeth would appear to be predicated on the proper conditioning of the enamel surface following prophylaxis. Although many substances have been tested as enamel conditioning agents, acids appear to be most effective. In this regard, phosphoric acid has been most extensively evaluated and employed in clinical studies.[130-137] Acid conditioning serves not only to clean the surface to render it more wettable and to markedly increase surface bonding area, but also to create microspaces in the enamel into which the adhesive can flow to provide mechanical retention.[138-140] Figure 10-3 shows a

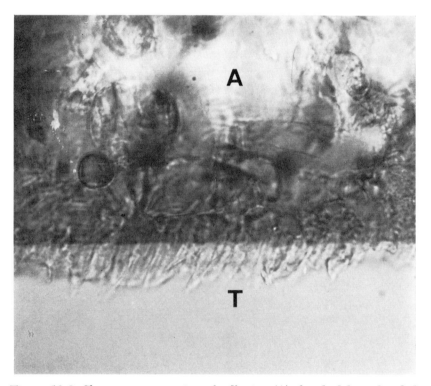

Figure 10-3. Shows a cross section of adhesive (A) that had been bonded to conditioned enamel. The enamel has been dissolved by HCl, leaving prism-like structures called "tags" (T) projecting from the surface of the adhesive that had previously been in contact with the enamel.

cross section of Nuva-Seal adhesive that had been bonded to conditioned enamel. The enamel has been dissolved away by hydrochloric acid, leaving prism-like structures called "tags" projecting from the surface of the adhesive previously in contact with the enamel. These "tags" are believed to represent a combination of adhesive and organic matter of enamel which was entrapped by the adhesive that penetrated the microspaces created in the enamel surface by acid conditioning. In this sense, the adhesive does not simply rest on the enamel surface but is also in it.

Presently available fissure sealants require that the tooth surface be thoroughly washed and dried. From experience with the ultraviolet light-polymerized adhesive, with which the authors are most familiar, there can be no compromise on this latter point. Failure to adequately dry the surface after conditioning will result in a poor bond. Warm, compressed air is recommended for drying as it would be less likely to cool the enamel surface; cooling would favor moisture condensation that could interfere with bonding. In addition, care should be exercised that the air line used for drying does not contain water or oil. The former will prevent adequate drying, while the latter is a particularly effective antibonding agent.

A conditioned enamel surface is quite reactive and will as avidly absorb and/or adsorb fluorides and salivary constituents,[141-144] etc., as it does the adhesive. Studies have shown that the acquisition of fluorides and proteinaceous material from saliva by a conditioned enamel surface results in the formation of reaction products that significantly lower bonding strengths.[145] Contact with such materials, therefore, should be avoided subsequent to conditioning and drying of the enamel surface. Hence, after conditioning of the enamel surface and washing, the patient should expectorate quickly and return to position immediately for isolation of the teeth with cotton rolls to avoid any additional salivary contact. The use of the rubber dam will largely eliminate the problem of salivary contamination of the conditioned surface. Subsequent to placing the adhesive, however, topical fluoride treatments can be employed to provide the usual benefits of fluoride to the smooth surfaces and to incorporate large quantities of fluoride into accidentally or inadvertently acid-conditioned enamel that is not subsequently covered by adhesive. The application of fluorides to etched enamel surfaces assures greater uptake and retention of fluoride; this finding has resulted in the recent recommendation to etch enamel with dilute phosphoric acid prior to the application of acidulated sodium fluoride.[146]

Research done in the authors' laboratory with a variety of fissure sealants indicates that thin layers of adhesive do not perform as well as thicker ones. Therefore, in applying adhesives to tooth surfaces, the maximum amount of material possible, consistent with occlusal clearance, should be employed. As one gains experience with the use of occlusal sealants, it becomes quite obvious that between opposing teeth there is considerable dead space that can be filled with an adhesive. Even with slight overfilling, the adhesive is generally quickly worn down by

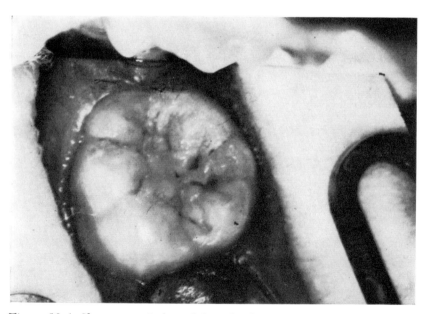

Figure 10-4. Shows a typical candidate for fissure sealing. Prophylaxis has not removed the brown stain at the orifices of the multitude of pits and fissures present, which are somewhat sticky but not considered carious.

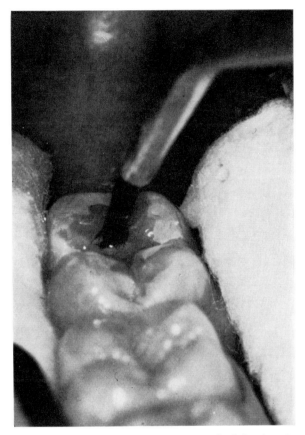

Figure 10-5. Shows a liquid adhesive being applied by brush to a conditioned enamel surface. The adhesive rapidly spreads over the surface.

masticatory forces so that occlusal interference appears to be a minor problem.

It is the authors' belief that adhesive sealing is not indicated for all teeth. Typical candidates for sealing should have well-defined, sticky, stained or unstained pits and fissures and/or deep fossae present in mouths in which decay already exists in other teeth. Teeth showing well-coalesced pit and fissure areas and/or smooth, saucer-shaped fossae in caries-free individuals are usually not treated since it is felt that natural protection exists in such cases. Treatment in these instances should be deferred until the situation indicates otherwise. Figure 10-4 shows a typical candidate for fissure sealing. Note that prophylaxis has not removed the stain at the orifice of the pits and fissures. This stain, moreover, will not be removed even with the conditioning solution. The orifice of stained pits and fissures is acid resistant and probably represents enamel that had previously been demineralized by oral acids and subsequently impregnated by protein and/or pigmented material. Although these resistant areas, usually called brown spots, are common on smooth, noncontacting proximal

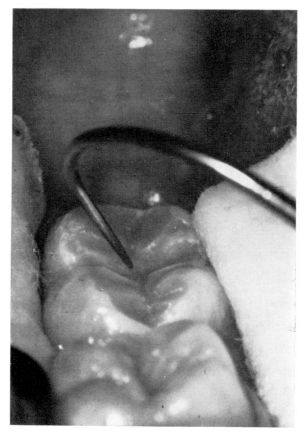

Figure 10-6. Shows an explorer point resting on the ultraviolet light-hardened adhesive which almost completely covers the occlusal surface. The adhesive bridges the central fossa between the cuspal inclined planes.

surfaces, they offer little protection against the type of caries characteristic of pit and fissure lesions. In such lesions, decay tends to progress more in depth than laterally, resulting in the rather common finding of an explorer point-sized hole in enamel that mushrooms in dentin to a large cavity. Figure 10-5 shows the liquid adhesive being carried by brush on to a dull, satiny appearing conditioned enamel surface. Note the spreading of the adhesive to form a small contact angle. Figure 10-6 shows an explorer point resting on the ultraviolet light-hardened adhesive, which almost completely covers the occlusal surface. While most sealant studies have been concerned with posterior teeth, pits and fissures present on the palatal surfaces of the upper anterior teeth are also candidates for adhesive sealing.

Questions have arisen, incident to the application of sealants, regarding the use of topical fluorides and/or fluoride prophylaxis pastes. As stated previously, fluorides and saliva should not be permitted to contact a conditioned enamel surface, as the reaction products formed will reduce bonding strengths. However, fluoride treatments may be given before conditioning the enamel surface or subsequent to application of the adhesive. The advantages of the latter approach have already been discussed in this section. There are potential advantages, however, to applying topical fluorides prior to acid conditioning. For instance, by applying topical fluorides such as sodium fluoride or stannous fluoride to an occlusal surface, the spaces in the pits and fissures will undoubtedly become flooded with the fluoride solution. Considerable amounts of fluoride may thus be acquired by the enamel walls of the pit or fissure since enamel in these areas commonly presents an incipient demineralization. In addition, the organic material present in the fissure may also pick up fluoride. A good part of this fluoride may be retained in these sites even after conditioning. If this is the case, the retained fluoride will be sealed in by the adhesive and may gradually become more permanently fixed in the enamel to afford protection when sealant applications are discontinued.

The fact that the adhesive appears to penetrate the enamel in depth (Figure 10-3) is an additional favorable aspect of fissure sealing. Even if the external bulk of adhesive is worn down completely by mastication, the possibility of protection could still exist due to the presence of adhesive deep in the enamel. In addition, the probability of in-depth impregnation of the enamel surface by adhesive supports application over interproximal surfaces where the external bulk of adhesive is contraindicated due to space limitations. Research presently in progress indicates that early carious lesions, which are represented by white spots, often occur in Class V locations and may also be impregnated by adhesive to render them resistant to acid dissolution.

It is felt that adhesive sealing of pits and fissures could be an important adjunct in a caries-preventive program since it is intended for those caries-susceptible areas least benefited by fluoride.

REFERENCES

1. B. G. Bibby, "The Use of Fluorine in the Prevention of Dental Caries. II. Effect of Sodium Fluoride Applications," *JADA*, *31*:317-321, 1944.

2. J. W. Knutson and W. D. Armstrong, "The Effect of Topically Applied Sodium Fluoride on Dental Caries Experience," *Public Health Rep*, *58*:1701-1715, 1943.

3. J. W. Knutson and W. D. Armstrong, "The Effect of Topically Applied Sodium Fluoride on Dental Caries Experience. II. Report of Findings for Second Year Study," *Public Health Rep*, *60*:1085-1090, 1945.

4. J. W. Knutson and W. D. Armstrong, "The Effect of Topically Applied Sodium Fluoride on Dental Caries Experience. III. Report of Findings for the Third Year Study," *Public Health Rep*, *61*: 1683-1689, 1946.

5. D. J. Galagan and J. W. Knutson, "The Effect of Topically Applied Fluorides on Dental Caries Experience. V. Report of Findings With Two, Four, and Six Applications of Sodium Fluoride and Lead Fluoride," *Public Health Rep*, *62*:1477-1483, 1947.

6. G. Bergman, "Topical Application of Sodium Fluoride Using School Children as Subjects," *Acta Odontol Scand*, 11, *supplement 12*:53 112, 1953.

7. F. E. Law, M. H. Jeffreys, and H. C. Sheary, "Topical Applications of Fluoride Solutions in Dental Caries Control," *Public Health Rep*, *76*:287-290, 1961.

8. P. Torell and Y. Ericsson, "Two-Year Clinical Tests With Different Methods of Local Caries-Preventive Fluoride Application in

Swedish School-children," *Acta Odontol Scand*, 23:287-322, 1965.

9. G. N. Davies, "Dental Caries Control and the General Practitioner," *NZ Dent J*, 46:25-31, 1950.

10. R. E. T. Hewat and F. B. Rice, "Control of Dental Caries by Topical Application of Sodium Fluoride. Experimental Study on 97 Children in Wellington," *NZ Dent J*, 45:215-219, 1949.

11. R. Harris, "Observations on the Effect of Topical Sodium Fluoride on Caries Incidence in Children," *Austr Dent J*, 4:257-260, 1959.

12. N. D. Martin, "The Scientific Evaluation of Fluoride as a Means of Preventing Dental Caries," *Austr Dent J*, 1:141-150, 1956.

13. M. G. Buonocore and B. G. Bibby, "Fluoride Dentifrices, Topical Fluorides and Fluoridation," In A. H. Kutscher, E. V. Zegarelli, and G. A. Hyman (Eds.), *Pharmacotherapeutics of Oral Disease* (New York, McGraw, 1964), pp. 222-231.

14. R. A. Downs and W. J. Pelton, "The Effect of Topically Applied Fluorides in Dental Caries Experience on Children Residing in Fluoride Areas," *J Colorado Dent Assoc*, 29:7-10, 1950.

15. D. J. Galagan and J. R. Vermillion, "Effect of Topical Fluorides on Teeth Matured on Fluoride-Bearing Water," *Public Health Rep*, 70:1114-1115, 1955.

16. V. H. Mercer and J. C. Muhler, "Comparison of a Single Application of Stannous Fluoride With a Single Application of Sodium Fluoride or Two Applications of Stannous Fluoride," *J Dent Child*, 28: 84-86, 1961.

17. C. W. Gish, C. L. Howell, and J. C. Muhler, "A New Approach to the Topical Application of Fluorides for the Reduction of Dental Caries in Children," *J Dent Res*, 36:784-786, 1957.

18. C. W. Gish, C. L. Howell, and J. C. Muhler, "A New Approach to the Topical Application of Fluorides in Children, With Results at the End of Two Years," *J Dent Child*, 24:194-196, 1957.

19. C. W. Gish, C. L. Howell, and J. C. Muhler, "Stannous Fluoride Versus Sodium Fluoride—A Progress Report," *J Dent Child*, 25: 177-179, 1958.

20. C. W. Gish, J. C. Muhler, and C. L. Howell, "A New Approach to the Topical Application of Fluoride in Children With Results at End of Four Years," *J Dent Child*, 26:300-303, 1959.

21. C. W. Gish, J. C. Muhler, and C. L. Howell, "A New Approach to the Topical Application of Fluorides for the Reduction of Dental Caries in Children: Results at the End of Five Years," *J Dent Child*, 29:65-71, 1962.

22. J. K. Peterson and L. Williamson, "Effectiveness of Topical Application of Eight Percent Stannous Fluoride," *Public Health Rep*, 77: 39-40, 1962.

23. R. Harris, "Observations on the Effect of Eight Percent Stannous Fluoride on Dental Caries in Children," *Austr Dent J*, 8:335-340, 1963.

24. H. V. Cartwright, R. L. Lindahl, and J. W. Bawden, "Clinical Findings on the Effectiveness of Stannous Fluoride and Acid Phosphate as Caries-Reducing Agents in Children," *J Dent Child*, 35: 36-40, 1968.

25. H. S. Horowitz and H. S. Lucye, "A Clinical Study of Stannous Fluoride in a Prophylaxis Paste and a Solution," *J Oral Ther*, 3:17-25, 1966.

26. W. D. Wellock, A. Maitland, and F. Brudevold, "Caries Increments, Tooth Discoloration and State of Oral Hygiene in Children Given Single Annual Applications of Acid Phosphate-Fluoride and Stannous Fluoride," *Arch Oral Biol*, 10:453-460, 1965.

27. W. A. T. Salter, F. McCombie, and L. W. Hole, "The Anticariogenic Effects of One and Two Applications of Stannous Fluoride on the Deciduous and Permanent Teeth of Children Age 6 and 7," *J Can Dent Assoc*, 28:363-371, 1962.

28. J. C. Muhler, "Stannous Fluoride Enamel Pigmentation—Evidence of Caries Arrestment," *J Dent Child*, 27:157-161, 1960.

29. V. H. Mercer and J. C. Muhler, "The Clinical Demonstration of Caries Arrestment Following Topical Stannous Fluoride Treatments," *J Dent Child*, 32:65-72, 1965.

30. J. C. Muhler, L. B. Spear, Jr., D. Bixler and G. K. Stookey, "The Arrestment of Incipient Dental Caries in Adults After the Use of Three Different Forms of SnF_2 Therapy: Results After 30 Months," *JADA*, 75:1402-1406, 1967.

31. R. R. Lobene, B. J. Zulgar-Nain, and J. W. Hein, "Masking of Enamel Caries by Topically Applied Stannous Fluoride: A Source of Error in Clinical Diagnosis," *J Oral Ther*, 3:35-43, 1966.

32. R. L. Glass, "Radiographic Evidence of Tin Uptake by Human Tooth Structure," *Arch Oral Biol*, 12:401-406, 1967.

33. J. C. Muhler, "The Effectiveness of Stannous Fluoride in Children Residing in an Optimal Communal Fluoride Area," *J Dent Child*, 27:51-54, 1960.

34. J. C. Muhler, "The Anticariogenic Effectiveness of a Single Application of Stannous Fluoride in Children Residing in an Optimal Communal Fluoride Area. II. Results at the End of 30 Months," *JADA*, 61:431-438, 1960.

35. H. S. Horowitz and S. B. Heifetz, "Evaluation of Topical Applications of Stannous Fluoride to Teeth of Children Born and Reared in a Fluoridated Community: Interim Report," *J Dent Child*, 34:290-295, 1967.

36. H. S. Horowitz and S. B. Heifetz, "Evaluation of Topical Applications of Stannous Fluoride to Teeth of Children Born and Reared in a Fluoridated Community: Final Report," *J Dent Child*, 36:355-361, 1969.

37. F. Brudevold, A. Savory, D. E. Gardner, M. Spinelli, and R. Spiers, "A Study of Acidulated Fluoride Solutions. I. *In Vitro* Effects on Enamel," *Arch Oral Biol*, 8:167-177, 1963.

38. W. D. Wellock and F. Brudevold, "A Study of Acidulated Fluoride Solutions. II. The Caries Inhibiting Effect of Single Annual Topical Applications of an Acidic Fluoride and Phosphate Solution. A Two-Year Experience," *Arch Oral Biol*, 8:179-182, 1963.

39. J. H. N. Pameijer, F. Brudevold, and E. E. Hunt, Jr., "A Study of Acidulated Fluoride Solutions. III. The Cariostatic Effect of Repeated Topical Sodium Fluoride Applications With and Without Phosphate: A Pilot Study," *Arch Oral Biol*, 8:183-185, 1963.

40. J. C. Muhler, G. K. Stookey, and D. Bixler, "Evaluation of the Anticariogenic Effect of Mixtures of Stannous Fluoride and Soluble Phosphates," *J Dent Child*, 32:154-169, 1965.

41. H. S. Horowitz, "The Effect on Dental Caries of Topically Applied Acidulated Phosphate-Fluoride: Results After One Year," *J Oral Ther*, 4:286-291, 1968.

42. H. S. Horowitz, "Effect on Dental Caries of Topically Applied Acidulated Phosphate-Fluoride: Results After Two Years," *JADA*, 78:568-572, 1969.

43. H. S. Horowitz and J. Doyle, "The Effect on Dental Caries of Topically Applied Acidulated Phosphate-Fluorides: Results After Three Years," *JADA*, 82:359-365, 1971.

44. H. M. Averill, J. E. Averill, and A. G. Ritz, "A Two-Year Comparison of Three Topical Fluoride Agents," *JADA*, 74:996-1001, 1967.

45. N. C. Cons, D. T. Janerich, and R. S. Senning, "Albany Topical Fluoride Study," *JADA*, 80:777-781, 1970.

46. P. F. DePaola, W. D. Wellock, A. Maitland, and F. Brudevold, "The Relationship of Cariostasis, Oral Hygiene, and Past Caries Experience in Children Receiving Three Sprays Annually With Acidulated Phosphate-Fluoride: Three-Year Results," *JADA*, 77:91-94, 1968.

47. F. Brudevold, "Recent Research on Topical Fluoride," *Ala J Med Sci*, 5:351-357, 1968.

48. E. T. Bryan and J. E. Williams, "The Cariostatic Effectiveness of a Phosphate Fluoride Gel Administered Annually to School Children. I. The Results of the First Year," *J Public Health Dent*, 28:182-185, 1968.

49. R. Q. Ingraham and J. E. Williams, "An Evaluation of the Utility of

Application and Cariostatic Effectiveness of Phosphate-Fluorides in Solution and Gel States," *J Tenn Dent Assoc, 50*:5-12, 1970.

50. L. F. Swejda, C. V. Tossy, and D. M. Below, "Fluorides in Community Programs: Results from a Fluoride Gel Applied Topically," *J Public Health Dent, 27*:192-194, 1967.

51. B. G. Bibby, H. A. Zander, M. McKelleget, and B. Labunsky, "Preliminary Reports on the Effect on Dental Caries of the Use of Sodium Fluoride in a Prophylactic Cleaning Mixture and in a Mouthwash," *J Dent Res, 25*:207-211, 1946.

52. B. G. Bibby, "Fluoride Mouthwashes, Fluoride Dentifrices and Other Uses of Fluorides in Control of Caries," *J Dent Res, 27*:367-375, 1948.

53. V. A. Sereto, N. O. Harris, and W. R. Hester, "A Stannous Fluoride, Silex, Silicone Dental Prophylaxis Paste With Anticariogenic Potentialities," *J Dent Res, 40*:90-96, 1961.

54. J. K. Peterson, W. A. Jordan, and J. R. Snyder, "Effectiveness of Stannous Fluoride-Silex-Silicone Prophylaxis Paste," *Northwest Dent, 42*:276-278, 1963.

55. F. P. Scola and C. A. Ostrom, "Clinical Evaluation of Stannous Fluoride When Used as a Constituent of a Compatible Prophylactic Paste, as a Topical Solution, and in a Dentifrice in Naval Personnel," *JADA, 73*:1306-1311, 1966.

56. F. P. Scola and C. A. Ostrom, "Clinical Evaluation of Stannous Fluoride When Used as a Constituent of a Compatible Prophylactic Paste, as a Topical Solution, and in a Dentifrice in Naval Personnel," *JADA, 77*:594-597, 1968.

57. D. Bixler and J. C. Muhler, "Effect on Dental Caries in Children in a Non-fluoride Area of Combined Use of Three Agents Containing Stannous Fluoride: A Prophylactic Paste, a Solution, and a Dentifrice," *JADA, 68*:792-800, 1964.

58. D. Bixler and J. C. Muhler, "Effect on Dental Caries in Children in a Non-fluoride Area of Combined Use of Three Agents Containing Stannous Fluoride: A Prophylactic Paste, a Solution, and a Dentifrice. II. Results at the End of 24 and 36 Months," *JADA, 72*:392-396, 1966.

59. C. W. Gish and J. C. Muhler, "Effect on Dental Caries in Children in a Natural Fluoride Area of: Combined Use of Three Agents Containing Stannous Fluoride: A Prophylactic Paste, a Solution, and a Dentifrice," *JADA, 70*:914-920, 1965.

60. J. K. Peterson, H. S. Horowitz, W. A. Jordan, and V. Pugnier, "Effectiveness of an Acidulated Phosphate Fluoride-Pumice Prophylactic Paste: A Two-Year Report," *J Dent Res, 48*:346-350, 1969.

61. V. Vrbic, F. Brudevold, and H. G. McCann, "F Uptake from Use of

F Containing Prophylaxis Pastes," *IADR Abstracts*, No. 171, 1967.
62. M. A. Zuniga and R. C. Caldwell, "The Effect of Fluoride-Containing Prophylaxis Pastes on Normal and "White-Spot" Enamel," *J Dent Child*, 36:345-349, 1969.
63. J. R. Mellberg and C. R. Nicholson, "*In Vitro* Evaluation of an Acidulated Phosphate Fluoride Prophylaxis Paste," *Arch Oral Biol*, 13: 1223-1234, 1968.
64. G. E. Kelley, G. K. Stookey, and J. C. Muhler, "Laboratory Studies Concerning the Development of a Stannous Fluoride Phosphate Prophylactic Paste," *J Dent Child*, 36:321-328, 352-354, 1969.
65. H. Berggren and E. Welander, "Supervised Toothbrushing With a Sodium Fluoride Solution in 5,000 Swedish School Children: Results and Analysis of Procedures," *Acta Odontol Scand*, 18:209-234, 1960.
66. H. Berggren and E. Welander, "The Caries-Inhibiting Effect of Sodium, Ferric and Zirconium Fluorides," *Acta Odontol Scand*, 22: 401-413, 1964.
67. D. C. T. Bullen, F. McCombie, and L. W. Hole, "One-Year Effect of Supervised Toothbrushing With an Acidulated Fluoride-Phosphate Solution," *J Can Dent Assoc*, 31:231-235, 1965.
68. D. C. T. Bullen, F. McCombie, and L. W. Hole, "Two-Year Effect of Supervised Toothbrushing With an Acidulated Fluoride-Phosphate Solution," *J Can Dent Assoc*, 32:89-93, 1966.
69. H. S. Horowitz and S. B. Heifetz, "A Review of Studies on the Self-Administration of Topical Fluorides," *Canad J Public Health*, 59: 393-398, 1968.
70. S. B. Heifetz, H. S. Horowitz, and W. S. Driscoll, "Evaluation of a Self-Administered Procedure for the Topical Application of Acidulated Phosphate Fluoride," *IADR Abstracts*, No. 257, 1968.
71. S. B. Heifetz, H. S. Horowitz, and W. S. Driscoll, "Evaluation of a Self-Administered Procedure for the Topical Application of Acidulated Phosphate-Fluoride; Results After Two Years," *IADR Abstracts*, No. 544, 1969.
72. P. W. Goaz, L. P. McElwaine, H. A. Biswell, and W. E. White, "Anticariogenic Effect of Sodium Monofluorophosphate Solution in Children After 21 Months of Use," *J Dent Res*, 42:965-972, 1963.
73. P. W. Goaz, L. P. McElwaine, H. A. Biswell, and W. E. White, "Anticariogenic Effect of Sodium Monofluorophosphate Solution in Children After 21 Months of Use," *J Dent Res*, 45:286-290, 1966.
74. J. C. Muhler, "The Clinical Demonstration of the Mass Treatment of Children With the SnF$_2$-ZrSiO$_4$ Prophylactic Paste. Initial Observations Concerning Conduct of the Study," *J Ind Dent Assn*, 47: 428-431, 1968.

75. V. H. Mercer and C. W. Gish, "The Self-Administered Stannous Fluoride Treatment Paste for Caries Prevention in a Community," *J Ind Dent Assoc, 47:*432-434, 1968.

76. R. G. Schimmele, "A Suggested Method for Mass Application of Self-Administered Prophylactic Paste Using Student Auxiliary Personnel," *J Ind Dent Assoc, 47:*435-436, 1968.

77. J. C. Muhler, G. E. Kelley, G. K. Stookey, F. I. Lindo, and N. O. Harris, "The Clinical Evaluation of a Patient-Administered SnF$_2$-ZrSiO$_4$ Prophylactic Paste in Children. I. Results After One Year in the Virgin Islands," *JADA, 81:*142-145, 1970.

78. J. C. Muhler, "Mass Treatment of Children With a Stannous Fluoride-Zirconium Silicate Self-Administered Prophylactic Paste for Partial Control of Dental Caries," *J Am Coll Dent, 35:*45-57, 1968.

79. L. A. Lang, H. G. Thomas, J. A. Taylor, and R. E. Rothhaar, "Clinical Efficacy of a Self-Applied Stannous Fluoride Prophylaxis Paste," *J Dent Child, 37:*211-216, 1970.

80. C. W. Gish and V. H. Mercer, "Child Self-Application of a Zirconium Silicate-Stannous Fluoride Anticariogenic Paste—Clinical Results After One and Two Years," *IADR Abstracts*, No. 552, 1969.

81. J. F. Roberts, B. G. Bibby, and W. D. Wellock, "Effect of an Acidulated Fluoride Mouthwash on Dental Caries," *J Dent Res, 27:*497-500, 1948.

82. P. Torell and A. Sibert, "Mouthwash With Sodium Fluoride and Potassium Fluoride," *Odontol Rev, 13:*62-72, 1962.

83. W. S. Weisz, "Two-Year Study of Efficacy of a Sodium Fluoride Mouthwash," *Pa Dent J, 15:*36-43, 1947.

84. W. S. Weisz, "The Reduction of Dental Caries Through Use of a Sodium Fluoride Mouthwash," *JADA, 60:*438-456, 1960.

85. B. Forsman, "Effect of Mouth Rinses With Sodium Fluoride in Schools at Vaxjo, Sverige," *Tandlakarforb Tid, 57:*705-709, 1965.

86. T. Kasakura, "Dental Observation on School Feeding. 3. Effect of the Dental Caries Prevention of Oral Rinsing With Sodium Fluoride Solution After School Feeding," *Odontology, 54:*22-32, 1966.

87. J. Kann, "Systemic Controlled Use of Mouth Rinses With Fluoride," *Tandlaegebladet, 69:*638-641, 1965.

88. G. Swerdloff and I. L. Shannon, "Feasibility of the Use of Stannous Fluoride Mouthwash in a School System," *J Dent Child, 36:*363-368, 1969.

89. G. Koch, "Caries Increment in School Children During and Two Years After End of Supervised Rinsing of the Mouth With Sodium Fluoride Solution," *Odontol Rev, 20:*323-330, 1969.

90. H. R. Englander, P. H. Keyes, M. Gestwicki, and H. A. Sultz, "Clin-

ical Anti-caries Effect of Repeated Topical Sodium Fluoride Applications by Mouthpieces," *JADA*, 75:638-644, 1967.

91. H. R. Englander, J. P. Carlos, R. S. Senning, and J. R. Mellberg, "Residual Anticaries Effect of Repeated Topical Sodium Fluoride Applications by Mouthpieces," *JADA*, 78:783-787, 1969.

92. H. R. Englander, L. T. Sherrill, B. G. Miller, J. P. Carlos, J. R. Mellberg, and R. S. Senning, "Incremental Rates of Dental Caries After Repeated Topical Sodium Fluoride Applications in Children With Lifelong Consumption of Fluoridated Water," *JADA*, 82:354-358, 1971.

93. J. R. Mellberg, H. R. Englander, and C. R. Nicholson, "Acquisition of Fluoride *In Vivo* by Deciduous Enamel from Daily Topical Fluoride Applications. A Preliminary Report," *J Oral Ther*, 3:330-334, 1967.

94. J. R. Mellberg, H. R. Englander, and C. R. Nicholson, "Acquisition of Fluoride *In Vivo* by Enamel from Repeated Topical Sodium Fluoride Applications Over 21 Months," *Arch Oral Biol*, 12:1139-1148, 1967.

95. J. R. Mellberg, C. R. Nicholson, B. G. Miller, and H. R. Englander, "Acquisition of Fluoride *In Vivo* by Enamel from Repeated Topical Sodium Fluoride Applications in a Fluoridated Area: A Preliminary Report," *J Dent Res*, 47:733-736, 1968.

96. J. R. Mellberg, C. R. Nicholson, B. G. Miller, and H. R. Englander, "Acquisition of Fluoride *In Vivo* by Enamel from Repeated Topical Sodium Fluoride Applications in a Fluoridated Area: A Final Report," *J Dent Res, 49, Suppl:* 1473-1477, 1970.

97. H. S. Dwyer, "A Study of the Liability to Decay of the Deciduous Teeth of School Children," *J Dent Res*, 12:911-918, 1932.

98. D. K. Hennon, G. K. Stookey, and J. C. Muhler, "Prevalence and Distribution of Dental Caries in Pre-school Children," *JADA*, 79:1405-1414, 1969.

99. R. W. Leigh, "Incidence of Caries, The Different Teeth and Their Respective Surfaces," *Milit Dent J*, 6:183-194, 1923.

100. T. P. Hyatt and A. J. Lotka, "How Dental Statistics are Secured in the Metropolitan Life Insurance Company," *J Dent Res*, 9:411-445, 1929.

101. J. P. Walsh and R. S. Smart, "The Relative Susceptability of Tooth Surfaces to Dental Caries and Other Comparative Studies," *NZ Dent J*, 44:17-35, 1948.

102. J. W. Knutson, H. Klein, and C. E. Palmer, "Dental Needs of Grade School Children of Hagerstown, Md.," *JADA*, 27:579-588, 1940.

103. C. D. M. Day and H. J. Sedwick, "Studies on the Incidence of Dental Caries," *Dent Cosmos*, 77:442-452, 1935.

104. O. Backer-Dirks, The Distribution of Caries Resistance in Relation to Tooth Surfaces. G. E. W. Walstenhome and M. Connor, *Ciba Foundation Symposium: Caries Resistant Teeth* (Boston, Little, 1965), pp. 66-83.

105. D. B. Ast, D. J. Smith, B. Wachs, and K. T. Kantwell, "Newburgh-Kingston Caries Fluorine Study. XIV. Combined Clinical and Roentgenographic Dental Findings After Ten Years of Fluoride Experience," *JADA*, 52:314-325, 1956.

106. T. G. Ludwig and E. I. F. Pearce, "The Hastings Fluoridation Project IV. Dental Effects Between 1954 and 1963," *NZ Dent J*, 59:298-301, 1963.

107. O. Backer-Dirks, B. Houwink, and G. W. Kwant, "The Results of Six and One-Half Years of Artificial Fluoridation of Drinking Water in the Netherlands. The Tiel-Culemborg Experiment," *Arch Oral Biol*, 5:284-300, 1961.

108. H. S. Horowitz and J. K. Peterson, "Evaluation of Examiner Variability and the Use of Radiographs in Determining the Efficacy of Community Fluoridation," *Arch Oral Biol*, 11:867-875, 1966.

109. T. P. Hyatt, "Prophylactic Odontotomy the Ideal Procedure in Dentistry for Children," *Dent Cosmos*, 78:353-360, 1936.

110. C. F. Bodecker, "Fissure Eradication," *NYS Dent J*, 30:149-155, 1964.

111. C. F. Bodecker, "The Eradication of Enamel Fissures," *Dent Items of Int*, 51:859-866, 1929.

112. C. F. Bodecker, "Dental Caries Immunization Without Filling," *NYS Dent J*, 30:337-339, 1964.

113. J. Miller, "Clinical Investigations in Preventive Dentistry," *Brit Dent J*, 91:92-95, 1951.

114. J. Miller, "Biannual Treatment With Silver Nitrate, Sodium Fluoride and Copper Cement in the Prevention of Dental Caries," *J Dent Res*, 1951 Abst.

115. D. B. Ast, A. Bushel, and H. C. Chase, "Clinical Study of Caries Prophylaxis With Zinc Chloride and Potassium Ferrocyanide," *JADA*, 41:437-442, 1950.

116. E. I. Cueto and M. G. Buonocore, "Adhesive Sealing of Pits and Fissures for Caries Prevention," *IADR Abstracts*, No. 480, 1965.

117. E. I. Cueto and M. G. Buonocore, "Sealing of Pits and Fissures With an Adhesive Resin: Its Use in Caries Prevention," *JADA*, 75:121-128, 1967.

118. L. W. Ripa, M. G. Buonocore, and E. I. Cueto, "Adhesive Sealing of Pits and Fissures for Caries Prevention: Report of Two Year Study," *IADR Abstracts*, No. 247, 1966.

119. L. W. Ripa, M. G. Buonocore, and E. I. Cueto, "An Approach to Occlusal Caries Prevention Utilizing an Adhesive Sealing Technique,"

Scientific Session, American Dental Association Convention, Dallas, Texas, Nov. 1966.

120. L. W. Ripa and W. W. Cole, "Occlusal Sealing and Caries Prevention: Results 12 Months After a Single Application of Adhesive Resin," *J Dent Res*, 49:171-173, 1970.

121. M. Takeuchi, T. Kizu, T. Shimizu, M. Eto, and F. Amano, "Sealing of the Pit and Fissure With Resin Adhesive. II. Results of Nine Months Field Work, an Investigation of Electric Conductivity of Teeth," *Bull Tokyo Dent Coll*, 7:50-59, 1966.

122. M. Takeuchi, M. Eto, and T. Kizu, "Studies on Caries Prevention by Sealing With Resin Adhesive and Certain Metal Fillers. I." *Shikwa Gakuho*, 66:2, 1966, and *Dent Abstracts*, Oct. 1966.

123. R. C. Parkhouse, and G. B. Winter, "A Fissure Sealant Containing Methyl-2-Cyanoacrylate as a Caries Preventive Agent," *Brit Dent J*, 130:16-19, 1971.

124. Council on Dental Materials and Devices, "Polymers Used in Dentistry: Part II Resins Containing BIS-GMA: Coating and Cementing Uses," *JADA*, 90:841-843, 1975.

125. R. H. Roydhouse, "Prevention of Occlusal Fissure Caries by Use of a Sealant: A Pilot Study," *J Dent Child*, 35:253-262, 1968.

126. Council on Dental Materials and Devices, "Recommended Standard Practices for Biological Evaluation of Dental Materials," *JADA*, 84:382-387, 1972.

127. Council on Dental Materials and Devices, "Nuva-Seal Pit and Fissure Sealant Classified as Provisionally Acceptable," *JADA*, 84: 1109, 1972.

128. Council on Dental Materials and Devices, "Additions to the List of Classified Materials and Devices," *JADA*, 87:381, 1973.

129. Council on Dental Materials and Devices, "Pit and Fissure Sealants," *JADA*, 88:390, 1974.

130. M. G. Buonocore, "A Simple Method of Increasing the Adhesion of Acrylic Filling Materials to Enamel Surfaces," *J Dent Res*, 34:849-853, 1955.

131. D. L. Mitchell, "Bandless Orthodontic Bracket," *JADA*, 74:103-110, 1967.

132. L. T. Swanson and J. F. Beck, "Factors Affecting Bonding to Human Enamel With Special Reference to a Plastic Adhesive," *JADA*, 61: 581-586, 1960.

133. G. V. Newman, "Epoxy Adhesives for Orthodontic Attachments," *Am J Orthod*, 51:901-912, 1965.

134. D. H. Retief and C. J. Dreyer, "Epoxy Resins for Bonding Orthodontic Attachments to Teeth," *JDA South Africa*, 22:338-346, 1967.

135. M. G. Buonocore, A. Matsui, and A. J. Gwinnett, "Penetration of

Resin Dental Materials into Enamel Surfaces With Reference to Bonding," *Arch Oral Biol, 13:*61-70, 1968.

136. A. J. Gwinnett and M. G. Buonocore, "Adhesives and Caries Prevention," *Brit Dent J, 119:*77-80, 1965.

137. R. D. Mulholland and D. O. de Shazer, "The Effect of Acidic Pretreatment Solutions on the Direct Bonding of Orthodontic Brackets to Enamel," *Angle Orthod, 38:*236-243, 1968.

138. A. J. Gwinnett and A. Matsui, "A Study of Enamel Adhesives: The Physical Relationship Between Enamel and Adhesive," *Arch Oral Biol, 12:*1615-1620, 1967.

139. G. V. Newman and L. H. Sharpe, "On the Wettability of Tooth Surfaces; Preliminary Investigation," *J NJ Dent Soc, 37:*289-291, 1966.

140. Z. Sheykholeslam, and M. G. Buonocore, "Resin Penetration into Enamel Surfaces of Permanent and Deciduous Teeth," *IADR Abstracts,* No. 238, 1970.

141. H. Myers, S. G. Hamilton, and H. Becks, "A Tracer Study of the Transfer of F18 to Teeth by Topical Application," *J Dent Res, 31:* 743-750, 1952.

142. E. Pearce and B. G. Bibby, "Protein Adsorption on Bovine Enamel," *Arch Oral Biol, 11:*329-336, 1966.

143. J. L. Hardwick and E. B. Manley, "Caries of the Enamel. II. Acidogenic Caries," *Brit Dent J, 92:*225-236, 1952.

144. F. Brudevold, "The Response of Intact and Experimentally Altered Human Enamel to Topical Fluoride," *Arch Oral Biol, 13:*543-552, 1968.

145. Z. Sheykholeslam, *Bonding of Adhesive Resins to Enamel Surfaces,* Master of Science Thesis, University of Rochester School of Medicine and Dentistry, 1970.

146. R. Assenden, F. Brudevold, and H. G. McCann, "The Response of Sound and Experimentally Altered Human Enamel to Topical Fluoride," *Arch Oral Biol, 13:*543-552, 1968.

147. W. P. Rock, "Results Obtained with Two Different BIS-GMA Type Sealants After One Year," *Brit Dent J, 134:*193-196, 1974.

148. W. P. Rock, "Fissure Sealants: Further Results of Clinical Trials," *Brit Dent J, 136:*317-321, 1974.

149. C. J. Wilson, G. M. Gillespie, and T. G. N. Williams, "Anticaries Effect of Sealants Placed by Dental Auxiliaries in Jamaica," *IADR Abstracts,* No. 834, 1973.

150. M. Buonocore, "Adhesive Sealing of Pits and Fissures for Caries Prevention, With Use of Ultraviolet Light, *JADA, 80:*324-328, 1970.

151. M. Buonocore, "Caries Prevention in Pits and Fissures Sealed With an Adhesive Resin Polymerized by Ultraviolet Light: A Two Year

Study of a Single Adhesive Application," *JADA,* 82:1090-1093, 1971.

152. R. J. McCune, H. S. Horowitz, S. B. Heifetz, and J. Cvar, "Pit and Fissure Sealants: One Year Results From a Study in Kalispell, Montana," *JADA,* 87:1177-1180, 1973.

153. H. S. Horowitz, S. B. Heifetz, and R. J. McCune, "The Effectiveness of an Adhesive Sealant in Preventing Occlusal Caries: Findings After Two Years in Kalispell, Montana," *JADA,* 89:885-890, 1974.

154. H. S. Horowitz, S. B. Heifetz, and S. Poulsen, "Retention and Effectiveness in Preventing Occlusal Caries of a Single Application of an Adhesive Sealant: Findings After Four Years in Kalispell, Montana," presented as part of a Sealant Symposium, American Association for Dental Research, New York, 1975.

155. R. E. Going, "Clinical Studies," presented as part of a Sealant Symposium, American Association for Dental Research, New York, 1975.

156. W. P. Rock, "Fissure Sealants, Results Obtained With Two Different Sealants After One Year," *Brit Dent J,* 133:146-151, 1972.

157. H. Luoma, J. Meurman, S. Helminen, and H. Heikkila, "Retention of a Fissure Sealant With Caries Reduction in Finnish Children After Six Months," *Scand J Dent Res,* 81:510-512, 1973.

158. J. H. Meurman, H. Luoma, A. H. Heikkila, and P. Rautio, "Carries Reductions 1.5 Years After Application of a Fissure Sealant as Related to Dietary Habits," *Scand J Dent Res,* 83:1-6, 1975.

159. J. Risager and S. Poulsen, "Fissure Sealing With Nuva-Seal in a Public Health Program for Danish School Children After 12 Months Observation," *Scand J Dent Res,* 82:570-573, 1974.

160. J. M. Gourley, "A One-year Study of a Fissure Sealant in Two Nova Scotia Communities," *J Can Dent Assoc,* 40:549-552, 1974.

161. J. M. Gourley, "A Two-year Study of Fissure Sealant in Two Nova Scotia Communities," *J Pub Health Dent,* 35:132-137, 1975.

AUTHOR INDEX

SUBJECT INDEX

A

Abscesses, 210, 244
 fulminating, 211
Achieved status, 57
Acidulated fluride phosphate
 advantage of, 327
 gell form, 318, 320
 mouthpieces with, 334, 341
 prophylaxis paste containing, 322,
 324
 topical application by toothbrushing
 with, 332
 topical application in dental office,
 315-318, 325-327
Acquired pellicle, 18
Acquired salivary pellicle, 180-181
Actinomyces, 184
Actinomyces israelii, 202
Actinomyces naeslundii, 189, 202
Actinomyces odontolyticus, 189
Actinomyces viscosus, 185, 189, 202,
 211, 216
Actions, 68
Acute necrotizing ulcerative gingivitis
 (ANUG), 155, 186, 219
 bacterial zone, 209
 identification of predominant spirochetes in, 209-210
 microbiology of, 209-212
 necrotic zone, 209
 neutrophile-rich zone, 209
 recurrence, 212
 spirochetal infiltration zone, 209
 transmissibility of, 211-212
 zones in tissue specimens, 209
Acute necrotizing ulcerative periodontitis (ANUP), 212
Acute oral necrosis, 155
Addison's disease, 148
Additives, 276

Adherent polysaccharides, 185
Adhesives for pit and fissure caries control, 341-352
 acids as bonding agents, 346-347
 bisphenol A and glycidyl methacrylate (BIS-GMA), 344-345
 candidates for, 349
 cryanoacrylate system, 343-345
 fluoride treatments prior to, 351
 preparation of tooth surface for, 346-
 348
 thickness of, 348
Adolescent conflicts, 161
Adults
 dental health education, 64-66
 methods of, 80-84
 habit formation in, 70
Aerobic glycolysis, 204
Age, 53, 60, 84, 152
Aging, 154
Agranulocytosis, 213
Alcoholism, 148
Alcohols, 218
Allergic manifestations, 147, 215, 217
Alveolar bone resorption, 171-174, 184,
 189-190, 197
 increasing resistance to, 214
American Dental Association, 45
 Class A dentifrices, 297, 302-303
 Class B dentifrices, 297, 302
Amino acid, caries in relation to, 261-
 262
Ammonia, 189
Anaerobic diphtheroids, 188
Anaerobic streptococci, 188
Anaphylactic reactions, 192
Anaphylatoxin, 194
Anaphylatoxin generation, 204
Anatomical lesions, 148
Angular cheilosis, 149
 oral manifestations of, 147